of Medicine.

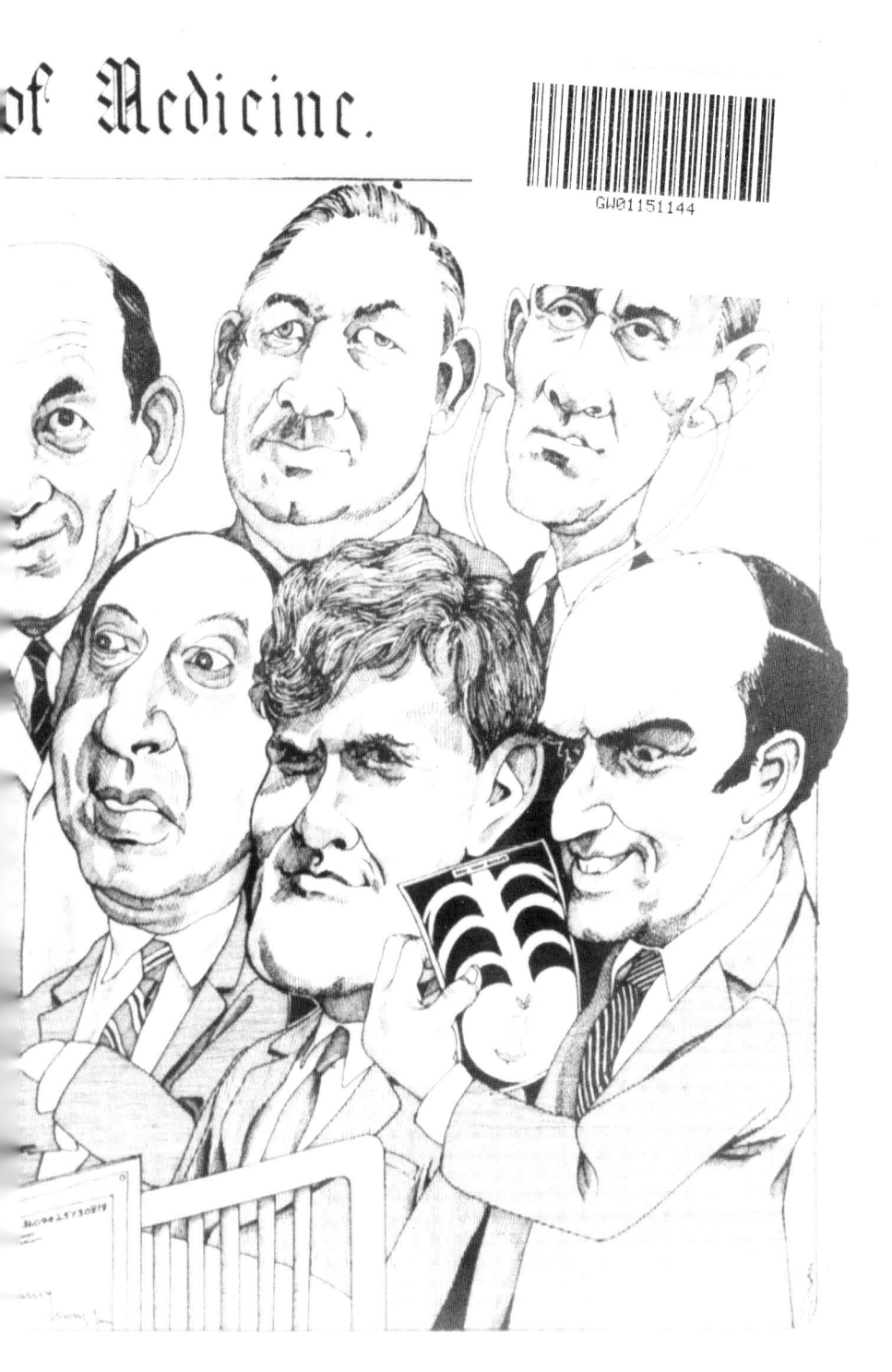

to right) Drs Seumas Gallen, Alan Thompson, Hugh Staunton, Billy O'Dwyer, Jim Cogan).

A Pride of Professors

By the same author

James Joyce and Medicine
Brief Lives of Irish Doctors
An Assembly of Irish Surgeons
'What Did I Die Of?'
Surgeon Major Parke's African Journey: 1887–89
William Henry Drummond: Poet in Patois
etc.

A Pride of Professors

The Professors of Medicine at the Royal College of Surgeons in Ireland 1813–1985

J. B. Lyons

A. & A. Farmar

© J. B. Lyons 1999

Published by
A. & A. Farmar
Beech House
78 Ranelagh Village
Dublin 6
Ireland

ISBN 1-899047-51-4

Designed and typeset by A. & A. Farmar
Index by Helen Litton
Printed in Ireland by βetaprint

To the Memory of William Doolin (1887–1962),
Surgeon, Editor, and Medical Historian

Acknowledgements

The Council of the RCSI made a generous grant to defray publication costs. The librarians of TCD, the RIA, the Colleges of Physicians and Surgeons tolerated my demands ungrudgingly. The staff of the Audio-Visual Department were equally supportive. Jim Cogan has permitted the use of his cartoon of the medical faculty.

The individuals who helped in various ways include C. S. Breathnach, C. Brennan, Alan Browne, Harold Browne, Davis Coakley, Harry Counihan, Bernadette Cunningham, Charles Dupont, Peter Gatenby, Richard Moore, Ms Moorhead, Ronald Nesbitt, Eoin O'Brien, Mary O'Doherty, Richard Pollard, Joseph Robins, Gillian Smith.

'This College, although called a College of Surgeons is just as much a College of Physicians.'
Arthur Jacob

'A teacher affects eternity; he can never tell where his influence stops.'
Henry Adams

'History should be a witness, not a flatterer.'
William Doolin

Foreword

The Royal College of Surgeons in Ireland opened its undergraduate medical school in 1786. The school is not actually mentioned in the charter given by King George III in 1784, but professorships of anatomy and surgery were created in 1785, and a chair of midwifery in 1789. The chair of medicine was established in 1813.

This book is a series of brief lives of the professors of medicine from 1813–1985—a hundred and seventy-two years. They are a remarkable group by any standard, and their names are evocative of much that is storied in Irish medicine.

As I write I am looking at what is probably the finest portrait in the college. It is of John Cheyne, the college's first professor of medicine, and the painter was Sir Henry Raeburn (1756–1823), Scotland's greatest portrait painter. The characterful face is of an era. Why is it, although there have been something in the order of 55,000 generations of homo sapiens, that some faces reflect a finite period in our evolution? Certainly this is one of them. It is wonderful to be able to start a book with the story of a man who has given his name (Cheyne-Stokes breathing) to a clinical sign in use to this day.

It will be recalled that up to 1900 a patient had only a 50/50 chance of benefiting from an encounter with a doctor; it is only since about 1950 that it could be shown, by controlled trials, that the doctor was doing some good. The man who came to the top had something extra: what was it? For some it was empathy, for others it was panache. Surgeons didn't have a monopoly on this quality. Lord Dawson of Penn, King George V's physician in the twenties and thirties, had two stethoscopes, one for the heart and one for the lungs. The meticulous, but pharmacologically useless prescriptions, 'to be taken in a wineglass full of warm water half an hour after meals', serve as reminders of the body's power of recovery and the power of suggestion, as well as the powerlessness of these distinguished men in the face of real disease.

They can't all have been colourful characters, but when you read Jack Lyons's account of them they come alive on the page, and I found it interesting to see the variety of personalities that were appointed.

On this day (11 March 1999), we are mourning the demise of the subject of the final chapter, Professor William ('Billy') O'Dwyer. He was a lively, vigorous stimulating personality; a top-class clinician, and a sought-after teacher. He was a man much in keeping with those other lively personalities.

This book seems like another triumph for Professor J. B. Lyons.

Barry O'Donnell,
President,
Royal College of Surgeons in Ireland

Contents

Introduction	1
Chapter 1: John Cheyne, 1777—1836	
Professor of Medicine 1813–19	11
Chapter 2: Whitley Stokes, 1763—1845	
Professor of Medicine 1819–28	47
Chapter 3: Sir Henry Marsh, 1790—1860	
Professor of Medicine 1828–32	81
Chapter 4: John Timothy Kirby, 1781—1853	
Professor of Medicine 1832–36	99
Chapter 5: Richard Tonson Evanson, 1806—71	
Professor of Medicine 1836–43	119
Chapter 6: Charles Benson, 1797—1880	
Professor of Medicine 1836–72	131
Chapter 7: James Little, 1837—1916	
Professor of Medicine 1872–83	151
Chapter 8: Arthur Wynne Foot, 1838—1900	
Professor of Medicine 1883–95	167
Chapter 9: Sir John William Moore, 1845—1937	
Professor of Medicine 1889–1916	179
Chapter 10: Thomas Gillman Moorhead, 1878—1960	
Professor of Medicine 1916–17	209
Chapter 11: Francis Carmichael Purser, 1877—1934	
Professor of Medicine 1917–26	223
Chapter 12: George Edward Nesbitt, 1882—1948	
Professor of Medicine 1926–30	237
Chapter 13: Victor Millington Synge, 1893—1976	
Professor of Medicine 1930–34	245
Chapter 14: Leonard Abrahamson, 1897—1961	
Professor of Medicine 1934–61	255
Chapter 15: Alan Thompson, 1906—74	
Professor of Medicine 1962–74	267
Chapter 16: William Francis O'Dwyer, 1916–99	
Professor of Medicine 1975–85	277
Sources	290
Index	294

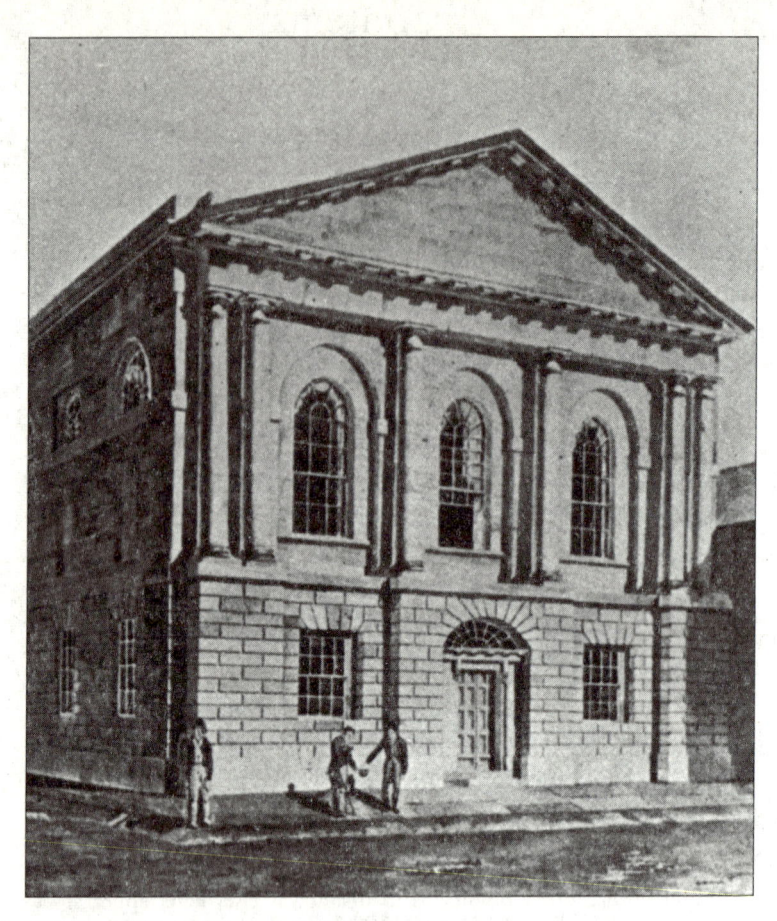

The Royal College of Surgeons in 1821

Introduction

The familiar barber's pole, striped red and white, is a token of a tradition linking barbers and surgeons, a reminder of an age when bleeding was a popular therapeutic procedure. The pole represents the phlebotomist's staff which the patient gripped to distend his veins; the red stripe symbolises the fillet placed to obstruct the veins; the white a bandage used when the bleeding was completed. In Dublin the barbers and surgeons were members of the guild of St Mary Magdalene established by Henry VI on 18 October 1446,[1] an association which persisted well into the eighteenth century to the disadvantage of the surgeons.

A college of physicians existed in Dublin since 1654. A school of physic was available in Trinity College (TCD) since 1711 but Europe's greatest medical teacher was a Dutchman, Herman Boerhaave, and there were many Irish students among his pupils in Leyden. Boerhaave did not subscribe to the centuries-old theory which attributed disease to excess or lack of one or other of the four humours—*blood, black bile, phlegm, yellow bile*—a theory which echoes in the words *sanguine, melancholy, phlegmatic* and *choleric*. The body, as he conceived it, had solid and fluid parts. The former 'are either membranous Pipes or Vessels including the Fluids . . . we find some of them resemble *Pillars, Props, Cross-Beams, Fences, Coverings . . .*' The body, as Boerhaave and his pupils saw it, was subject to mechanical laws, attention to which should direct their therapies.[2]

Eighteenth-century physicians in Ireland, as elsewhere, appear to us to reflect a measure of complacency, permitting a self-satisfied regard while they energetically purged, cupped and bled their patients. Surgeons occupied a subsidiary position. The apothecaries stood at the lowest level of a rigid hierarchy. They were incorporated in the Guild of St Luke in 1745, and opened an apothecaries' hall in Mary Street in 1791.[3]

Looking at these men (their ranks as yet closed to women), our backward glances should not be derisory, or our comments scathing. Anaesthetics, antisepsis, diagnostic devices and antibiotics are missing from the medical armamentaria, but many appurtenances of modern living are also missing. It was a candle-lit world; the horse, the stage-

---

[1] Stanley McCollum, 'The roots of the Royal College of Surgeons in Ireland: the barber/chirurgeons of Dublin', *J. Irish Colls. Phys. & Surgs.* (1994); 23: 53–9.
[2] G. A. Lindeman, *Herman Boerhaave* (London: Methuen, 1968), *passim*.
[3] Sir C. Cameron, *History of the Royal College of Surgeons in Ireland*, 2nd ed. (Dublin: Fannin, 1916), p. 99.

coach and the sailing-ship were the regular means of transport; the penny-post and the internal combustion engine were uninvented; the medical enlightenment had not yet dawned.

Two corner-stones of the modern temple of healing were in position: scientific anatomy, and the discovery of the circulation of the blood, were the gifts of Andreas Vesalius and William Harvey respectively; a third was to be laid by Morgagni, an Italian pathologist in 1761, when *De sedibus et causis morborum* was published. The fourth corner-stone could not be fashioned until the germ theory was validated by Louis Pasteur, Robert Koch and others in the mid-nineteenth century. The profession's moral duties were stated by Hippocrates in antiquity, and Voltaire was moved to say: 'Men who are occupied in the restoration of health to other men . . . are above all the great of the earth.' The French philosopher said, too, and more characteristically: 'The efficient physician is the man who successfully amuses his patients while Nature effects a cure.'

College of surgeons

The need to establish a college of surgeons in Ireland was clearly articulated in 1765 by a Limerick surgeon, Sylvester O'Halloran (1728–1807), who, impressed by the Académie Royale de Chirurgie in Paris, founded by Georges Mareschal, the son of an Irish emigrant, demanded: 'That a decent and convenient edifice be created in the capital . . . That an exact list be taken throughout the kingdom of all reputable surgeons.' Professors were to be appointed. Public examinations were to be held for all who wished to have their names included in the annual register, and he added the Utopian recommendation that courses of instruction should be provided free to any Irishman.[4]

The Dublin Society of Surgeons was founded on 29 March 1780, its main object to obtain a royal charter separating the surgeons from the barbers, and enabling them to establish 'a liberal and extensive system of surgical education.' This was granted on 11 February 1784 by George III. The monarch's mind was then still unaffected by madness, but it will be appreciated that a local matter concerning a group of obscure surgeons would have been handled by the chief secretary, Sir Thomas Pelham, and the lord lieutenant. The latter, Robert Henley, second Earl of Northington, was thirty-six and a bachelor when he came to Dublin in June 1783. He had been described as unwieldy in person and lacking grace, but well disposed to this country and determined 'to do something that may appear to have been obtaining boons, however trifling, for Ireland'. Not the least of these was the surgeons' charter, the granting of which was final-

---

[4] J. B. Lyons, 'Sylvester O'Halloran (1728–1807)', *Irish J. Med. Sc.*, (1963): 217–32, 279–88.

INTRODUCTION

ised on the last day of his term of office. The governors' minute permitting the new college (which had no premises) to meet in the board room of the Rotunda Hospital on 2 March 1784, was signed by the Duke of Rutland, his successor.

This was a temporary measure. Planning for that 'decent and convenient edifice' envisaged by O'Halloran went ahead, and an old house 'lately occupied by the Charity Children of the Parish of St Peter in the City of Dublin', in Mercer Street to the rear of Mercer's Hospital, was leased[5] and adapted for teaching purposes without government aid. It had access to a narrow lane through which bodies might be taken privily to the dissecting room, for in those days anatomists purchased their subjects from the 'sack'em-up' men, the ghoulish 'resurrectionists' who robbed the graves of their dead.[6]

The Duke and Duchess of Rutland brought with them complete dinner-services of gold and silver plate, to do justice to their vice-regal eminence in a city where the upper classes entertained lavishly. The duke's own habits were such that he was thought to have been sent over 'to drink the Irish into good humour'. The brevity of his vice-royalty suggests that they were more than a match for him, but the duke's death in 1787 was attributed to fever.

Many noblemen lived on St Stephen's Green, and Lord Powerscourt had a mansion in William Street, close to Mercer's Hospital and the new Schools of Surgery—use of the plural indicated that schools of both anatomy and surgery were available but both forms are encountered. These foundations were well sited, but the eighteenth-century elegance depicted by Gainsborough had its counterpart in Hogarth's cartoons. Inescapable realities of wretchedness and ill-health were the *raison d'être* of the hospital and the schools.

The Royal College of Surgeons (RCSI) opened its doors in October 1789. It was a two-storey building which in addition to the dissecting room had a lecture theatre, a museum and some offices. Its schools of

---

[5] The college's agent in this transaction was a Dublin bookseller, Patrick Byrne, later a member of the Society of United Irishmen and an advocate of Catholic emancipation. Byrne was to suffer for his political views, being committed to Newgate Prison in 1798; subsequently he settled in Philadelphia.

[6] After considering the report of the committee appointed in 1828 to inquire whether the porters employed by the school of anatomy were connected with the traffic of exporting dead bodies, the court of examiners laid down Janitor Dixon's duties carefully: 'He is answerable for any riotous conduct on the part of resurrection men or others frequenting the College yards or passages whether by day or night . . . He is not to allow any subject on pain of Dismissal to be removed from the College . . . without permision of the Professors.' Should Dixon be detected supplying other establishments with subjects, he was to be fined in accordance with the amount he had received. The gate porter should not allow any to enter but the pupils attending lectures and dissections. (Court of examiners minutes, 20 March 1828.)

surgery prospered beyond expectation owing to the Napoleonic Wars, and by 1804 it was apparent that a larger premises was needed. The government, by now aware that the schools provided a succession of military and naval surgeons, gave a grant of £6,000 in 1805. An old Quaker burial-ground on St Stephen's Green was purchased for £4,000, and here the building of a new and more commodious college was completed in 1810, with further government support. The architect was Edward Parke whose creation had the character 'of a Roman Temple raised on a heavy "podium"'. Its striking façade 'must have served to bring the relatively new professional body to the public attention and enhance its prestige'.[7]

The student body grew in size; the number of candidates for the letters testimonial increased, augmenting the income of the college which was now self-supporting.[8] By the 1820s an expansion of the museum seemed desirable. A minority, as we shall see, suggested that the available funds should be expended on a national surgical hospital, but finally it was decided that enlargement of the museum must take precedence, even though this would entail major alterations.

The first stone of the new extension was laid on 25 August 1825, and the work went ahead so speedily that in April 1826 the building committee issued the following note of progress: 'That the present hall door being about to be closed up permanently your committee beg leave to suggest the propriety of having a temporary door made in the wall in York Street.' The existing premises was preserved in the new one whose lofty pediment supports statues of three Greek deities, Asclepius, Athena and Hygeia, gods who have survived in an iconoclastic Dublin where effigies of the mighty rest on insecure perches.[9]

Keen rivalry existed between the RCSI and TCD, a rivalry into which the unchartered or private schools also entered. Competition increased when the Queen's University of Ireland—with medical schools in Belfast, Cork and Galway was established—to be replaced later by the Royal University of Ireland (RUI). The Catholic University Medical School in Cecilia Street was opened in 1855; its survival was ensured when its lectures were 'recognised' by the RCSI.

A project to enlarge the library and provide a pathology museum was completed in April 1878. At the inauguration of the extension, Philip Smyly, PRCSI, referred jokingly to a subject 'which had given them a world of trouble, and that was the admission of ladies to the profession'. His comments evoked laughter, but evidently the RCSI's attitude to-

---

[7] Colin Brennan, 'Architectural History (1805–1997) of the RCSI', MA thesis UCD; Dublin, November 1997, pp. 8–9.
[8] Cameron, *RCSI*, (note 3), p. 167.
[9] A. D. H. Browne and B. Doran, 'The external statuary of the RCSI', *J. Irish Colls. Phys. & Surgs.* (1988); 17: 177–9.

INTRODUCTION

wards women was less liberal than that of its sister college, the King and Queen's College of Physicians of Ireland (KQCPI) in Kildare Street, which admitted women in 1876

At a meeting of council on 16 December 1884, the motion of the vice-president Dr (later Sir) Charles Cameron, proposing the admission of women to the college licence was finally discussed and passed by 7 votes to 4. But Sir George Porter, who had opposed the motion, remained dissatisfied and handed in the following motion: 'That the question of admitting women to the License of this College be reopened and discussed.' As Sir George was absent on 8 January 1885, his motion lapsed. A clause in the second supplemental charter (1885) granted women access to education and examinations. Later in the year it was agreed to make appropriate arrangements for 'the accommodation of Female Students in the School'.[10]

Amalgamation of the Ledwich and Carmichael Schools with the RCSI proposed first in 1884 became effective in November 1888. In view of the larger numbers attending the college additional use was made of the Carmichael School's premises, conveniently situated in Aungier Street.

The rapid evolution of the modern medical school in the post-Second World War period is described by Harry O'Flanagan and W. A. L. MacGowan in *The Irresistible Rise of the RCSI* (1984). Colin Brennan, in his recent thesis, provides a valuable analysis of the architectural accretions: 'To the east lies the formal beauty and dignity of the early 19th-century Neo-classicism, erected at a time when medical science languished in a primitive condition. To the west is the Medical School of the late 20th century, its repetitive and business-like precast concrete panels seeming to reflect an age which has more important matters on its mind than elaborate theories of aesthetics.'[11]

Chair of medicine

Turning now to academic matters,[12] O'Halloran's demand for three professorships should be recalled—'one for anatomy, a second for the disorders of surgery and midwifery, and the third for the operations of surgery'. An application for the professorship of midwifery received from Thomas Costello, dated 15 August 1784, was declined. John Halahan's offer on 30 November 1785 to deliver lectures on anatomy and physiology in a theatre to be fitted up by himself was accepted (1785–99).

---

[10] For a fuller account of the acceptance of women by Dublin's medical schools see Lyons, *Irish Medical Times*, (Supplement, January 1992): pp 38–40.

[11] Brennan, 'Architectural History', (note 7), p. 53.

[12] The first examination was held on 12 and 14 August 1784; the successful candidate, John Birch, was awarded letters testimonial, and practised for many years in Roscrea.

Halahan had an established reputation as an anatomist, and many years previously was included in Gilborne's *Medical Review*:

> John Hallahan [sic] our just Esteem deserves,
> His curious Art dead bodies long preserves
> Entire and sound, like Monuments of Brass;
> Embalm'd Aegyptian Mummies they surpass,
> Surpass the Labours of the famous Ruysch,
> He does injections to Perfection push.

William Dease's offer to lecture on surgery was also accepted. The professors were unsalaried, in accordance with a principle laid down by Adam Smith who held that if teachers were given a stated salary they might or might not, as it pleased them, be active workers.[13] They were allowed to charge a fee of two guineas to registered pupils, and three guineas to others. When the Mercer Street premises was established a guinea was deducted by the college from the fee paid by each student but after 1793 the professor of anatomy, who supplied demonstrators and subjects for dissection, was permitted to retain the full fee.

Halahan briefly held a second professorship (1789–93)—the chair of midwifery—but was soon succeeded by Sir Henry Jebb.[14] A chair of surgical pharmacy (later designated materia medica) was instituted in 1789, and held by Clement Archer (1789–1803). Walter Wade was professor

---

[13] J. D. H. Widdess, *The Royal College of Surgeons in Ireland and its Medical School 1784–1984*, 3rd ed. (Dublin: RCSI, 1984), p. 18.

[14] The sons of a Boyle apothecary, Edward Jeeb, Frederick and Henry, were destined to flourish in Dublin, becoming master of the Rotunda Hospital and president of the Royal College of Surgeons respectively. At the outset of their professional careers in the city they replaced the second 'e' in their name by 'b', probably influenced by the enviable success in London of Sir Richard Jebb, physician to the king.

Frederick Jebb studied in Paris, returning to Dublin in 1764 to practise as a man-midwife. He lived at 20 St Andrew Street, residing in the Rotunda Hospital during his mastership (1773–80). Author of an important paper entitled 'Physiological Enquiry into the Process of Labour' (1770) he turned later to politics. Under the biblical pseudonym 'Guatimozin' he wrote six articles in the *Freeman's Journal* (1779), condemning the proposed parliamentary union between England and Ireland. His writings were influential, and the lord lieutenant directed that he should be offered an annual pension of £300 to support the government. The bribe was enticing, and the man who had changed his surname with an eye to personal advancement now changed his politics. He supported the government until his death in 1782.

Henry Jeeb may have served an apprenticeship to his father in Boyle, before studying at the Rotunda Hospital during his elder brother's mastership. He practised as a surgeon and man-midwife at 22 North Anne Street, moving to William Street and finally to Grafton Street. He had a remunerative practice, and it was for services in obstetrics, rendered at Dublin Castle, that he was granted a knighthood in 1782. Sir Henry Jebb, surgeon to Mercer's Hospital (1778–1811), was PRCSI in 1800. As a side-line he engaged in commercial building. Dublin's North Frederick Street is named for his son, a surgeon in the Peninsular War, and at Waterloo.

INTRODUCTION

of botany (1792–1825).

The decision to establish a chair of the theory and practice of medicine was strongly influenced by the army medical board which wrote to the college on 23 April 1813, stating that the board required proof of a medical education as well as a surgical one. Candidates for posts as first-class hospital attendants should have had the benefit of at least two sessions of medical lectures, and have spent a year in a hospital.

The college responded promptly, and on Monday 3 May 1813 resolved 'that the Court of Examiners be requested to consider if it be advisable to annex a professorship of the practice of physic to the Schools of Surgery—and in case such a measure shall be deemed expedient, that the court shall be and they are hereby empowered to elect a person to that office.'[15]

On Thursday 27 May the secretary reported from the court of examiners 'that the Court, in compliance with the request of the College, having taken into consideration the expediency of annexing a professorship of the practice of physic to the School of Surgery in the College, had come to the following resolution':

> Resolved, that it is the opinion of the Court that in order to facilitate the Education of Surgeons and Assistt. Surgeons for the Army and Navy, it is highly expedient that a professorship of the practice of physick be annexed to the School of Surgery in the College, and that no person shall be deemed eligible to such professorship who is not a regularly educated and practising physician.[16]

The court was empowered to elect a professor 'on the third Tuesday in June next', and the secretary was instructed to insert an official notice of this intention 'in two of the Dublin Newspapers'. A Scotsman, John Cheyne, MD, who held a post on the honorary staff of the Meath Hospital was appointed to the chair of medicine on 15 June 1813, the first of a line of distinguished physicians to serve the college as professors of medicine.[17]

---

[15] College minutes.
[16] *Ibid.*
[17] The court of examiners consisted of the president and six censors, one of whom was the vice-president. They held an entrance examination in the Greek and Latin classics for prospective pupils, and a qualifying examination for letters testimonial. The latter was a two-day affair: the first day for anatomy and physiology; the second for theory and practice of surgery, surgical pharmacy and mode of prescriptions. Medicine was not an examination subject until 1834.
 Perusal of the records of the court of examiners shows that the examinations held for letters testimonial were by no means a formality: quite a number of candidates were

These worthies are the subject of my book, which presents in outline the careers of the men who have held the chair of medicine in a surgical college, which college, however, as Arthur Jacob was at pains to point out, has always been 'just as much a College of Physicians'.

Through the interstices, individual careers are linked by an invisible web of progress, which throughout two centuries transformed a dubious art into a highly-equipped clinical science, changing the prescriber of coloured water to a purveyor of potent (and possibly toxic) specifics, transforming the physician's aspirant beneficence towards his/her patient (client) to an imperious demand from the latter for relief that if not instant shall at least be rapid.

Sadly, in the course of production of this book, William F. O'Dwyer (1975–85)—in whose company the present author has heard the chimes at midnight—died suddenly, on 8 March 1999. He is survived by his wife, a daughter and a son. The two other contemporary physicians who have held the chair, J. Stephen Doyle (1975–93) and John Fielding (1982–96) are not included here, for there is a convention which ordains such decisions, tending to avoid periods of service too close for comment.

Dr Doyle, though retired from clinical practice, is still active in many areas. He remains an *éminence grise*—sometime medical director of the Ibn al Bitar Hospital, Baghdad; a former president of the Royal College of Physicians of Ireland (RCPI); an ex-president of the Irish Medical Council and an extremely influential member of his profession.

Dr Fielding resigned his chair unexpectedly; he remains in practice though no longer at Beaumont Hospital, and much can still be expected from his considerable and varied talents.

Both Doyle and Fielding are gastro-enterologists; skilled endoscopists, they were active in research and having many publications to their credit are fully representative of modern twentieth-century medicine. John is an erudite musicologist, especially knowledgeable about operas. Stephen's avocations relate to equine matters.

Since January 1998 the chair of medicine has been held by Gerard McElvaney, consultant respiratory physician to Beaumont Hospital. Gerry is a graduate of UCD (1982). He has worked in Vancouver at the University of British Columbia; in the respiratory division of the National Heart, Lung and Blood Institute, Bethesda, Maryland; and at the

---

rejected.

A licentiate of the college was expected to be 'fully qualified and authorized to practise Surgery and to be elected to fill the situation of Surgeon to a public institution as a Member—The Licentiate is also eligible to become a Member upon payment of an additional fee, and submitting to a ballot for his admission, but is not required to pass any additional examination, or perform any additional exercise for that purpose.' The fellowship (for which an examination is required) was substituted for membership in 1844. (Court of examiners minutes, 26 June 1833.)

INTRODUCTION

New York Hospital in Manhattan.

Professor McElvaney has a major interest in applications of basic science to clinical medicine. He is entrusted with the guidance of his students through the millenium towards the expected new developments of the twenty-first century. Quite a challenge! But no greater, perhaps, than that which each of his predecessors has faced; so many of them striving to make bricks without straw, to cure diseases they could not expect to understand. Yet which of them did not hope for epoch-making discoveries?

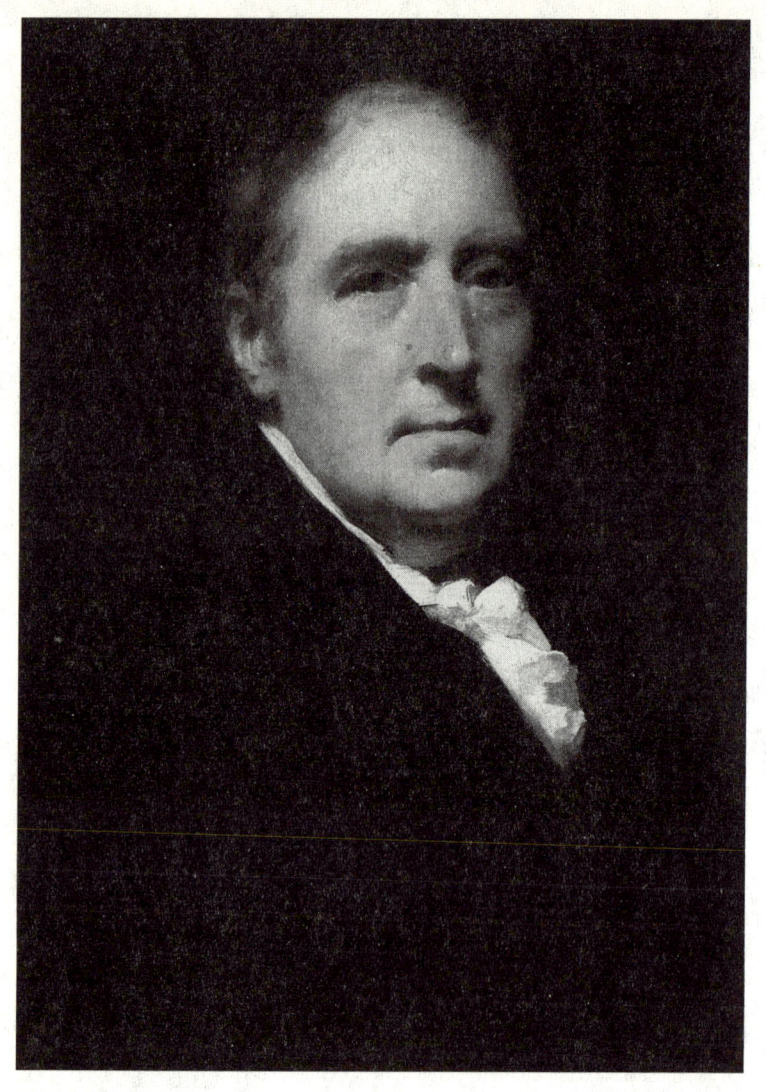

John Cheyne, 1777–1836 Professor of Medicine 1813–19 (portrait by Charles Raeburn, courtesy RCPI)

Chapter 1: John Cheyne, 1777–1836

John Cheyne was born on 3 February 1777 at Leith, Scotland, where his father—'a man of great cheerfulness, benevolence, good sense, and singleness of mind'[1]—practised medicine, and provided for a family of sixteen children. The mother of this large family, a daughter of William Edmonton, a fellow of the College of Surgeons of Edinburgh, was ambitious for their advancement.

At the age of ten John passed from Leith Grammar School to the High School in Edinburgh, where the standard was beyond him, and he often feigned illness to avoid his classes. Eventually he was placed in the care of a tutor, an idle and dissipated clergyman. 'Both master and pupil', Cheyne recalls in his 'Autobiographical Sketch', had 'more relish for frivolous talk than for Homer or Virgil.' Little work was done and although the lessons continued for two years, the additions to the boy's knowledge of Greek or Latin were meagre.[2]

Apprenticeship

Apprenticed to his father at thirteen, young Cheyne was duly impressed by his mentor: 'He would visit the poor as promptly as the rich, and his half-crown was as freely given to those who had no means of procuring food, as his prescription.'[3]

Before long, and rather prematurely, the youngster was attending lectures at the University of Edinburgh where his teachers included Alexander Monro[4] (*secundus*) in anatomy, Andrew Duncan in the Institutes of Medicine (physiology), and Alexander Hamilton in midwifery. Joseph Black, discoverer of 'fixed air' (carbon dioxide) held the chair of chemistry until 1795. Benjamin Bell was Edinburgh's leading scientific surgeon,

---

[1] The principal biographical source is the 'Autobiographical Sketch' included in John Cheyne's *Essays on Partial Derangement of the Mind* (Dublin: Curry, 1843); see also Sir C. Cameron, *History of the Royal College of Surgeons in Ireland*, 2nd ed. (Dublin: Fannin, 1916), pp. 583–86; Lambert H. Ormsby, *History of the Meath Hospital* (Dublin: Fannin,1888); J. D. H. Widdess, *A History of the Royal College of Physicians of Ireland* (Edinburgh: Livingstone, 1963), pp. 150–55; Eoin O'Brien, 'John Cheyne (1777–1836)', *J. Irish Colls. Phys. & Surgs.* (1974); 3: 91–3; Davis Coakley, *Masters of Irish Medicine* (Dublin: Town House, 1992), pp. 65–71; J. B. Lyons, 'John Cheyne's classic monographs', *J. Hist. Neurosci.* (1995); 4: 27–35.
[2] Cheyne, 'Autobiographical Sketch', (note 1), p. 4.
[3] *Ibid.*, p. 1.
[4] Discoverer of the intra-ventricular foramen ('foramen of Monro') which was first observed in dilated form in a case of hydrocephalus which Monro and R. J. Whytt had seen in consultation in 1764.

author of a six-volume *System of Surgery*.

William Cullen resigned his chair in medicine in 1789. He died in the following year but Cheyne senior would have been familiar with his *Nosology* and *First Lines in Physic,* and the concept of a 'sympathetic' action between parts of the body connected by nerves was widely accepted. Cullen was succeeded by James Gregory (1753–1821), remembered today for 'Gregory's Powder' (*Pulv. Rhei Co.*), and generally agreed by his contemparies to have been 'a great physician, a great lecturer, a great Latin scholar and a great talker'.

Gregory engaged unremittingly in professional controversies; 'a disposition towards personal attack was his besetting sin'. The assaults did not always remain verbal, and he was obliged to pay damages of £100 to Professor James Hamilton whom he had beaten with his walking-stick. His example influenced Cheyne in at least two directions: the latter became determined to remain on good terms with his colleagues; he accepted, too, the need to act vigorously in the field of therapy.

Army surgeon

Having taken a diploma at Surgeons' Hall, Cheyne obtained a medical degree in June 1795. Because of his height, 'big John Cheyne' (as he was sometimes called), looked older than eighteen. He secured an appointment as assistant-surgeon to the Royal Regiment of Artillery, and having served in various parts of England he was promoted surgeon, and accompanied a brigade of horse-artillery under Lieut-Col. Howorth to Ireland. With part of the brigade commanded by Lord Bloomfield he 'was present at the actions with the rebels which took place at Ross, Vinegar Hill, &c. in June 1798'.[5]

While in the army, Cheyne frittered his leisure time away playing billiards, shooting and reading books supplied by the circulating libraries, until disillusion finally set in and he realized that he was studying nothing but the manners of his superiors, and learning nothing but ease and good manners, a way of life that was leading him nowhere. 'At last I became dissatisfied with my prospects, anxious to distinguish myself in my profession, and persuaded that unless I made a strenuous effort I must be content with a subordinate station, which my vanity would not have permited me tamely to occupy.' He left the army in 1799, took an appointment at the Ordnance Hospital in Leith Fort, and returned to his father's practice as assistant.

The importance of keeping records, and of performing autopsies on fatal cases, was clear to him, and in this he was helped by Mr (later Sir) Charles Bell, a future professor of surgery who was a few years his senior. 'He opened most of the bodies which I obtained permission to dissect,

---

[5] Cheyne, 'Autobiographical Sketch', (note 1), p. 6.

taught me many things which I might not otherwise have learned, and confirmed my taste for distinction.'

Ambition

Cheyne's ambition was to be a leading physician in a large city, and he set about equipping himself for this position. He was particularly interested in the diseases of children, and in epidemic fevers, and he made a point of carefully studying any unusual case he encountered, by obtaining 'the best monograph I could on the subject', and seeking the opinions of his most skilled colleagues.

> Thus, by means of observation, reading, and the experience of others, my mind was made up on the most important points of practice, and I acquired a facility of prescription, especially in acute diseases, which proved of great advantage to me, particularly in dispensary practice.[6]

He also drew on a sheaf of written opinions obtained from Edinburgh's most eminent physicians over many years, and carefully preserved by his grandfather, grand-uncle and father. These may have included the detailed but undated instructions sent by Alexander Monro (*secundus*) to Surgeon Cheyne of Leith for the management of 'that dreadfull [sic] Distemper of Water in the Head'.[7]

Cheyne's eventual decision to leave Scotland, where so many of his kin[8] had prospered, may have been the unforeseen outcome of his friendship with Charles Bell. The latter's brother, Surgeon John Bell, outstanding among Edinburgh's 'extra-academical' teachers of anatomy, had earned the enmity of James Gregory who did not scruple to say that any sick person 'should as soon think of calling in a mad dog, as Mr John Bell'. It is likely that Professor Gregory's disfavour extended to friends of the Bells, militating against their local preferment. Be this as it may, being more anxious 'for an opportunity of distinguishing myself' than in pecuniary reward (a claim not easily reconciled with his later tendency to

---

[6] *Ibid.*, p. 9.
[7] 'That some Leeches shall immediately be applied to his Temples; 2. I would, at the same time, give him a purgative, with Two or Three grains of Calomel, observing whether he passes any Worms; 3. Shave the top of his head & apply to it a Blister, to be kept open as an Issue; 4. Give him Morning & Evening Two Mercurial Pills, rubbing in also a Scruple of the Ointment each time till the gums become sore; and increase or diminish the dose occasionally, so as to keep up a constant soreness of the gums; 5. If costive give him occasionally a Pill composed of Calomel & dried Scilla.' (R. E. Wright-Sinclair, *Doctors Monro*, London: Wellcome, 1964, p. 80.)
[8] His family lent large sums of money which were never repaid to the Stuarts' agents. His great-grandfather, grandfather and father were members of the College of Surgeons of Edinburgh. His mother was the granddaughter of Alexander Bayne, professor of Scots law in the University of Edinburgh.

equate a large income with success), Cheyne sought a position in a proposed army medical school at Woolwich. He wrote to Dr Rollo, surgeon-general to the Artillery, offering his services as instructor to the junior officers, but got no reply to his letter.[9] He next considered where he might settle in England, until hearing certain comments about 'the state of the medical community in Dublin' his mind turned to the Irish capital which he visited in March 1809, leaving his wife, Sarah, in Antrim with her father, the Rev. Dr George Macartney.[10]

Dublin

What Cheyne saw of Dublin evidently pleased him. He learned that during the preceding fifty years many eminent doctors had flourished there; the profession was respected—'the field was extensive and the labourers liberally rewarded'. The first decade of the nineteenth century had been a period of change in the Irish capital. The Act of Union became effective on 1 January 1801, resulting in predictable social changes. 'The closing of parliament meant the exodus of people of wealth and fashion and the gradual fading of Dublin's brilliance.'[11] The parliament house was sold to the Bank of Ireland, a transaction Shelley described in 1812 as the conversion of the fane of Liberty into a temple of Mammon. Many of the nobility dispensed with their Dublin houses, and the value of property fell. Elegant Georgian dwellings suffered the fate of transformation into lodging-houses or tenements.

Paradoxically, professional men gained in status. With a population of approximately 200,000, the city was well supplied with hospitals. The oldest were the Charitable Infirmary (1718), Dr Steevens' (1733) and Mercer's Hospitals (1734). The Rotunda Lying-in Hospital was celebrated both medically and artistically, for its obstetrical expertise and its decorative plaster-work. The Meath and Hardwicke Hospitals had yet to experience the glory of the 'Golden Age'. The Richmond Hospital was planned but as yet unbuilt. The Lock Hospital for syphilis, and the Royal Hospital for Incurables, catered for special problems. The Fever Hospital in Cork Street, which opened in 1804, was a sadly needed amenity. The west wing of Sir Patrick Dun's Hospital was completed in 1809, and the first clinical lecture at Dublin's first purpose-built teaching hospital was delivered in that year.

The leading physicians at the time of Cheyne's arrival included Ed-

---

[9] John Rollo, MD St Andrew's, army surgeon, served in the West Indies; promoted surgeon-general 1804; d. Woolwich 1809. Author of *Diabetes* (1797), etc. At the time of Cheyne's application, Rollo was declining in health and ambition.

[10] Sarah Cheyne bore her husband nine sons and seven daughters. A daughter, Selina, married Charles Graves, Lord Bishop of Limerick, whose son was the author of the popular song, 'Father O'Flynn'.

[11] Constantia Maxwell, *Dublin Under the Georges* (London: Faber, 1956), p. 92.

ward Hill, William Harvey, Francis Hopkins, James Cleghorn, Whitley Stokes and John Crampton. The prominent surgeons were Richard Dease, Abraham Colles, Philip Crampton and others. Medical practice was largely in the hands of surgeons and Cheyne did not doubt that with his experience he would be more successful than they could ever be in the management of acute diseases.

By now he was the author of three books published in Edinburgh: *Essays on the Diseases of Children* (1801–8);[12] *Essay on Hydrocephalus Acutus, or Dropsy of the Brain* (1808); *The Pathology of the Membranes of the Larynx and Bronchia* (1809). He set up in practice in Dublin towards the end of 1809, taking a house in Ely Place and moving later to 6 Merrion Square West. Like any newcomer he found the going difficult— 'from the 9th of November, 1810, to the 4th of May, 1811, a period of nearly six months, I received only three guineas'.[13] This situation changed in 1811, when thanks to the goodwill of 'some of the most respected of my professional brethren',[14] he was appointed physician to the Meath Hospital (then in the Coombe and small, mean and gloomy), as successor to G. F. Todderick.[15] His fees amounted to £472 in 1812, and as if to confirm that success breeds success, he was elected in the following year to a chair of medicine established in the schools of surgery of the RCSI at the request of the British army medical board.

At a meeting of the court of examiners on 15 June 1813 the secretary 'laid before the Court a letter from John Cheyne Esq MD—offering himself as a Candidate for said office—together with a prospectus of the Course of Lectures he proposed to deliver—'. As there was no other applicant and Cheyne's qualifications were 'highly satisfactory' the court resolved:

> That Doctor Cheyne be and he is hereby appointed Professor of the Theory and practice of Physic, in the School of Surgery under the direction of the Royal College of Surgeons in Ireland for one year from the 14th day of September next.[16]

---

[12] The copy of *Essays on the Diseases of Children, With Cases and Dissections* (Edinburgh: Mundell, Doig & Stevenson; London: Murray; 1801–8) in the RCPI contains 'Essay I, On Cynanche Trachealis' (1801); 'Essay II, On the Bowel Complaints more immediately Connected with the Biliary Secretion, and particularly of Atrophia Ablactatorum, or Weaning Brash' (1802); 'Essay III, On Hydrocephalus Acutus, or Dropsy in the Brain' (1808).
[13] Cheyne, 'Autobiographical Sketch', (note 1), p. 14.
[14] *Ibid.*, p. 14.
[15] For accounts of the Meath Hospital see Lambert H. Ormsby, *History of the Meath Hospital* (1888); P. B. Gatenby, *Dublin's Meath Hospital*, (Dublin: Town House, 1996), *passim*.
[16] RCSI council minutes.

He lectured in full detail on military surgery and medicine, for the Napoleonic Wars had brought prosperity to the college, and the surgeons of the garrison were encouraged to attend his classes gratis.

House of Industry Hospitals

Cheyne became physician to the House of Industry Hospitals in October 1815, in succession to Alexander Jackson, an appointment within the gift of the lord lieutenant.[17] He had four wards in the Hardwicke Fever Hospital and a double ward in a nearby building, with charge of seventy-four beds in all. Many of his patients were local labourers, servants and the like, wasted by fever but basically strong. A significant number, however, were in a different category, broken and infirm from age and intemperance, or grossly disabled and diseased. 'In the House of Industry there are also depots for incurable lunatics, epileptics, and idiots.' The Bedford Asylum for homeless children was another source of clinical cases.

After settling in Cheyne took steps to re-organize the nursing service.

> To every ward there is a nurse and a deputy-nurse or ward-maid, neither of whom is allowed to leave the hospital, without special permission. The deputy is required to scour the ward, at least once a week, and to mop it daily, and this service is never dispensed with. The nurses are charged with the ventilation of the hospital, and made responsible for any irregularity on the part of the patients, and they are expected to conduct themselves in conformity with regulations which have been issued by the governors, a copy of which is hung up in every ward. And each nurse and deputy has a printed copy of the following instructions, which I drew up for their guidance.[18]

These instructions, however rudimentary, established a routine. According to J. D. H. Widdess, they are of prime importance in the history of nursing—'the first recorded attempt at education of nurses in this country'.[19]

The nurses were 'to instruct the visitors and patients in such things as

---

[17] For accounts of the House of Industry Hospitals (the Hardwicke, Richmond and Whitworth Hospitals were named for viceroys under whose rule they were constructed) see W. Thornley Stoker, 'The Hospitals of the House of Industry', *Dublin J. Med. Sc.* (1885); 80: 469–86; E. O'Brien, Lorna Browne and K. O'Malley, (eds.) *The House of Industry Hospitals 1772–1987* (Dublin: Anniversary Press, 1987). Later called St Laurence's Hospital, it closed in 1987, its staff amalgamating with that of the Charitable Infirmary, Jervis Street, at Beaumont Hospital which opened to receive patients on 29 November 1987.

[18] Cheyne, 'Medical Report of the Hardwicke Fever Hospital for the Year Ending 31 March 1817', *Dublin Hosp. Reps.* (1817); 1: 5.

[19] J. D. H. Widdess, *The Royal College of Surgeons in Ireland and its Medical School 1784–1984*, 3rd ed., (Dublin: RCSI, 1984), p. 128.

relate to their conduct'; the deputy nurse must wash the 'face and neck, hands and arms, and feet and legs' of each patient who arrived in the ward, supplying him with a hospital shirt and night-cap, and put him to bed.[20] Detailed instructions are given relating to the care of the bowels; 'the nature of the patient's stools and urine' will be reported to the physician at every visit. A daily examination of the backs 'of all patients who are in a stupid state' shall be made, and the state of the patient's mouth should be watched.

She shall frequently supply him with drink, when he is not able to assist himself, and take care, when he is, that the vessel from which he drinks is placed commodiously within his reach, and is never empty; and when his tongue and gums are covered with a brown or dark crust, she must have them wiped with a bit of fine flannel, moistened with salt and water, two or three times a day; or, if this cannot be accomplished, she must put a thin slice of lemon, without the rind, in his mouth.[21]

A deranged patient was to be calmed, without forcible restraint. 'She must wrap his legs in a blanket, put on his bed-gown, and permit him to sit on his bed, or even go to the fire, till the violence of his derangement shall abate.' The assistance of the apothecary is to be sought in the event of sudden pain or convulsive attacks, and if there is an alarming deterioration a clergyman should be summoned. In the event of a death, the corpse is to be screened and lie untouched for two hours, and an order sent to the apothecary for a coffin.

Cheyne praised the nurses. They were 'kind, handy and faithful to their trust', but he hesitated to give them charge of the patients' punch—'more may be ordered than can be taken by a patient, which is often the case with cordials, when the patient is dying, and the surplus will be a temptation which a nurse, exhausted by watching, might find it difficult to withstand.'[22] Nevertheless, he prescribed porter generously for nurses who seemed delicate.

His private practice flourished; he made £1,710 in 1816, and so that this carefully cultivated pecuniary success should not be at risk he withdrew from the college, and from the Meath Hospital. The House of Industry Hospitals offered a distinct possibility of academic development and with a colleague, Dr Edward Percival, also a newcomer to Dublin, he planned to establish there a clinical school and a museum of morbid anatomy. They both recognised the institution's enormous potential; the House of Industry had an endless supply of indigent patients.

---

[20] Cheyne, 'Hardwicke Fever Hospital 1817', (note 18), p. 6.
[21] *Ibid.*, p. 8.
[22] *Ibid.*, p. 62.

Their plans included an annual report of the diseases they treated; *The Dublin Hospital Reports* materialized in due course but the other projects fell through when Percival left Dublin and settled in Bath.[23] His departure benefitted Cheyne, nevertheless, for the latter's soaring ambition was not yet fully satisfied. A glittering prize was still to be won, the post of physician-general to the army in Ireland, a situation for which he had already applied unsuccessfully. It was held by Percival and now became vacant. Cheyne was already acting as Percival's deputy, so on 7 October 1820 he was appointed to the post he coveted, which was agreed 'to confer on the possessor the highest medical rank in Ireland'.[24] He had now reached the summit of his expectations; he had an annual income of £5,000 but he was not at all a happy man.

Eponym

Turning now to Cheyne's contributions to clinical science, it is convenient to mention first the eponym, 'Cheyne-Stokes breathing', shared with William Stokes, his younger but better-known colleague; that ominous waxing and waning of the respiration which one cannot listen to without a certain dread, for it is a harbinger of death. Cheyne described it in the *Dublin Hospital Reports* in 1818, having observed it two years earlier in a gouty man, one of those well-to-do patients who provided his ample income: 'A. B. sixty years of age, of a sanguine temperament, circular chest, and full habit of body, for years had lived a very sedentary life, while he indulged habitually in the luxuries of the table.'

In offering his description of a single case, Cheyne was really at pains to record an instance 'of the conversion of the fleshy part of the heart into fat'. Almost by chance, it would appear, did he bother to mention the memorable and important detail of the clinical picture.

> The only peculiarity in the last period of his illness, which lasted eight or nine days, was in the state of the respiration: For several days his breathing was irregular; it would cease for a quarter of a minute, then it would become perceptible, though very low, then by degrees it became heaving and quick, and then it would gradually cease again: this revolution in the state of his breathing occupied about a minute, during which there were about thirty acts of respiration.[25]

In a footnote, Cheyne added that he had observed similar breathing

---

[23] See T. P. C. Kirkpatrick, *An Account of the Irish Medical Periodicals* (Dublin: Falconer, 1916).
[24] Cheyne 'Autobiographical Sketch', (note 1), p. 19. He was the 14th physician-general in Ireland, and the last. The appointment was abolished in 1833.
[25] Cheyne, 'A Case of Apoplexy in which the Fleshy Part of the Heart was converted into Fat', *Dublin Hosp. Reps.* (1818); 2: 216–23.

in a relative of his patient, but an autopsy had been refused. His paper was recalled by William Stokes in 1846 when the latter described abnormal breathing in a patient under his own care:

> For more than two months before his death, this singular character of respiration was always present, and so long would the periods of suspension be, that his attendants were frequently in doubt whether he was not actually dead. Then a very feeble, indeed barely perceptible inspiration would take place, followed by another somewhat stronger, until at length high heaving, and even violent breathing was established, which would then subside till the next period of suspension. This was frequently a quarter of a minute in duration.[26]

This 'ascending and descending respiration' was labelled 'the Cheyne-Stokes phenomenon' by Ludwig Traube of Berlin, and one is hardly surprised to learn that it is recognisable in the Hippocratic writings: 'The respiration throughout like that of a man recollecting himself, and rare and large . . .'[27] Cheyne-Stokes respiration has been shown to be accompanied by cyclic changes in blood gases and is the outcome of brainstem dysfunction.

Dublin Hospital Reports

Cheyne was helped in the production of the *Dublin Hospital Reports* by Edward Percival, Abraham Colles and Charles Hawkes Todd, but according to Mr (later Sir) William Wilde, it was Cheyne who possessed 'the art of eliciting the knowledge and bringing forth the powers and acquirements of others, together with a stern honesty of purpose, and suavity of manner—qualities rare, but very requisite in the editor of a periodical'.[28]

The second, third and fourth volumes were edited by Cheyne and Colles, who then relinquished the editorial chair to Robert J. Graves, then in his prime. T. P. C. Kirkpatrick has supplied an author index to the *Dublin Hospital Reports*, which he saw as 'a valuable record of the work of the Irish Medical School', selecting for special mention John Shekelton's paper, 'Dissection of Aneurism', and John Houston's 'Observations on the Mucuous Membrane of the Rectum', with the first description of 'Houston's valves'.[29] Did he overlook a paper by Robert Adams ('Cases of Diseases of the Heart Accompanied by Pathological Observations', 1827, IV, 396) which created the eponym 'Stokes-Adams

---

[26] William Stokes, 'Observations on Some Cases of Permanently Slow Pulse', *Dublin Quart. J. Med. Sc.* (1846); 2: 73–85.
[27] Ralph H. Major, *Classic Descriptions of Disease* (Springfield: Thomas, 1945), p. 548.
[28] [William Wilde] 'The Editor's Preface', *Dublin J. Med. Sc.*, 1846; 1: xxxvii.
[29] Kirkpatrick, *Periodicals*, (note 23), pp. 14–23.

syndrome'? One wonders if Cheyne, as he edited this paper, saw its relevance to his monograph on apoplexy. 'What most attracted my attention [Adams wrote] was, the irregularity of his breathing, and remarkable slowness of pulse, which generally ranged at the rate of 30 in a minute.'[30] During the previous seven years there had been 'not less than twenty apoplectic attacks' from which there was recovery without paralysis.

Essays on the Diseases of Children

'Children are not admitted into public hospitals, and their diseases are ill understood, and superficially treated, or slurred over, by those who profess to teach medicine.' This neglect prompted Cheyne's *Essays on the Diseases of Children*; his first subject being 'croup' which he saw as a single entity of varying severity, not to be confused with the acute asthma of Millar. 'In croup, the cough . . . is constantly ringing in our ears; in acute asthma there is little or no cough.'

Croup tends to affect children between weaning and puberty, and a graphic description is offered:

> The disease generally comes on in the evening, after the little patient has been much exposed to the weather during the day, and after a slight catarrh of some days standing. At first his voice is observed to be hoarse and puling; he shuns his play-fellows, and sits apart from them, dull, and, as it were, foreseeing his danger. His illness, indeed, does not prevent him from going to sleep, but soon he awakes with a most unusual cough, rough and stridulous. And now his breathing is laborious, each inspiration being accompanied by a harsh shrill noise, most distressing to the attendants: His face is swelled and flushed, and his eye bloodshot; and he seems in constant danger of suffocation: His skin burns, and he has much thirst; he labours more and more in breathing; still the ringing noise is heard, and the unusual cough: he tries to relieve himself by sitting erect; no change of posture, no effort gives him relief.[31]

When favourable, croup 'terminates in various ways' but not uncommonly the patient succumbs—'weakened by the violence of his illness, with purpled lips and leaden countenance, he dies in two or three days'.

The pathology of croup, as Cheyne envisaged the disorder, was tracheal inflammation causing a secretion which becomes 'a white membrane of considerable tenacity'; it seems likely that some of his cases were diphteritic. According to Osler, in most cases of membranous laryngitis

---

[30] Robert Adams, 'Cases of Disease of the Heart Accompanied by Pathological Observations', *Dublin Hosp. Reps.*, 1827; 4: 396.
[31] Cheyne, *Diseases of Children*, (note 12), pp. 15–16.

the Klebs-Loffler bacillus is present.³²

The treatment Cheyne advises is to let blood freely from the tumid jugular veins with a lancet, following this with an emetic and a warm bath. If the physician hesitates to use the lancet a second time he can apply leeches to the neck.

Jaundice and 'The Weaning Brash' are dealt with in the second essay. The former includes 'Icterus Infantum' caused by complete obstruction of the bile duct, and the jaundice which develops a few days after birth and ends in marasmus—'It is a disease peculiar to some families.' Do we have here an early reference to icterus neonatorum resulting from Rh incompatibility?

'Atrophia Ablactatorum' was the term coined by Cheyne to dignify a condition attributed to sudden or inopportune weaning, and ushered in by green diarrhoea. Occurring 'in sultry seasons', it was seldom fatal before the sixth or seventh week. Was it a manifestation of low-grade intestinal infection?

The third essay, 'On Hydrocephalus Acutus', was revised in a second edition (1819) which is discussed later.

Cases of Apoplexy

The bibliography added to *Garrison's History of Neurology* includes Cheyne's *Essay on Hydrocephalus Acutus* (1808), and *Cases of Apoplexy and Lethargy* (1812), which McHenry refers to as 'The first noteworthy monographs on neuropathology to appear in the Nineteenth Century'.³³ While preparing the first edition of *Hydrocephalus Acutus* for the press, Cheyne was struck by the lack of information on diseases of the brain in the British literature, and finding the treatment of apoplexy a matter for dispute he decided to take notes on every case of nervous disease he encountered. Though acquainted with what Wepfer, Morgagni, Matthew Baillie and other pioneers had written on apoplexy, he felt that many questions remained unanswered, and that certain facts deserved to be re-established.³⁴ He confirms, for instance, that haemorrhage is found in the hemisphere opposite to the side of the hemiplegia. He also described intra-cerebellar haemorrhage: 'It has been thought, that extravasation of blood is only to be found in the cerebrum. This opinion, however, is erroneous: I have observed extravasation in the cerebellum in three, if not in four instances.'

---

³² William Osler, *The Principles and Practice of Medicine*, 7th ed. (London: Appleton, 1909), p. 202.

³³ Lawrence C. McHenry, *Garrison's History of Neurology* (Springfield: Thomas, 1969), p. 248.

³⁴ Cheyne, *Cases of Apoplexy and Lethargy: with Observations upon the Comatose Diseases* (London: Underwood, 1812), p. 11.

He mentions theoretical causes of apoplexy and dismisses them as 'mere expressions of opinion in abstract terms'. Discussing 'The Anatomy of Apoplexy', Cheyne describes both subarachnoid and intracerebral haemorrhage, and he was the first to publish an illustration of the former. He was painstaking in his endeavours to discover the precise mechanism of haemorrhage, and, using a syringe or a camel's hair pencil, spent hours examining 'the seat of the extravasation', but these minute inspections led him into error.

He cites alterations noted by Matthew Baillie in the internal carotid arteries and their branches:

> The disease consists in a boney [sic] or earthy matter being deposited in the coats of the arteries, by which they lose a part of their contractile and distensile powers, as well as of their tenacity. The same sort of diseased structure is also found in the basillary artery and its branches. The vessels of the brain, under such circumstances of disease, are much more liable to be ruptured than in a healthy state. Whenever blood is accumulated in unusual quantity, or the circulation is going on in them with unusual vigour, they are liable to this accident; and accordingly, in either of these states, ruptures frequently happen.[35]

He will not, however, accept Baillie's reasonable conclusion that this 'diseased structure' leads to haemorrhage, which, Cheyne believes, 'generally proceeds not from one considerable vessel, but from a number of the smaller vessels . . .' He claims to have seen in his dissections of extravasations, 'many vessels, not larger than a human hair, ending in small clots of blood . . .'

> Hence it seems that the bleeding does not depend on erosion, (which, indeed, could not be considered as an ultimate cause, for we should have to explain the origin of the eroding matter,) nor is it owing to aneurism, nor ossification, but to a great and simultaneous action of the smaller arteries of a hemisphere, or of the whole brain; an action which, strong as these arteries are, they, in general, are unable to bear without a rupture of their coats.[36]

McHenry points out that 'The first idea that anaemia of the brain rather than vascular congestion might be the cause of apoplexy is to be found in the work of John Cheyne.'

An arresting passage merits quotation in full if only for its candour:

> Our knowledge of the brain is still circumscribed within very narrow bounds: we do not know with certainty any thing beyond the form, consis-

---

[35] *Ibid.*, p. 36.
[36] *Ibid.*, pp. 39–40.

tence, and colour of its various eminences, depressions, and cavities, and the origin of the nerves and distribution of the blood vessels, which connect this organ with the rest of the system. We indeed know, from the effects of obstruction in the course of a nerve, and the uniform effects of similar diseases of the brain, that sensation and volition are functions of this organ; but we are as much in the dark with regard to the use of most of its parts, its ultimate structure, and the kind of influence which it exerts over the body and most of the circumstances upon which the origin and transmission of that influence depends, as we are with respect to the nature of impressions made by external objects upon our organs of sense, or the sensations associated with these impressions.

While his knowledge of the mechanism and functions of the brain is so limited, perhaps the physician ought to confine himself to careful and minute observation, and accurate description, of the alterations of action or of structure which are produced in it by disease.[37]

Cheyne saw blood-letting as the sovereign remedy for apoplexy—'The first and second blood-letting ought to be large', and if necessary followed by a third. He disagreed vehemently with the contrary teaching of John Fothergill: 'Every one [he wrote] who respects the memory of this excellent man, must regret the publication of his remarks on apoplexy.'

The blood may be taken from the temporal artery, or a large vein in the arm, or from the jugular vein; although, as the latter sometimes requires a ligature to make the vein swell, or to stop the bleeding, I generally prefer the arm or the temple. Two pounds of blood ought to be removed as soon as possible after the attack.[38]

If for any reason direct bleeding is not practicable, the head should be shaved and leeches applied, 'or the cupping glasses, with extensive scarification used'. He drew the line at 'scarification within the nostrils'.

He did not favour emetics but believed that an active purgative should be given as soon as the patient can swallow, preferably calomel.

To secure a speedy operation, it ought to be followed by a dose of some of those cathartics, which operate chiefly on the upper part of the alimentary canal, as rhubarb, jalap, or scammony; or a draught of the infusion of senna, in half an hour after the calomel has been swallowed, may be administered, to secure and quicken its operation.[39]

---

[37] *Ibid.*, pp. 30–1.
[38] *Ibid.*, p. 61.
[39] *Ibid.*, p. 77.

Hydrocephalus Acutus—tuberculous meningitis

Robert Whytt's *Observations on the Dropsy in the Brain* (1768), based on twenty cases, divides the illness into three stages. The *first* is characterised by anorexia, vomiting, lassitude and weight loss; there is headache, fever and a quick pulse. 'They cannot easily bear the light, and complain when a candle is brought before their eyes.'[40] The pulse 'becomes slow and irregular' in the *second* stage and Whytt saw this as 'the surest *diagnostic*'. There may be a delirium, squint and double vision. 'They moan heavily, yet cannot tell what ails them.' The pulse 'rises again to a feverish quickness' in the *third* stage, some days before death.

The 'Dropsy within the Brain' must be distinguished, Whytt points out, from other cranial disorders, from worms, 'a foulness in the stomach and bowels, or from a slow fever ending in a coma'. Appreciation of the pattern of the illness, he believes, will permit recognition of *hydrocephalus*.

> When therefore, with a slow and irregular pulse we meet with thirst and a feverish heat, watching, a *strabismus*, or double sight, a *delirium*, and screaming, succeeding the symptoms mentioned in the first stage, we may strongly suspect water in the ventricles of the brain. But this is still more evident, when soon after the patient grows comatose, the pupil dilates and loses its motion, the pulse becomes quick, the cheeks are flushed, the tendons start, and convulsions follow.[41]

The second edition of Cheyne's *Essays on Hydrocephalus Acutus; or Water in the Brain* (1819) opens with an introduction which discusses a disorder known to many generations of physicians, but subjected to examination in terms of morbid anatomy only in the eighteenth century, 'a fatal kind of fever, incident to children, attended with strabismus, dilatation of the pupil, coma, and convulsions'. He reviews the British literature crediting Dr St Clair, professor of medicine at Edinburgh, with the first modern clinical description in 1733 and recognising John Paisley, a Glasgow surgeon, as the first to submit cases to autopsy. Robert Whytt regarded the disease as 'always incurable' but a Dr Watson described a case with recovery in 1768.[42]

'With respect to medical practice', Cheyne affirms, 'pyrrhonism is a

---

[40] Robert Whytt, *Observations on the Dropsy in the Brain* (Edinburgh: Balfour, 1768), p. 13.
[41] *Ibid.*, p. 30. Whytt (1714–66) was professor of medicine at Edinburgh, where he studied before graduating MD Rheims (1736). Active in research, his publications included *Essay on the Virtues of Lime-water and Soap in the Cure of the Stone* (1743), *An Essay on the Vital and other Involuntary Motions of Animals* (1751), and *Physiological Essays* (1755). Appointed physician to the king in Scotland (1761); elected president of the Royal College of Physicians at Edinburgh (1763).
[42] Cheyne, *Essays on Hydrocephalus Acutus: or Water in the Brain*, 2nd ed. (Dublin: 1819), p. v.

much more dangerous extreme for a Physician to fall into than credulity.' Consequently he is prepared to see the introduction of mercury (1775), and the recommendation of blisters and opium (1777), as important steps in therapy. William Withering, who enjoyed such success with digitalis in dropsy secondary to heart failure, tried it for hydrocephalus but lacked 'a sufficient number of cases to enable him to ascertain its powers'.[43]

Dr Charles William Quin of Dublin is cited for introducing 'a new doctrine of the disease, founded upon the basis of dissection', and for ascribing its basic cause to inflammation. Four of Quin's post-mortem examinations disclosed, in addition to a considerable quantity of fluid in the ventricles, turgid bloodvessels and thickened and opaque meninges 'coated with coagulable lymph'.[44]

The body of Cheyne's work consists of two essays followed by descriptions of his own cases, and finally an account of the 'dissections' or autopsies. The first essay presents the clinical features of hydrocephalus acutus (HA) which may be preceded for days or weeks by non-specific symptoms; these are apt to be disregarded until such time as it is suspected that the brain is disordered.

> When the attention is more particularly excited by these symptoms, the headach [sic] or pain in the forehead will be observed returning at shorter intervals. The child often affectingly complains of his head; he sighs frequently, is dull, his head requires to be supported; he complains of weariness in his eyes; the pupils appear unusually contracted, and he has an aversion to light, but in the dark he sometimes fancies he sees flashes of light. The pulse becomes quick ... the child complains not of headach only but of pains in different parts of the body ... he will lie long on his mother's knee, restless and whining ... These disorders cannot last long without impairing the child's strength; and accordingly, in ten days, or a fortnight ... his appearance is altered; his manner becomes peevish; his hand tremulous; and his gait tottering.[45]

Or the disease may present more acutely:

> After the child has been in a drooping state for a short time ... there is a sudden change to a fever ... but we are led to suspect some deeply-seated evil, from his frantic screams, and complaints of his head and belly, alternat-

---

[43] *Ibid.*, p. xi.
[44] *Ibid.*, p. x. Charles William Quin (son of Henry Quin, FKQCPI and president in 1758) was the author of the first published record of the use of digitalis in Dublin. President of the College of Physicians in 1788, he was physician-general to the army in Ireland with charge of the Royal Hospital, Kilmainham, and the Military Hospital.
[45] *Ibid.*, p. 3.

ing with stupor, or rather lowness and unwillingness to be roused.⁴⁶

In a third form, which Cheyne describes as 'an instance of conversion of disease', HA develops in the wake of 'an indifferent state of health, as for example, after there has existed a scrofulous disease which has subsided . . . 'The first form has the best prognosis; the acute form might have an equally favourable outlook were early diagnosis possible; recovery from the third form is rare.

With some reluctance, Cheyne accepts Whytt's division of the illness into three stages: 'I shall venture to present them under some changes of character. The first, as the stage of increased sensibility; the second, as the stage of diminished sensibility; the third, as distinguished by palsy or convulsions.' But regularity in these stages is not to be expected. Hurried breathing may indicate that death is imminent; profuse sweating at the back of the neck has occasionally heralded recovery. Commonest in 'the middle years between weaning and puberty', the disease in infancy lacks 'the decided character which it assumes in childhood and youth'.

Cheyne regarded HA as a development secondary to 'irritation in the abdominal viscera, and especially in the liver'.⁴⁷ He disagrees with 'the late Dr. Parr of Exeter' who postulated the existence of 'an original defect in the brain itself', and scolds Parr for holding that the disease is incurable, a belief which 'must obstruct the progress of inquiry and improvement', and may be used 'as an apology for indifference, by all who are without inclination for the study of their profession'.

Always an energetic therapist, Cheyne outlines his therapeutic practice in the second essay: his method was to apply leeches over the liver, draw blood from a vein or from the temporal artery, administer cathartics, especially the mercury containing calomel. He favoured James's powder, the nostrum based on antimony which has been blamed for the death of Oliver Goldsmith. ('Antimony and mercury owe their wonderful powers of relieving the febrile complaints of children to their influence over the stomach and liver, in reducing action and restoring secretion.') Clysters, blistering and ice-packs, were also used and opiates relieved distress.

Cheyne saw Whytt's *Observations on the Dropsy of the Brain* as 'a highly valuable monograph' but outmoded—'the author has applied the theories which prevailed half a century ago, of the formation of dropsy to the disease in question'.⁴⁸ The judgement is not unfair: Whytt held that the immediate cause of the excess fluid was 'such a state of the parts as makes the exhalent arteries throw out a greater quantity of fluids than

---

⁴⁶ *Ibid.*, p. 3.
⁴⁷ *Ibid.*, p. 49.
⁴⁸ *Ibid.*, p. iv.

the absorbent veins can take up'.[49]

This in turn could have several causes: 'an original laxity or weakness in the brain'—and here Whytt ventured to draw an analogy between infantile hydrocele, easily cured by supporting the testicles with bandages, and hydrocephalus which might possibly be cured, too, if discovered at a comparable age—birth trauma, a pituitary tumour compressing the veins, 'a too thin or watery state of the blood'.[50]

The inference that the clinical features are those of tuberculous meningitis was made by others, for nowhere does Whytt consider tuberculosis as an aetiological factor. Cheyne noted a relationship between scrofula and HA but, although some of his dissections showed miliary and caseous intra-abdominal lesions, he failed to draw the direct aetiological conclusion. Dr William Patterson, of Londonderry in the north of Ireland, went nearer than most to recognise the exact cause in a book published in 1794 but not read by Cheyne until many years later. Patterson saw the disease as an instance of inflammation affecting diaphanous membranes (pleura, peritoneum, pericardium, meninges were diaphanous membranes), among the causes of which 'the scrophulous virus is justly accounted one'.[51] The clinical features Cheyne and others described were certainly those of 'meningitis', a word the *Oxford English Dictionary* credits to Abercrombie in 1828 though Osler says that Guersant used the name 'granular meningitis' in 1827; Papavoine showed the nature of the granules in 1830; W. W. Gerhard of Philadelphia placed the disease on a firm clinical and pathological basis in the early 1830s.[52]

Cheyne also took exception to the prognosis offered by Whytt, who stated: 'I freely own that I have never been so lucky as to cure one patient who had those symptoms which with certainty denote this disease.'[53] But even in the present century, Osler was equally lacking in hope: 'I have neither seen a case which I regarded as tuberculous recover, nor have I seen post-mortem evidence of past disease of this nature.'[54] Twenty cases are described by Cheyne who claimed ten recoveries (presumably ten misdiagnosed cases, a slur he would have bitterly resented); the monograph supplies the details of eight autopsies.

The disease remained a death-sentence until streptomycin, the first anti-tuberculous medication, became available in the 1940s. With the general reduction in the incidence of Koch's infection tuberculosis meningitis is now a rarity in Ireland. Few doctors are familiar with the clini-

---

[49] Whytt, *Dropsy*, (note 40), p. 32.
[50] *Ibid.*, pp. 32–6.
[51] William Patterson, *Letters Concerning the Internal Dropsy of the Brain* (Dublin: 1794), p. 22.
[52] Osler, *Principles*, (note 32), p. 301.
[53] Whytt, *Dropsy*, (note 40), p. 47.
[54] Osler, *Principles*, (note 32), p. 304.

cal picture; it has been reported that in the recent case of a County Waterford woman, who died after two months in hospital, the diagnosis was established at autopsy.

Reports from the Hardwicke Hospital

Cheyne contributed ten articles to the five volumes of the *Dublin Hospital Reports*. These included reports for the Hardwicke Fever Hospital for the years 1816–17, 1817–18; an account from the Whitworth Hospital of a dysentery epidemic; a long report 'On the Feigned Diseases of Soldiers' based on his attendance at military hospitals. His other subjects were melena, jaundice, the virtues of James's powder, erethism of the stomach, and venesection in early phthisis.

Fifty-three of 780 patients admitted to Cheyne's beds in the Hardwicke Hospital between 1 April 1816 and 31 March 1817 died. Whenever possible, post-mortem examinations were performed. Cheyne's report aimed at describing prevailing fevers rather than naming them, for 'what one would call typhus or synochus, another might call a pituitous or bilious fever; and a third . . . might denominate a gastric, pulmonic or cephalic fever'.[55]

His pages resemble a graphic Hogarthian frieze: 'Mary Graham. Squalid, and although only fifty, she had all the appearance of old age'; 'John Toole, a soldier who had served in Spain . . . Countenance flushed, livid and swoln; eyes glassy'; 'Richard Gibson. Tongue foul . . . Hippocratic face—insensible. He died in the night.'

Patients who 'had lingered in their own miserable dwellings, under a load of filthy bedclothes', frequently benefitted immediately following their admission to the hospital. 'In many instances, the ablution of [a] great part of the body, change of linen, the common purgatives of the hospital, the pure air of the ward, and the supply of cold diluting drinks, were productive of a crisis in the course of the first night.'[56] Defending his use of the lancet as the first line of therapy for fevers, Cheyne invoked the authority of Sydenham—'While he recommends the patient to be let blood early and largely, he affirms that blood-letting will be injurious, if sparingly or tardily performed'—but does acknowledge that at the hands of Francis Home, a regimental surgeon serving in the Low Countries, the practice fell into disrepute.

> Dr. Home sometimes had patients in fever let blood, to the scandal of his clinical pupils, who were convinced that fever was sustained by a spasm of the minute vessels, or that all its symptoms were symptoms of mere debility. Hence they thought the learned Professor a Homicide, whose hands

---

[55] Cheyne, 'Hardwicke Fever Hospital 1817', (note 18), p. 13.
[56] *Ibid.*, p 19.

ought to have been tied up by the managers of the Royal Infirmary, and they admired the skill of those physicians who, while they gave their patients in fever three or four pints of wine a day, forced them to swallow a reasonable quantity of the shop cordials in addition.[57]

Yet during his lifetime, Home had seen blood-letting return to favour and Cheyne was suitably impressed by Beddoes' wish to apply leeches 'by relays of dozens', and convinced all the more by the results he saw Dr Mills obtain at Cork Street Fever Hospital.

Cheyne insisted, however, that he was not 'an advocate for indiscriminate bleeding'. Cathartics, the second-line of treatment, were to be used cautiously: 'in the administration of purgatives, the bridle is often more wanted than the spurs'. Cordials were given with great moderation but they were not withheld from motives of economy. Emetics were given only to cases of threatened relapse, or at an advanced period of the illness ('to resuscitate secretion') when the tongue was dry and shrivelled.

Cheyne's second report from the Hardwicke Hospital dealt mainly with an epidemic which gripped Dublin in the summer of 1817. The disease was deemed contagious as it frequently affected a number of persons belonging to the same family. 'Between the beginning of April and end of August there were twenty-two or twenty-three houses, or perhaps more properly speaking, lodgings in different parts of the city, which yielded from two to six patients each.'[58]

The illness usually began with a period of dejection followed by headache, rigors, constipation and anorexia; severe pains in the back and loins, debility and fever soon presented. In the early stage, the tongue was white with florid edges 'and several declared that the smell of their own breath was insufferable'. Chest pain with expectoration of bloody mucus was common and in severe cases the patients became confused and delirious towards the end of the first week or at the beginning of the second.

In many cases the delirium was of a very troublesome kind; first it was only occasional, then it continued all night, then it was uninterrupted. We had many patients who created a great disturbance by wandering about the wards all night, prying into the closets, and looking under the beds. Some of these were full of their usual occupations: one man, by trade a cooper, endeavoured to pull his bed to pieces, in order to make a tub of the spars.[59]

Stupor with subsultus tendinum often supervened and the patient was unable to protrude a black, shrivelled tongue.

---

[57] *Ibid.*, p. 58.
[58] Cheyne, *Dublin Hosp. Reps.* (1818); 2: 4.
[59] *Ibid.*, p. 6.

As the soporose state went off, the blackness and dryness of the tongue went off also ... The expression of the patient daily improved. The temperature gradually approached the point of health, the flushing subsided and the inflammation of the eyes, also the complexion became clearer as well as paler, and the eye more expressive ... The patient turned upon his side, and about the end of the second week, in many cases, began to attend to external circumstances, and to call for food ...[60]

Petechial haemorrhages were frequently seen towards the end of the summer and many physicians believed they were dealing with a typhus epidemic. Cheyne, on the other hand, saw it as 'only the common continued fever, which generally prevails, more or less during the summer, in many of the great towns in these countries'. The steward of the House of Industry and several doctors fell ill. 'Most of the unseasoned nurses took the disease.' The servants who undressed patients on admission seemed particularly at risk, a fact that gains significance now that typhus is known to be louse borne.

Was Cheyne's interpretation incorrect? He admitted, as we have seen, the uncertainty of diagnosis in fever cases, nor did he claim to be an authority. 'I confess that I never saw Typhus epidemic, save in the military hospitals in the South of England, where I chanced to be at the time [1809] when Sir John Moore's army landed from Corunna.'[61]

Between April and August, 289 patients were admitted to the Hardwicke Hospital. On 31 May and the four succeeding days, the admissions averaged nine daily, double the expected intake. When fifteen patients sought admission on 1 September the governors of the House of Industry reported the epidemic to the lord lieutenant who decided that the Whitworth Hospital should be used for fever cases.

To combat the epidemic, the city was divided into districts, each with a medical inspector to ascertain the prevalence of fever, to select houses of rooms for whitewashing, and to supervise the cleansing operations. 'For a considerable time there were two hundred persons in separate gangs, employed by the Governors of the House of Industry in cleansing the city, and in removing from those parts of it, which were not under cognizance of the Paving Board, the accumulated filth of years.'[62]

When the wards of the Hardwicke and Whitworth Hospitals were full, the lord lieutenant ordered that the Richmond General Penitentiary be used as a temporary fever hospital. Cases were also sent to Sir Patrick Dun's Hospital, and the City Bridewell, capable of containing 400 cases,

---

[60] *Ibid.*, p. 8.
[61] *Ibid.*, p. 3.
[62] *Ibid.*, p. 41.

was held in readiness should the need arise. The House of Industry and its hospitals were well sited, commanding an extensive view of the city and of the Dublin Mountains, but the insalubrity of the neighbourhood is indicated by a report made by two of the medical inspectors, Dr Peebles and Mr Macdowell, concerning conditions they found in the vicinity of nearby Church Street:

> Foul lanes, courts and yards are interposed between this and the adjoining streets. A few respectable shop keepers excepted, the entire street is inhabited by persons of the lowest order. There are many cellars which have no light but from the door, which, in several, is nearly closed by bundles of rags, vegetables and other articles exposed to sale. In some of these cellars the inhabitants sleep on the floors, which are all earthen; but in general they have bedsteads. Most of the courts are crowded and filthy. Nicolson's court, which immediately joins the Root-market, contains 151 persons in 28 small apartments, of whom 89 are unemployed; their state is very miserable, there being only two bedsteads and two blankets in the whole court.[63]

The street nearest Dublin's principal barracks supplied more cases than any other part of the city—'the disease affected many of the women of the town, whose haunts are in that street'. The soldiers' relative immunity was attributed to their excellent living conditions, good food and clothing. Pawnbrokers, huxters and shopkeepers were not spared but the disease never involved the well-to-do.

The desirability of proper ventilation, cleanliness, cooling drinks and purgatives was not in question but the indications for 'blood-letting, mercury, opium, and wine' were discussed with a bias that varied from author to author in the best books on fevers. Cheyne ventured to remind 'the young, inexperienced and ardent practitioners', that patients must be considered individually: 'the perfection of our art consists in knowing the exact point at which expectation should yield to action.' Nor should the operations of nature be interfered with lightly.[64]

Wine was never withheld if it appeared at all likely to be of help, and not uncommonly he gave it without a specific indication 'to those who greatly longed for it'. Punch was to be avoided—'a physician who wishes to maintain discipline will not introduce punch into his wards'—and Cheyne acknowledged personal dislike of both the smell and sight of it, 'from having so often witnessed the ruin that ardent spirits, unmixed or diluted, brings upon the health and morals of the poor of the country.'[65]

His general clinical observations included an account of a scrotal abscess resulting from undetected urinary retention with overflow. He em-

---

[63] *Ibid.*, p. 48.
[64] *Ibid.*, p. 64.
[65] *Ibid.*, p. 71.

phasised that the complication could have been avoided had he not neglected to carry out a routine inspection for a distended bladder in an apparently incontinent patient. This was the physician's duty, rather than the nurse's. 'The patient died on the 27th of June, in a miserable way; for no sooner was a dressing applied than he tore it off. Indeed he was consistent in no part of his conduct but in his efforts to baffle every endeavour which was made to save his life.'[66]

An Account of the Fever Lately Epidemical in Ireland (1821), edited by Barker and Cheyne, supplied a fuller account of the epidemics of 1817, 1818 and 1819, drawing on material provided by contributors from the provinces. Dr Francis Barker was physician to Cork Street Fever Hospital and held a chair of chemistry in TCD for forty-one years.

Opinion was the divided as to the cause of fever epidemic: to some they were the outcome of a miasma that corrupted the air; others (the contagionists) held that fever was spread by sick-persons and fomites. Both groups incriminated meteorological factors and undernourishment, either directly or indirectly.

Cheyne and his co-author accumulated evidence that recent epidemics were spread by contagion.

> It attacked those persons who were sufficiently exposed, whatsoever might be their condition in life; on the contrary those who were secluded from the sick or their effluvia, escaped. Like other contagious disorders, it was communicated by fomites, and the agency of this cause has been confirmed by various reports, announcing that the disease broke out in families after the visits of mendicants and vagrants, although these visitors at the time, were not labouring under fever.[67]

They did not, however, speculate on the means by which spread from person to person was effected. Detailed attention, on the other hand, is devoted to social aspects of the epidemics, the 'sufferings of the lower classes in Ireland'; the economic disruption, with lowered wages and high prices for goods. They recorded that many medical practitioners 'fell a sacrifice to fever', and recognised the courage of clergymen of all denominations.

> The Roman Catholic Clergymen, in general, evinced that disregard for danger in the discharge of their functions, for which they are distinguished in this country. The Roman Catholic Priest was often to be seen leaning over the bed of the poor, ministering comfort to the dying, regardless of the

---

[66] *Ibid.*, p. 28.
[67] F. Barker and J. Cheyne, *An Account of the Fever Lately Epidemical in Ireland* (Dublin: Dublin University Press, 1821), vol. I, p. 144.

infectious exhalations arising from the sick, by whom he was often surrounded.[68]

In a report submitted by Cheyne and other physicians from the House of Industry's fever hospitals, the recruitment of additional cleansing inspectors was recommended. These should extend their attention 'to the bedding and persons as well as to the houses of the poor'. Active co-operation should be encouraged, too, 'between the servants of the Paving Board and the scavengers employed by the governors of the House of Industry'.

Observing that many rural patients spent a night or two in the city before entering a hospital—'leaving, in the lodging which they had occupied their germ of disease'—it was easy to account for 'the obstinancy' with which fever persisted 'in some streets in the line of the great western and northern roads'.

To counteract this evil, fever hospitals should be established 'in those districts in the neighbourhood of Dublin from which some patients come'.[69]

Dysentery

Cheyne had intended to work for a third year in the fever wards but when Dr Percival resigned he moved to the Whitworth Hospital and availed of an opportunity to study ninety-eight cases of dysentery.

> I had often witnessed obstinate cases of dysentery, but I had not formed an adequate conception of the horrors of that disease, until I saw the patients who were congregated in the wards of the Whitworth Hospital: every successive visit more strikingly exemplified, in the hopelessness of the second stage of dysentery, the infinite consequence of treating its first stage with skill. The lower orders in this country, it is true, generally exhibit a very patient endurance of suffering, when they feel death approaching, yet to their physician, from whom they still hope for relief, their situation is only the more affecting, from the extraordinary calmness with which they prepare themselves for death, when it seems inevitable.[70]

Fifteen cases had occurred during the course of a fever, thirty-three in the recovery period; fifteen were caused from cold and wet, four by indigestion; the cause of the remainder was unclear. Cheyne was prepared to accept Sydenham's dictum that 'dysentery is a febris introversa, that is fever turned in upon the intestines'.

---

[68] *Ibid.*, p. 101.
[69] *Ibid.*, vol 2, p. 262.
[70] Cheyne, 'Report of the Whitworth Hospital, containing an account of Dysentery as it appeared in Dublin in the latter end of 1818 . . . ' *Dublin Hosp. Reps.* (1822); 3: 1–90.

When the disease continued without relief for twelve or fourteen days, a degree of emaciation usually became observable, much more rapid in some than in others, and which was always an alarming symptom; when, added to emaciation, a patient in the second or third week of dysentery acquired a haggard look, when he had a quick pulse, and an abdomen impatient of pressure, we had little hope of his recovery.[71]

Although castor oil was the accepted treatment, Cheyne's experience convinced him that its virtues 'had been too hastily conceded'. Venesection, on the other hand, although often cautioned against, he found 'the most uniformly useful' of the therapeutic measures he used in the Whitworth Hospital. 'It results from a consideration of the cases in my possession that venesection, calomel, and opium, followed by the capivi mixture, with farinaceous diet, proved more successful than any other method which was adopted in the severest cases.'[72] Extensive colonic ulceration was found in many of the post-mortem examinations.

Malingering

The 'Medical Report on the Feigned Diseases of Soldiers' took the form of a letter from the physician-general to George Renny, MD, director-general of military hospitals in Ireland. Cheyne had treated sick soldiers throughout his professional life and felt entitled to speak authoritatively of malingering, and the difficulty of detecting it. Barrack-room traditions prevented 'the exemplary from exposing the worthless'; informers were universally detested and it was hard to come to an understanding of methods used to simulate disease.

Malingering was a form of deceit that Cheyne pronounced to be 'an intolerable nuisance'. With the intention of collecting information about commonly feigned diseases, the methods used to mislead the medical officers, the best means of detecting the fraud, and the most successful way of dealing with malingerers, he circulated the staff and regimental medical officers on the Irish establishment in 1823.

From his researches he learned that factitious ophthalmia resulted from irritation with quicklime, tobacco infusion, silver nitrate, cantharides ointment, a gonnorheal discharge etc. A rupture could be simulated by puncturing the scrotum with a corking pin, blowing it up with air by means of a piece of tobacco pipe and reducing inflammation with a warm poultice. Paralysis was readily feigned. 'It is not uncommon for soldiers to pretend that they had suddenly been struck DEAF and DUMB, while all the faculties of the mind continue unimpaired.'[73] Amaurosis was

---

[71] *Ibid.*, p. 23.
[72] *Ibid.*, p. 45.
[73] Cheyne, 'Medical Report on the Feigned Diseases of Soldiers', *Dublin Hosp. Reps. (1827)*;

feigned with the aid of belladonna. Some soldiers learned how to quicken their pulse when the surgeon approached. Vomiting, enuresis and faecal incontinence were troublesome and difficult to expose.

Wonderful indeed is the obstinacy which some malingerers evince. Night and day they will remain with the endurance of a fakir, in a position the most irksome. For weeks or months many men have, with surprizing resolution, sat and walked with their body bent double. Some have continued to irritate sores in the leg until the case became so bad as to require amputation of the limb, and many instances have occurred, in Military and Naval hospitals, of factitious complaints ending fatally.[74]

Vertigo was complained of frequently, the malingerer describing his giddiness volubly but 'silent respecting the symptoms which attend the genuine complaint'. Epilepsy was often successfully simulated, but genuine epilepsy was sometimes regarded as feigned by inexperienced medical officers. 'It is obvious that the more we know of the disease by reading and observation, the more patience and temper we possess, the more successful shall we be in the detection of imposture.' The robust measures used to expose feigned epilepsy included 'applying a hot poker to the ear or hip, putting snuff, Cayenne pepper, or hartshorn up the nose; plunging the individual into a cold bath; drenching him with cold water...'[75]

Persistent air swallowing, or the ingestion of chalk and vinegar, could produce grotesque abdominal distention with tympany. If detected it was speedily controlled by glauber salts in weak tobacco water, a detestable compound known to Cheyne as 'Infusum Benedictum'. Diarrhoea was self-induced by inserting soap into the rectum, or swallowing a mixture of vinegar and burnt cork.

The incidence of malingering was related to the discipline of a corps: the better the discipline the less frequently was disease simulated. Cheyne felt he could judge discipline by the behaviour of the sick in hospital, contrasting 'the manly demeanour' during pain and suffering of the men of some regiments with 'the uncivil, sulky, lounging manner' characteristic of others. 'Among those who counterfect [sic] disease, the Irish are the most numerous and expert, the lowland Scotsman comes next to the Irish, and what he wants in address, is supplied in obstinacy.'[76]

English soldiers were the most straightforward, but malingerers generally were men of bad character. Their aim was to be discharged from the service, possibly with a pension, and Cheyne believed every effort

---

4: 123–81.
[74] *Ibid.*, p. 131.
[75] *Ibid.*, p. 154.
[76] *Ibid.*, p. 127.

should be made to frustrate them, for should they succeed not merely was 'a reward granted to fraud' but a premium was 'held out to future imposition'.

Cheyne realized military surgeons could be guilty of 'no small degree of caprice and irregularity'; he appreciated, too, the danger of making a mistaken diagnosis of malingering, which was a tragic error, and supplied several instances. 'Thus in the year 1804 or 1805, a soldier of the name of Smith, of the Ninth Foot, who complained of great uneasiness of the loins, was treated as a malingerer, and was sent to punishment drill, at which he was kept till a tumour appeared in his back, symptomatic of a lumbar abscess, of which the poor fellow died.' A strong, active hussar, becoming careless and listless was discharged from his regiment as a 'skulker', but his life ended with coma and convulsions. The post-mortem examination revealed two tumours in the right cerebral hemisphere.

Shortly after becoming physician-general, Cheyne himself had discharged two soldiers because of repeated vomiting, a serjeant of infantry and a new recruit. Before long he met the former in Barrack Street in the best of health, and realized he had been manipulated; the recruit, being destitute, 'threw himself on the establishment, wherein he died in a few days'. The post-mortem examination showed advanced gastric disease, 'the mucus membrane being everywhere varicose and pulpy'.[77]

When malingering was suspected, the medical officer should conceal his suspicions until they were either confirmed or removed. During the observation period, he should prescribe the treatment ordinarily appropriate to the disease suspected to be feigned. If finally convinced that the complaint was unreal, the case should be reported to the commanding officer. The surgeon should never, on his own authority, resort to punishment, nor should he apply any painful remedy unless that cure was actually called for by the disease in question.

> I am well aware, that the strait waistcoat, the log, and the solitary cell, have often been used by medical officers of character; nay, I rather think they are still sometimes employed without any warrant from higher authority, but certainly those who thus act, very gratuitously expose themselves to censure. There used to be the greatest coarseness and severity in the treatment of men in hospital, nay military as well as medical officers frequently treated common soldiers as if they belonged to an inferior order of beings. In former times, I have often heard soldiers called the greatest villains on the face of the earth, only to be kept in subjection by the lash. This was folly in the extreme and happily it has become obsolete.[78]

---

[77] *Ibid.*, p. 168.
[78] *Ibid.*, 136.

Cheyne insisted, in conclusion, that the suppression of malingering was essential to the maintenance of the discipline of a corps, but the medical officer should always be guided by just principles. 'He must avoid all harsh, arbitrary, and unauthorized proceedings' and the final responsibility rested with the commanding officer.

The Prince of Hohenloe

We have John Cheyne's own assurance that he was 'more generally employed as a consulting than an attending physician', and early in his career he had observed the importance of punctuality ('which is not much practised in Ireland') in a consultant.

> Punctuality precludes the necessity of explanations and excuses . . . Punctuality is considered by junior and subordinate members of a profession as manifesting respect for their feelings and occupations; it is felt to be a compliment; and it is a compliment in which there is no surrender of truth. When a case of disease was assuming an unfavourable aspect, and when the question was mooted—to whom shall we apply for further help? it has, in a multitude of instances, been decided in my favour solely by the consideration that I would appoint the earliest hour for a meeting, and that I might be expected to appear within five minutes of the appointed time.[79]

Prudence, and attention to the feelings of colleagues, had also, he believed, contributed to his success. He made a practice of returning to his house at appointed times during the day to form new engagements, but refused to say by what route he would go from point to point in case he was 'obliged to yield to an unexpected requisition' which might upset his routine, and impose delays. The frequency with which he was summoned to see members of medical families he calls 'a painful distinction', but such an attendance, though a cause of great anxiety, could not be declined. He avoided mentioning the names of those who had been his patients, and never made a second visit unless requested to do so. His 'closeness' was proverbial, his deportment 'as little assuming as possible'.

Cheyne realized that, merely through his established reputation, a physician could find himself in a position 'to effect improvements in the health of his patients which appear to the ignorant almost miraculous'. This was so, particularly, where prolonged mental depression had made recovery seem unlikely.

> In such cases a physician, unless he obtains dominion over his patients, so far from affording relief, fails in every prescription; nay, prescriptions un-

---

[79] Cheyne, 'Autobiographical Sketch', (note 1), p. 21.

exceptionable in all respects appear uniformly to aggravate the symptoms which in general they alleviate. The Physician is felt to be a chief cause of the patient's suffering; but instead of looking to those influences which improve the general health—such as a proper regimen, air and exercise, change of scene, and amusements which do not exhaust the spirits—he is led by disappointment to the exhibition of medicines more and more active, till the patient in despair refuses all further aid, or seeks help from some other quarter, or very generally, if affluent, goes to the metropolis to consult the Radcliffe or the Mead of his day. A popular physician with a composed yet decided and rather unyielding manner, to such a patient appears almost like a ministering angel.[80]

Cheyne knew he had cured many patients in Dublin, using exactly 'the same means which have signally failed in the country'. He compared his successes with the relief of the so-called *'Hohenlohe cases',* Maria Lalor and Mary Stuart, who were a recent cause of controversy in Ireland.

After a long illness, Maria Lalor had been deprived of her speech in her eleventh year, remaining mute during the next six years despite the efforts of local doctors and consultations with eight Dublin physicians. At the request of her father, the Right Rev. Dr Doyle, Bishop of Kildare and Leighlin, communicated in 1823 with a German priest and supernatural healer, Alexander Emmerich, Prince of Hohenlohe. Emmerich agreed to offer his intercession on 10 June; at the same time Mass was celebrated in Maryborough, Queen's County, on behalf of Maria who after receiving communion heard a voice saying, 'Mary, you are well'. She was then able to speak 'in an agreeable, clear, and distinct voice, such as neither she nor her mother could recognise as her own voice.'[81]

Two months later, in Dublin, a similar cure was obtained for Mary Stuart, a nun who was paralyzed and unable to speak. Bishop Doyle and Archbishop Byrne issued pastoral letters pronouncing the cures to be authentic miracles, a contention disputed by surgeon-general Crampton, physician-general Cheyne and others.

Cheyne's patients in 1824 included James Henry, a recent medical graduate of TCD, a brilliant young man who had fallen ill with typhus, and after his recovery regularly availed of Cheyne's expertise in consultation in his own growing practice. But subsequently Dr Henry was to publish a critical pamphlet, *Strictures on the Autobiography of John Cheyne, M.D.*, which will be considered below.

---

[80] *Ibid.*, p. 25.
[81] W. J. Fitzpatrick, *The Life, Times and Correspondence of the Right Rev. Dr. Doyle*, vol. I (Dublin: Duffy, 1880), pp. 246–54. See also S. J. Connolly, *Priests and People in Pre-Famine Ireland* (Dublin: Gill and Macmillan, 1982), p. 116.

JOHN CHEYNE

Depression and retirement

Cheyne's account of his own career betrays his obsessional nature; one is not surprised to find that he was affected early in 1825 by what he calls 'a species of nervous fever'. This was probably an affective disorder. In the previous autumn there had been an epidemic of dysentery in Dublin and a number of his patients had succumbed. There were additional anxieties unconnected with his profession. 'I became so weak that I was not able to dress in the morning till I had had coffee, and when I returned from a day of toil at seven or eight o'clock in the evening I was obliged to go to bed to obtain rest before I was able to dine.'[82]

Having struggled on unavailingly, he went to England for a complete rest. Whatever benefit he may have obtained was lost when, on his return, he found a close friend, Charles Hawkes Todd, one of the surgeons to the House of Industry, mortally ill. 'He had awaited my return, in order to put himself under my care. His sufferings proved an incubus on my spirits, which strangled every cheerful thought.' Todd died on 19 March 1826 at his residence, 3 Kildare Street, subsequently the site of the Kildare Street Club. Two of his nine sons (he had six daughters) attained distinction: the Rev. James Henthorn Todd is remembered for 'Todd's roll' of the alumni of TCD and for his Gaelic scholarship; Dr Robert Bentley Todd, one of the founders of King's College Hospital, created the eponym 'Todd's paralysis'.

Cheyne had left the Meath Hospital long before the arrival there of R. J. Graves and William Stokes, but they were well aware of his contributions to medicine and dedicated *Clinical Reports of the Medical Cases in the Meath Hospital*, a small book published in 1827, to their senior colleague. On 25 March 1827, Cheyne, keenly interested in the latest methods, invited Richard Townsend, who had mastered the use of the stethoscope, to examine an ailing dragoon at the King's Infirmary. Townsend diagnosed a cavity in the left lung. and a right-sided pneumothorax due to a broncho-pleural communication; a few days later the changed signs indicated a pleural effusion. Death was followed by a post-mortem examination and Cheyne was impressed when Townsend's diagnosis was confirmed.[83]

Consumption was the commonest cause of death among soldiers

---

[82] Cheyne, 'Autobiographical Sketch', (note 1), p. 28.
[83] Davis Coakley, *The Irish School of Medicine* (Dublin: Town House, 1988), p. 34. See also Samuel Bell Labatt's fee-book which contains the following entry for Mrs Rothwell who paid him one guinea on 16 October 1829: 'Consult[ation] w[it]h Cheyne—abd-[ome]n & mamma swelled but no uterine tumour nor areola round ye nipples. Catam[eni]a reg[ula]r as to period but rather scanty in quant[it]y—no morning sickness —rather more fulness & some soreness in region of left ovarium . . . I do not think her pregnant but I apprehend dropsy of left ovarium'.

serving in Ireland; Cheyne recommended 'mediate auscultation, to which percussion of the thorax should be added', for every army recruit whose chest was poorly developed, before his acceptance for service. 'The stethoscope would also appear applicable to those persons in hospital who are simulating pulmonary consumption, or organic disease of the heart.'[84]

He puzzled out the nature of his own problem—'a climacteric disease was forming, which ever since has been slowly executing its appointed mission'.[85] By dint of relaxation, reduction of his undertakings, 'sleeping out of town', and arranging for a co-operative colleague to act as his deputy at the military hospital, he managed to remain in practice. Between 1 February and 31 May 1829 he took £2,230 in fees, more than he had ever received in a similar period.

He put pen to paper on 13 July 1830, to confirm views he had expressed verbally to Robert Graves on the effectiveness of 'small bleedings, frequently repeated' in incipient consumption and haemoptysis. The 'Letter to R. J. Graves', published in the *Dublin Hospital Reports*, mentions that he rarely sent consumptive patients to the continent of Europe but favoured 'short residences at Mallow, or the Cove of Cork . . . Diet as generous as the state of the lungs will permit, in some cases a glass or two of claret, and small bleedings.'

> In haemoptysis venesections act rather as an alterative than a styptic, mere hemorrhage from the lungs does not justify the measure. Bleeding, however, is amply justified by the existence, during haemoptysis, of pain, hurried respiration, or any other symptom of parenchymatous or of membranous inflammation.[86]

He struggled on with his upper-class practice until 1831, when he retired. This decision resulted in appreciative addresses from Dublin's physicians and apothecaries. Forty-five eminent fellows and licentiates of the College of Physicians acknowledged the qualities underlying his success.

> We cannot but deeply lament the absence of one who, whilst occupying for many years the very first rank in his profession, equally maintained its respectability and protected *our* interests. In you we have witnessed the enlightened practitioner and experienced the disinterested friend. Faithful alike to your patients and your colleagues, you became pre-eminent without exciting jealousy. Your extensive information and sound practical judgement, the candour and kindness which you have ever shown to your brethren, and the sterling integrity and dignified deportment which have always been conspicuous in your intercourse with every member of the profession, have so

---

[84] Cheyne, 'Feigned Diseases', (note 73), p. 163.
[85] Cheyne, 'Autobiographical Sketch', (note 1), p. 29.
[86] Cheyne, 'Small and Repeated Bleedings in Incipient Phthisis, Recommended in A Letter to R. J. Graves, Esq. M.D.' *Dublin Hosp. Reps.* (1830); 5: 350–64.

fully commanded our highest esteem and unlimited confidence, that we should hail with sincere pleasure your return to that important station amongst us which you have so long and so deservedly occupied.[87]

Dublin's apothecaries were no less eloquent:

> Permit us . . . to express as our unanimous opinion, founded on the long acquaintance with you which we have had the pleasure of enjoying, that amongst those who within our recollection have occupied the prominent station of head of the Profession of Medicine in this metropolis, not one has ever ranked higher in acquirements, in professional integrity, or in those qualifications which constitute the gentleman.[88]

As a therapeutic exercise—'when it was desirable to find such occupation as would divert him from anxious thought'—Cheyne wrote *Essays on Partial Derangement of the Mind in Supposed Connexion with Religion*. He wished to show that mental upsets 'are invariably connected with bodily disorder', and that the 'moral treatment for the insane' then favoured was unlikely to succeed until attention was directed to the postulated physical cause.

Cheyne objected to the division of mental disorders into *melancholia* and *mania*, and while arguing the point he offers a prime example of what has come to be termed manic-depressive psychosis.

> Again, interchanges between melancholy and raving madness are frequent: an individual who may have been seen as dark, silent and motionless as Cibber's statue—his mind long engaged in brooding over expected misery—will sometimes start into action, and at once be filled with the wildest and most impracticable projects; happiness and prosperity will reel before him, his countenance will beam with gaiety and hope, and he will obtain a degree of bodily strength to execute his insane purposes, which nothing can restrain but fetters and manacles.[89]

His acceptance of the literal truth of *Genesis* influenced his concept of the human constitution, which he saw as flawed and weakened by the disobedience of Adam and Eve. An inheritance of disease and death is a consequence of eating the forbidden fruit which led to the loss of the uprightness of our first parents' original nature.[90]

---

[87] Cheyne, 'Autobiographical Sketch', (note 1), p. 30.
[88] *Ibid.*, p. 31.
[89] Cheyne, *Partial Derangement*, (note 1), p. 44.
[90] Stumbling towards a scientific analogy, Cheyne cites the ill-fated dissector's contaminated abrasion as an example of how a deleterious substance is absorbed into the system from a cadaver.

It seems that the mind can now perceive and think and act only by means of the bodily organs: compress the nerves which convey sensation and all perception of the qualities of bodies will be interrupted; compress the brain, and thought will be suspended; compress the nerves of motion, and the mandates of the will can no longer be executed. If we suppose that at the fall the body was first corrupted, it could no longer be a fit recipient for a soul created to reflect the image of God. Through the injury sustained in the first instance by the physical constitution of man, we might conceive that his mental constitution was injured, and his judgement and affections became depraved. Every fresh inroad which is made on the mind—every instance of amentia, delirium, or insanity—is connected with superadded disorder of the body.[91]

Most of the affections of perception selected by Cheyne for comment—vertigo, diplopis, tinnitus, disorders of the body-image—have an organic cause, and he advances a useful rule of thumb. 'The moment an individual believes in the reality of his false perception, he becomes insane.' He goes on, however to explain suicidal ideas and the not infrequent obsessional compulsions, often attributed to demonical possession by those afflicted by them, to disordered states of the digestion affecting the nervous system and meriting alkaline bitters, mild cathartics and country air. 'In a word, we must cure the choler, and choleric operations of the devil will cease.'[92]

He was familiar with what was later called 'pyschosomatic': 'The contemplation of a contingency which is full of responsibility or danger will cause a sense of anxiety identical with that angina which is symptomatic of several diseases of the heart.'[93] He recognised the possible effects of the menses on the emotions: 'A young lady for several years was uniformly reduced to the lowest dejection before the end of the month, and continued so for a week.'[94]

He made no claim to knowledge of the mind other than that gained 'from having long witnessed the drama of life from behind the scenes . . . [and] from having been for some years in superintendance of a considerable number of insane persons', in addition to his personal experience of 'lowness of spirits, arising from dyspeptic nervousness'. He placed menal derangements into five groups, those arising from: (1) the organs of sense; (2) the intellectual faculties; (3) natural affections and desires; (4) the moral affections; (5) derangement of the whole mind.

Naturally he was familiar with the tragic disability which Broca later called 'aphemia' and Trousseau 'aphasia', a disorder in which neither the

---

[91] Cheyne, *Partial Derangement*, (note 1), p. 156.
[92] Ibid., p. 77.
[93] Ibid., p. 159.
[94] Ibid., p. 239.

tongue that is stilled, nor the hand that can no longer write, is at fault—'it is the power of language in the mind, if we may so speak, which is destroyed'.

Attacks of aphasia may be repeated, a misfortune that Cheyne recalled was suffered by the widow of the poet Robert Burns; she had five episodes of palsy, the last rendering her unconscious: 'from that time [according to the *Dumfries Courier*] till the hour of her death, her situation was that of a breathing corpse—and thus passed away "Bonny Jean".' In a different context, Cheyne refers to Dr Samuel Johnson whom he deems to have been 'often on the very brink of insanity'.[95]

Death

He settled at Sherington, near Newport Pagnell, a Buckinghamshire village where one of his sons lived, and having decided it was better 'to wear out than to rust out' he made his services available to the locals on three mornings in the week. 'On the fourth morning the sick came to me from distant parts of the country, for whom I prescribed; and, as there was no physician within twelve miles of the post town nearest to my house, I was occasionally consulted by some of the more respectable families in the neighbourhood.'[96] He contributed to *The Cyclopaedia of Practical Medicine*, until in 1833 a cataract in his right eye prevented this occupation.[97] One of his articles deals with 'Wakefulness', of which he had bitter personal experience. He had several beds in his room, and would move restlessly from one to another in his quest for a deep and dreamless sleep.

Cheyne suffered from arterial disease which caused 'mortification of the extremities'. The six weeks prior to his death on 31 January 1836 were spent 'On a bed of languishing . . . .' He left detailed instructions regarding his funeral: this should be unostentatious, costing as little as possible and there was to be no sermon. 'I would pass away without notice from a world which with all its pretentions is empty.' His death was to be announced as follows in the Irish newspapers: '"Died at Sherington, Newport Pagnel, Bucks, on the—day of—Dr. Cheyne, late physician-general to the forces in Ireland." Not one word more; no panegyric.' The funeral should be attended by his sons only, with six villagers to bear his remains. There was to be no tolling of bells, but so that the bell-ringers should not feel deprived they might be given an order for bread equal to the sum due to them; they should not be given money, for they would

---

[95] *Ibid.*, p. 118.
[96] Cheyne, 'Autobiographical Sketch', (note 1), p. 32.
[97] Cheyne's subjects in J. Forbes, A. Tweedie and J. Conolly (eds.) *The Cyclopaedia of Practical Medicine* (London: Sherwood, Gilbert and Piper, 1834), are croup, epilepsy, epidemic gastric fever, laryngitis and insomnia.

spend it in the ale-house.[98]

John Cheyne's headstone carries his initials, J. C., three biblical texts and a pious admonition:

> Reader! the name, profession and age of him whose body lies beneath, are of little importance; but it may be of great importance to you to know, that, by the grace of God, he was brought to look to the Lord Jesus, as the only Saviour of sinners and that this 'looking into Jesus' gave peace to his soul.

His instructions were attended to scrupulously, but in Dublin his colleagues were not prepared to let him pass without a contemporary record which praised his writings for their elegance and sound precepts, and stated that he had treated them, young and old alike, with equal courtesy. 'No man ever maintained, in the circle in which he practised, more respect and confidence from his professional brethren, or a higher character with the public as a skilful physician.'[99]

Many years later, Cheyne's *Essays on Partial Derangement of the Mind* (1843) fell into the hands of Dr James Henry, who had forsaken medicine for his obsessive quest of Virgilian manuscripts, and was an inveterate pamphleteer and polemicist. He devoted the morning of 9 November 1859 to the perusal of the curious book, and dashed off *Strictures on the Autobiography of the late John Cheyne M.D.* which charged Cheyne with materialistic astuteness, finding it impossible to reconcile such unremitting ambition in a person who had embraced the cross of Christ. 'At one and the same time a worldling and a Christian, equally greedy of the treasure which perishes and of the treasure which perishes not . . . .'.[100] But then, as Henry points out, modern civilization has succeeded in blending 'the spiritual with the carnal, the eternal and the temporal'; it is adept in the pursuit of both God and mammon, 'or, as it may with greater propriety be called, Mammon in God'.

James Henry condemns Cheyne for publishing, as an exemplar rather than a confession, an autobiographical sketch which lauds an ambitious career that ended, spent and exhausted, at fifty-four in broken health, depriving himself of the restful years with his family in which he should have enjoyed the fruits of his exertion.

The pamphlet is gratuitous. Not only does Dr Henry fail to honour the golden rule *de mortuis nil nisi bonum*, but he overlooks, and may have been unaware of, the importance of Cheyne's speculation—doubtless influenced by Sir Charles Bell's demonstration of the separation of func-

---

[98] Cheyne, 'Autobiographical Sketch', (note 1), p. 38.
[99] Obituary, *Dublin J. Med. Sc.* (1836); 9: 171.
[100] James Henry, *Religion, Worldly-Mindedness and Philosophy being Strictures on the Autobiography of the late John Cheyne, MD*, (Dresden: 1860).

tions, motor and sensory, of the spinal nerve roots—as to whether the mind, 'whatever unity of essence it may have, operates as though it were an aggregate of distinct faculties'.[101] Late-nineteenth-century physiologists were to confirm the localization of particular functions in certain brain areas, confirming an idea to which Cheyne had at least given tentative consideration.

---

[101] Cheyne, *Partial Derangement*, (note 1), p. 44, p. 50.

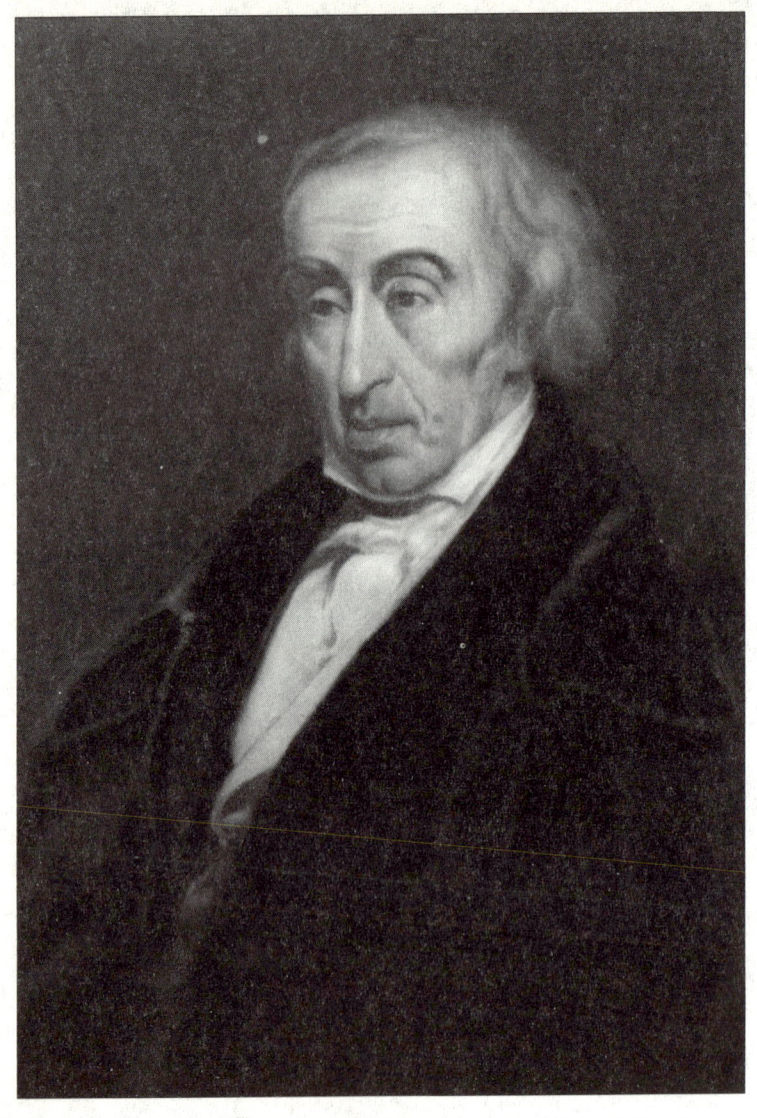

Whitley Stokes, 1763–1845 Professor of Medicine 1819–28 (portrait by Charles Grey, courtesy TCD)

Chapter 2: Whitley Stokes, 1763–1845

> *I am sure it will not hurt the self-love of any of the friends whose names I have recorded, when I say that, in the full force of the phrase, I look upon Whitley Stokes as the very best man I have ever known.*
>
> Theobald Wolfe Tone, Memoirs

The portrait in Trinity College, Dublin, of Whitley Stokes, painted surreptitiously by Charles Grey in 1840, is dismissed by Professor Anne Crookshank as 'nearly a caricature'.[1] And yet, whoever sees the deeply-lined, desiccated countenance of this remarkable-looking man wishes to know more about him. 'Never was the triumph of the soul in its tracings and impressions upon the temple of its abode, more manifest than in the physiognomy of Dr Stokes', wrote his younger contemporary, 'Erinensis'.[2] He was Cheyne's successor in the chair of medicine in the Royal College of Surgeons in Ireland, where he taught for nine years.

Birth and ancestry

Whitley Stokes was born in Waterford in 1763, son of Gabriel Stokes, DD (1732–1806), chancellor of the cathedral and master of Waterford endowed school, an ex-fellow of TCD.[3] His grandfather, Gabriel Stokes (1682–1768) resided in Essex Street, Dublin, and was deputy-surveyor general.[4] The minutes of the Ballast Office Committee contain the following extracts: *16 August 1725*—'Ordered that Mr Stokes be desired to make what haste he can with the map of the river [Liffey] and to consult with Captain Burgh and Captain Perry from time to time.' *2 February 1726*—'Mr Stokes this day petitioned the Committee that he may be paid for his trouble and care in drawing a new plan of the river and harbour of Dublin.' *23 May 1726*—5 'Ordered that Mr Gabriell [sic] Stokes be paid the sum of fifty pounds in full for surveying and drawing maps of

---

[1] See Eoin O'Brien and Anne Crookshank (eds.) *A Portrait of Irish Medicine* (Dublin: Ward River Press, 1984), p. 18.
[2] 'Erinensis' was the pseudonym of Dr Herries Greene, Dublin correspondent to *The Lancet*. See Martin Fallon, *The Sketches of Erinensis* (London: Skilton & Shaw, 1979), p. 40.
[3] *Alumni Dubliniensis* and Henry Boylan's *Dictionary of Irish Biography* give Dublin as his birth-place. Before taking a college living the Rev. Gabriel Stokes was professor of mathematics. He edited *Hippolytus* and *Iphigenia in Aulis* and was author of essays on Newcome's 'Harmony of the Gospels' and 'Subscription to the Thirty-Nine Articles'.
[4] He was the author of *A Scheme for Effectually Supplying Every part of the City of Dublin with Pipe water* (Dublin: 1735), and *The Mathematical Cabinet of the Hydrostatical Ballance unlock'd: or an easy key to All its Uses*.

47

the bay and harbour of Dublin.'

After a primary education at his father's school in Waterford, Whitley Stokes entered TCD in 1779, and was joined there two years later by Theobald Wolfe Tone with whom he became friendly.[5] Elected scholar in 1781 he commenced BA in 1783, proceeding MA in 1789. Meanwhile he had faced the task of obtaining a fellowship, a distinction gained at the time by competitive examination held in public over four days, and for which it was necessary to have attained the highest standard possible in mathematics, logic, natural and moral philosophy, chronology, history and the classical languages. Young Stokes had wide interests, and prepared himself so assiduously that he became physically weak and emaciated; he had to be carried into the examination hall in 1788, but he was rewarded with success. At his own request, though lacking a medical degree, he was given the medical fellowship in 1789, being designated 'Medicus'.

On 22 June 1793, having laid before the board certificates of his attendance on the several professors of medicine, and a thesis in Latin on 'Respiration', the degrees MB and MD were conferred on Stokes at the summer commencements. He was granted £50 by the board 'for the purpose of Prosecuting his studies in Edinburgh', and one wonders if the somewhat unworldly Irishman encountered 'big John Cheyne' in the Scottish capital.

Polymath

Like most inexperienced doctors of his time, his first ventures as a medical practitioner took him into the slums where he studied his patients' environments as intently as their ailments. Since 1795, incidentally, he had been a member of the committee of trustees of The Sick and Indigent Roomkeepers Society (1790–1990).

> A small room sets for three or four guineas a year; the family who take it have lodgers, who pay them sixpence-halfpenny per week to lay down a bed of straw if they have it. Thus, nine or ten people live in a room ten foot square; thirty is a low average for such houses. In Charles-street I understand, they run up to ninety.[6]

---

[5] A surprising friendship in two men so temperamentally different. In his *Memoirs* Tone recalls that at seventeen: 'I began to look on classical learning as nonsense; on a fellowship in a Dublin college as a pitiful establishment; and, in short, regarded an ensign in a marching regiment as the happiest creature living.' He was obliged, however, at his father's insistence, to enter Trinity College in Feb. 1781. He graduated BA in 1786 having meanwhile consummated his romantic ardour in a runaway match.

[6] Whitley Stokes, *Projects for Re-establishing the Internal Peace and Tranquility of Ireland* (Dublin: 1799), p. 27.

The lodgings of the poor were floored with a permanent layer of dirt, the windows often unglazed, the roof unrepaired, and at the rear a dunghill. The stairs were used as an ash-pit, the passageway so narrowed by refuse that Stokes found difficulty in moving from one level to the next.

> Sickness in Dublin [he wrote] arises very much from the filth and closeness of the lodgings; an infectious fever is the principal disease, and it is well known to prevail most in the dirtiest lanes: thus in the neighbourhood of the College and Park-place is more continually exposed to it than any other part. Indeed, I believe, there has not been a day since I began to practise, when the spot was clear of fever. I have seen there, three lying ill of a fever in a closet, the whole floor of which was literally covered by a small bed, and when I opened the door, an effluvia issued, from which, accustomed as I am to such things, I was obliged to retire for a moment.[7]

He believed that the well-to-do residents of Merrion Square would be horrified to know that nearby, in the area between Mount Street and Holles Street, he had found a room with ten occupants, of whom eight had fever.

Not confining himself to medical practice, Stokes, with the assurance of a polymath, became Donegall Lecturer in Mathematics in 1795, and was admitted licentiate of the College of Physicians without examination. He married Mary Anne Picknell, daughter of John Picknell, JP, a land owner of Loughgall, County Armagh, and Seatown House, Swords, County Dublin, in 1796 and in the following year he was appointed King's Professor of the Practice of Medicine.[8]

A young friend from Edinburgh called on him when visiting Dublin in the summer of 1797. This was Robert Jameson (1774–1854), a future professor of natural history at Edinburgh University, who noted their meeting in his journal, and tells how he found Stokes in good health, was given supper and fixed up with lodgings.[9] Next morning Jameson was taken by Stokes to the home of Richard Kirwan, the chemist, to deliver a letter of introduction and arrange a meeting. This done, Stokes took him on to Trinity College.

> Went to the College Museum with Dr Stokes [the journal continues]. It

---

[7] *Ibid.*, p. 32.
[8] Sir C. Cameron, *History of the Royal College of Surgeons in Ireland*, 2nd ed. (Dublin: Fannin, 1916), p. 501–4; see also T. P. C. Kirkpatrick, *History of the Medical Teaching in Trinity College Dublin and of the School of Physic in Ireland* (Dublin: Hanna & Neale, 1912); Constantia Maxwell, *A History of Trinity College Dublin 1591–1892* (Dublin: The University Press, 1946).
[9] See Jessie Sweet, 'Robert Jameson's Irish Journal 1797', *Ann. of Sci.* 1967; 23: 97–126.

is a large elegant room, with a few trifling fossils, some Indian dresses [collected by Captain Cook] &c. The new chapel is fine. Called upon Dr Mitchell but found he was in the country. Dined with Stokes.[10]

The following evening was spent at Kirwan's, where Jameson was joined by Stokes and George Mitchell. 'We had a great deal of interesting conversation.'[11]

Stokes is thus pictured as a figure already of consequence in scientific centres, but the glow of achievement surrounding his academic progress was to be diminished in April 1798 when the alarm over revolutionary activities, and rumours concerning the infiltration of the college, led to a visitation of Dublin University. This event necessitates some information to clarify Stokes's connection with the Dublin Society of United Irishmen.

The United Irishmen

According to Kirkpatrick's *History of the Medical Teaching in Trinity College Dublin*, Whitley Stokes withdrew from the society in 1791 (the year it was established),[12] but the author does not mention that Stokes accompanied Tone to Belfast in July 1792 to commemorate the fall of the Bastille.[13] It is clear from Dr William Drennan's letters to his brother-in-law, Samuel McTier of Belfast, that Stokes was elected to the Society of the United Irishmen of Dublin at its first meeting on 9 November 1791, one of eighteen persons balloted for in their absence.[14] Subsequently, with Thomas Russell and Tone, Stokes opposed the proposed solemn declaration or test as too rhetorical, argumentative and indeterminate.

Stokes left the meeting before the test was administered, and on 2 December Drennan expressed the hope to McTier that Stokes would 'be brought to attest, and some others who strain at gnats'. Towards the end of the month, however, Drennan confided to McTier his impression that Stokes and some others would form their own society—'but I should imagine they will scarcely get a Catholic to enter.'[15]

Nothing further is heard of this matter. It is evident, however, that

---

[10] *Ibid.*, p. 100.
[11] George Mitchell (1766–1803), BA, MB (Dublin), was awarded £100 by the Dublin Society for translating from German into English the catalogue of the Leskean cabinet of minerals.
[12] (Note 8), p. 225.
[13] For one reason or other, Stokes was poor company in the coach and Tone avoided him in Belfast for the next few days. See Marianne Elliott, *Wolfe Tone: Prophet of Irish Independence* (New Haven: Yale University Press, 1989), p. 172.
[14] D. A. Chart, ed., *The Drennan Letters* (Belfast: HMS Stationery Office, 1931), p. 62.
[15] *Ibid.*, p. 74.

his official membership of the Dublin Society of United Irishmen was brief, but he did not break fully with the radicals and when a committee was appointed in January 1793 to draw up a scheme of parliamentary reform he submitted a plan. This recommended that Ireland, a country with a population of about 4,200,000, should be divided into 300 districts, each returning one member to parliament. 'If the number was smaller, argument would have more weight, and violence less; men's conduct would be more observed, and the public expence diminished. On the other hand, they would be more apt to fall into juntos.'[16] The qualification for franchise required by Stokes was residence for one year in the district; age, twenty-one; property—occupying, say, five acres of arable land, or, in a town, a house of a certain rent, say, £10. 'Liberty is only as good as the means of virtue and happiness, and more may be lost in these, than gained in point of liberty, by the voting of the very lowest class.'[17]

He had ended his official connection with the Dublin Society long before its suppression in 1794, when it became an underground movement. He continued to have something more than a sympathetic interest, however, and in a letter to Thomas Russell on 5 March 1796 said that his brother Gabriel, a lawyer, 'is likely to have about two guineas for Tone but not more at present'. 'Do send me some of the letters you get from Tone', he requested on 12 April 1796.[18]

The visitation

The visitation at Trinity College lasted three days, the visitors being Lord Clare (the former 'Black Jack' FitzGibbon), and Dr Paddy Duigenan who represented the Protestant Archbishop of Dublin.[19] The entire college assembled in the dining hall, and in response to a roll-call each

---

[16] Whitley Stokes, cited by R. B. McDowell, 'United Irish Plans of Parliamentary Reform, 1793', Irish Historical Studies 1942; 3: 39–59.

[17] Ibid., p. 50.

[18] The letters are reproduced by Séamus Ó Casaide in *The Irish Language in Belfast and County Down* (Dublin: Gill, 1930), pp. 14–18. Cameron states: 'he retired from active participation in these operations about 1792, at which period they began to assume a revolutionary aspect', RCSI, (note 8), p. 502; Widdess is equally vague—'he resigned, about 1791', J. D. H. Widdess, *The Royal College of Surgeons in Ireland and its Medical School 1784–1984*, 3rd ed. (Dublin: RCSI, 1984), p. 225.

[19] Patrick Duignan, LL D, was MP for the City of Armagh. Responding to Dr Duignan's Representation of the Present Political *State of Ireland*, 'A Catholic Burkist' (possibly Theobald MacKenna), felt there was no laurel to gain: 'His learning is what no man of sense would wish to retain.—His facts, both ancient and modern, are detailed with a profligate regard to truth.—His inferences are the feeble operations of a mind, either naturally narrow, or pretending blindness from dissimulation. Where he attempts to sport in sarcasm, his wit, like the playfulness of a sea-monster, even to persons beyond its gripe, creates an impression of horror . . .' *An Argument Against Extermination* (Dublin, 1800), p. 3.

member answered his name, was sworn and interrogated regarding his knowledge of unlawful societies existing in the college.

When called, Stokes said he had been a member of the United Irishmen before the year 1792, but had withdrawn owing to the increasingly militant revolutionary tendency. He had subscribed to a fund to assist two impecunious United Irishmen who were in prison; and he had treated a sick member professionally, as the man was poor. He also claimed to have urged students to withdraw from treasonable associations, and to join the college corps established to guard the canal bridges and suppress rebellious manifestations. His *Reply to Mr Paine's Age of Reason*, for which the board had thanked him, was further proof of his orthodoxy.

An account of the inquisitorial proceedings written by an involved eye-witness, Lieutenant Colonel William Blacker, then a twenty-year-old student, has survived.

> At length to our great surprise Dr. Whitley Stokes, a fellow, and a captain of the College Corps was called forward. He took the oath and one of the first questions put to him was touching the knowledge of any secret society in the College. He said 'there was one Mr. Blacker a Fellow Commoner, who commanded a regiment of Orangemen in the North who he had heard was a leading member of such a society in the college.' It happened that I was seated close to the railing ... In one instant I was on the rail 'here was Mr. Blacker, my lord, to answer for himself. I am one of the oldest Orangemen in Ireland and ready to maintain it.' Such as well as I remember were the exact words, which uttered in a tone loud enough to be heard throughout the Hall in a manner electrified both Visitors and Fellows, while a burst of approbation which continued some minutes made the old walls ring again. Whether it was the surprise of the thing or the delight of seeing the feelings of the lads so unequivocally manifested I cannot say, but it was sometime before Lord Clare rose and commanded silence. The struggle between [amusement and] grim gravity which Paddy Duigenan's smug phiz exhibited was worth any money. Stokes on his examination being resumed steered clear of further allusion to Orangemen and having avowed republican sympathies was suspended from his situation as a Fellow and soon after removed from being a captain in the corps. He had been in rather bad odour with his company before this, for on some occasion of alarm, when he was under the necessity of issuing out some ammunition he accompanied the ball cartridges with an expression of hope that the lads would not use them against their countrymen.[20]

Witnesses appeared on behalf of Stokes, to testify that his influence among the students was beneficial—a pupil, Mr Kerns, said that Stokes

---

[20] William Blacker, cited by Constantia Maxwell, *History of TCD*, (note 8), p. 270.

had induced him to remain in the college corps rather than join a treasonable society, and Richard ('Pentateuch') Graves, DD, believed that his pamphlet was the earliest and best answer to Paine's *Age of Reason*—but Lord Clare listened sceptically, and decreed that he must be chastened. He was unfit to hold office as a College tutor; he was not to be elected to a senior fellowship for three years, nor sit on the board.[21]

A plea for clemency on behalf of Stokes left Lord Clare unmoved:

> I am favoured with your letter and memorial, very respectably signed by some of the Fellows of Trinity College in favour of Dr. Stokes. It is quite unnecessary I hope, to assure you that it will always give me great pleasure to comply with any request which may come so forcibly urged to me. In the present instance, however, the thing is impossible as what has been done at the last Visitation is, in my opinion, irrevocable; and even if it were not, I am sorry to be obliged to state to you that, from my knowledge of Dr. Stokes, he is a most improper person to be entrusted in any degree with the government or direction of any College. If I had been at liberty to act at the last Visitation on perfectly well-grounded private conviction, I must have expelled him.[22]

Kirkpatrick sees Stokes as a man whom Lord Clare 'could neither buy nor bully', and suggests that this explains the visitors' harsh sentence. Be that as it may, Clare[23] today is generally remembered as a man who sold his nation into political subjugation, with enduring and agonizing consequences, while Whitley Stokes emerges as a saintly man, thoughtful for the wellbeing of his countrymen.

Having heard of Stokes's punishment, Tone, in Paris, attributed Clare's animosity to the fact that the physician had reported to the lord lieutenant an account of 'some atrocious enormities' committed by British troops in the south of Ireland.

> Far less than that would suffice to destroy him in the Chancellor's opinion, who, bye-the bye, has had an eye upon him this long time; for I remember he summoned Stokes before the Secret Committee long before I left Ireland. I do not know whether to be vexed or pleased at this event as it regards Whitley. I only wish he had taken his part more decidedly; for, as it is he is destroyed with one party, and I am by no means clear that he is saved with the other.[24]

---

[21] 'Nineteen students have been expelled, and Stokes, the fellow, suspended for three years.' Chart, *Drennan Letters*, (note 14), p. 272.

[22] Cited by Kirkpatrick, *Medical Teaching*, (note 8), p. 226.

[23] Ann C. Kavanaugh, 'Lord Clare and his Historical Reputation', *History Ireland*, 1993; 1: 22–26.

[24] Richard R. Madden, *The United Irishmen, their Lives and Times* (London: Catholic Publishing Co., 1860), Vol. I, p. 104.

Tone inscribed the famous, and often quoted encomium in his journal on 20 May 1798:

> With regard to Stokes, I know he is acting rigidly on principle, for I know he is incapable of acting otherwise; but I fear very much that his very metaphysical unbending purity, which can accommodate itself neither to man, time, nor circumstances, will always prevent his being of any service to his country, which is a thousand pities; for I know no man whose virtues and whose talents I more sincerely reverence. I see only one place fit for him, and, after all, if Ireland were independent, I believe few enlightened Irishmen would oppose his being placed there—I mean at the head of a system of national education. I hope this last specimen of FitzGibbon's moderation may give him a little of that political energy which he wants; for I have often heard him observe himself that nothing sharpened men's patriotism more than a reasonable quantity of insult and ill-usage; he may now be a living instance and justify his doctrine by his practice.[25]

Non-medical writings

At the risk of a dislocation of chronology his non-medical interests are considered here together. *A Reply to Mr. Paine's Age of Reason Addressed to the Students of Trinity College, Dublin* (1795) was followed by *Projects for Re-establishing the Internal Peace and Tranquility of Ireland* (1799) and *Observations on the Necessity of Publishing the Scriptures in the Irish Language* (1808). He bore the expense of providing an English–Irish dictionary (1814), and in *Observations on the Population and Resources of Ireland* (1821) he charged Robert Malthus with errors.

'I believe in one God', wrote Tom Paine, 'and no more; and I hope for happiness beyond this life.' He rejected the possibility of divine revelation and belonged to no church, saying 'My own mind is my own Church.' He stigmatized 'the book called the Bible' as 'a history of the grossest vices and a collection of the most paltry and contemptible tales'. These statements must have saddened Stokes, secure in his own beliefs but immediately fearful for the students, many of whose young minds were defenceless against the arguments offered in easily-read, seductive prose by a person enjoying popularity in the Irish capital since the publication in 1791 of cheap Dublin editions of *The Rights of Man*.[26]

R. B. McDowell has referred to *A Reply* as 'a sensible little work in which [Stokes] explained that recent research on oriental manuscripts

---

[25] *Ibid.*, p. 104.
[26] Paine was proposed for honorary membership of the United Irishmen on 8 June 1792. See David Dickson, 'Paine and Ireland' in *The United Irishmen*, ed David Dickson, Dáire Keogh and Kevin Whelan (Dublin: Lilliput Press, 1993), p. 135.

had confirmed the Mosaic story, that the doctrines of the fall and the redemption were analagous to what we know in nature, and that the scriptural text was established on a number of very early manuscripts.'[27]

Stokes considered in sequence Paine's objections to the scriptures: that human language is too imperfect to have been been used by God to communicate His will; the inadequacy of miracles and prophecies as proof of a system of religion; the authenticity of the scriptures; the representation in the Old Testament of cruelty and injustice; the incredibility of the accounts of the fall and redemption of man; that the human race is too trifling for God's attention; that the study of nature is adequate to teach religion.

'What is Paine's objection to revelation by words?' he asks. 'That it has not certainty—'But if it had there would be a greater objection for then it would overpower our wills, removing us from a state of probation which benefits us.'

Stokes argued in favour of miracles and prophecies, held by Paine to be unfit for their object and incapable of proof. The function of miracles is 'to obtain authority to the teacher'; their occasional occurence is indubitable.

> Will any one in his senses suppose, that human power could restore wasted limbs to their full strength, and to that vigorous exertion which practice only could give, by a word in a moment? Will any one believe, that human power could give to the eyes, which have been sightless from birth, that wonderful arrangement of parts and powers, which in the ordinary course of nature grows from exercise itself . . . Can we believe, that human power can cure diseases, at a distance, with a word? Is it not more likely, that God might have done these things than that man could?[28]

The authenticity of the scriptures, Stokes insisted, is established far more securely than, say, Caesar's commentaries, or many of the classics—'the last five books of Livy, the first three Annals of Tacitus, and some epistles of Cicero, depend on a single manuscript.'

Paine's depiction of the Old Testament as a chronicle of criminality is countered by the explanation that all histories, in some measure, are histories of vice: 'because vices make the greater part of human actions'. Had the scriptures not recorded sordid events, the picture of the world as it then stood would have been incomplete. It is, moreover, a regrettable fact that the innocent are not spared in any public calamity. 'The convulsions of nature make no distinction between the virtuous, and vicious,

---

[27] McDowell, 'United Irish Plans', (note 16), p. 175.
[28] Stokes, *A Reply to Mr. Paine's Age of Reason* (Dublin: Byrne, 1795), pp. 13–14.

and innocent children continually suffer from the profligacy of their parents.'[29]

He accused Paine of having 'wonderfully perverted the Scripture doctrine of the fall and redemption of man' but was willing to accept that this was done unintentionally—'he had no Bible, and he took his account from some one who knew little more of it than himself'. History amply confirms that the world had become corrupt at the time when Jesus Christ was born, and Stokes asks is it incredible that our heavenly Father, having decided to remove this evil, should have done it through the intervention of another?

> Is not all nature a system of agency? God does not pour on our eyes the glory, which man cannot behold and live, but gives the greater light to rule the day, and the lesser light to rule the night; he cloaths the earth with plants for the use of animals, and gives them for our use.—Is it improbable, that a being of an exalted nature should submit to evil for our sakes, when we, unfeeling as we are, do it for one another? . . . The man who can say, it is unnatural to suppose our Saviour should have died for us, says that compassion and benevolence are unnatural; he has no heart, and shall never be my friend nor my adviser.[30]

He regarded as of little importance Paine's suggestion that the human race was too insignificant to merit divine favour, or that inhabitants of Jupiter and Saturn had an equal claim on the Deity. While agreeing that the study of nature is an excellent means 'of instruction in the wisdom and goodness of the Creator', he felt it had little effect except on cultivated minds:

> How many are there to whom the earth, clothed with grass, or buried in snow, the firmament beaming with morning light or sparkling with stars, scarce suggest any ideas but those of varying labour or returning rest. Nature instructs the wise: To the poor the Gospel is preached.[31]

The final pages of *A Reply* caution students that the defence was written by 'a man whose time is extremely occupied in other pursuits'. They refer to Paley's *Views of the Evidences of Christianity,* and urge regular reading of one of the gospels and the *Acts of the Apostles*: 'If then, even in a Deist not to examine the Scriptures be foolish, in a Christian it is highly criminal.' Thus on 26 March 1795, Stokes concluded his self-imposed task and turned to one or other of his multiple interests.

Projects for re-establishing the Internal Peace and Tranquility of Ireland appeared in 1799; it is mentioned by W. E. H. Lecky who did not doubt

---

[29] *Ibid.*, p. 25.
[30] *Ibid.*, pp. 32–33.
[31] *Ibid.*, pp. 39–40.

that Stokes joined the United Irishmen 'through the purest motives of philantrophy'. Lecky cites his estimation of the population of Ireland as something in excess of 4,500,000.[32]

Stokes deplored the loss of life, and destruction of property, caused by the rebellion. Equally serious the shock given to the nation's moral and religious principles: 'Those great and sweeping passions, which civil war excites, bear down the barriers of ordinary virtues.'[33] In *Projects for Peace* he finds a parallel between the poverty which caused Roman revolutions in the time of Catiline, and the pitiable plight in Ireland of the rural and urban poor. Therein lies the remedy:

> Take them out of the hands of men, who are leading them to resistance, and do some good to them yourselves, and they will soon become your subjects, instead of theirs; what their leaders impotently promised, do you actually perform for them; what they held out to them to be pursued through blood, and desolation, and the destruction of moral and religious principles, and of the very property they proposed to divide; do you give them without loss to any, with every prospect of encrease of moral and religious principles. Depend upon it, this country is not lost to feeling, or virtue, but that you will soon find, that you have acquired confidence, and support, by such conduct. Your friends will be cheered, and rendered active; your enemies disappointed.[34]

Having analysed the causes of poverty, Stokes offers schemes for its alleviation. He discusses the need to relieve general ignorance, and the desireability of religious instruction. Injurious books, purchased and removed from circulation, should be replaced by books on natural history, farming, gardening, domestic animals etc. The scriptures should be made available in the Irish vernacular.

Above all, it is necessary to secure the favour and protection of God's mercy and forgiveness:

> Look to this, lose not a moment, omit no means to secure his favour. If you cannot do so, how can you hope, with such peculiar sources of danger, to escape the fate which seems to hang over Europe? Whatever you think in your conscience is likely to attain his protection should be done instantly! If you cannot attain it, you are lost! If you can, you are safe. If God be with us, who shall be against us![35]

Through his connection with the United Irishmen, Stokes was intro-

---

[32] W. E. H. Lecky, *Ireland in the Eighteenth Century*, (London: Longman, Green, 1892), vol. v, p. 80.
[33] Stokes, *Projects for Peace*, (note 6), p. 1.
[34] *Ibid.*, p. 50.
[35] *Ibid.*, p. 51.

duced to Patrick Lynch of Loughlinisland, County Down, by Thomas Russell, in the early 1790s. He engaged Lynch to prepare a phonetic Irish version of the *Gospel of St Luke* and the *Acts of the Apostles*. Stokes lent him a copy of the printed Irish translation of the New Testament by O'Domhnuill (1602–3) to facilitate his task.

Two thousand copies in double columns were printed in 1799 of *An Soisgeal Do Reir Lucais, Agus Gniovarha Na Neasbal. The Gospel According to St Luke, And The Acts of the Apostles*. The Dublin Association for Discountenancing Vice, of which Stokes was a member, gave ten guineas towards the cost of publication.

In 1806 Stokes published in two volumes *Na Ceithre Svisgeula Agus Gniomhartha na Neasbal: A Ngaoidheilg Agus A Mbearla* printed in the Roman character and following O'Domhnuill's text. The Association for Discountancing Vice contributed £80. With the assistance of the board of Trinity College, he published in 1815 *Seanraite Sholaimh A Ghaoidheilge Agus Mbearla*. Séamus Ó Casaide thought it unlikely that Lynch was connected with the publications of 1806 or 1815, on neither of which does Stokes's name appear. 'They were the first successful attempts to print as separate publications sections of the Bible translated into Irish.'[36]

Stokes had no intention of proselytizing when writing *Observations on the Necessity of Publishing the Scriptures in the Irish Language*, a pamphlet which opens with the following incontrovertible statement: 'Every person who believes christianity to be true, must admit the general importance of having its precepts and records conveyed in every language that is spoken on the earth'. If it is praiseworthy to translate the scriptures into the languages of distant tribes in India, why not do the same 'for a great nation, with whose happiness or misery our own is so intimately connected'? There need be no fear that publishing in Irish can ever lead the Irish language to flourish to the exclusion of English, 'or to such a degree as to form an increasing barrier between the two races of men that inhabit Ireland'.[37] His investigations showed that in Leinster, Irish is mostly spoken in Louth, Meath and Westmeath; 'in Dublin, Kildare and Wicklow scarcely any'. Few spoke Irish in the King's and Queen's Counties, but it was spoken in south-west Carlow, and 'in Kilkenny, the language prevails greatly'.

> In all the counties of Munster the Irish language prevails beyond comparison, if we except the large towns . . . The native language is more prevalent in Connaught than in the rest of Ireland; in this province even the gentlemen often find it convenient to acquire the language, in order to be able

---

[36] Ó Casaide, *The Irish Language*, (note 18), p. 18.
[37] Stokes, *Observations on the Need for Publishing the Scriptures in the Irish Language* (Dublin: 1808), p. 3.

to deal with the pesantry without an interpreter. In Ulster, there is a greater proportion of Irish speakers than is generally supposed . . . [38]

A decline in the language had been noticed in certain districts—'This principally happens where the corn trade has found its way.' The farmers, embarrassed by difficulties 'on the conduct of their money dealings, from not being able to read and write', have been attentive to their children's education. Those who settled in towns discontinued the use of Irish, 'while no instance could be found of persons laying aside the English language'.

This did not in any way diminish the need to publish the scriptures in Irish, for while the language continued to exist 'it should be used as the only or best vehicle of instruction, and we know the decline of a language is always slow'. He calculated that 2,000 Irish catechisms were sold annually and discussed the possibity of revising the old translation of the bible by O'Donnell (London, 1690)—'in which, as Irish scholars inform me, there are many obsolete words and phrases'—and recommended that this revision should be made in two dialects, one for the north and one for the west and south.

He believed that the co-operation of the Catholic clergy would not be lacking.

> It may be supposed by some that the Catholic clergy would obstruct the distribution of the Scriptures in Irish. That some may do so I will not take on me to deny, but from various and extensive enquiries I can assert that a very considerable proportion will not.[39]

Stokes did not expect that the availability of the scriptures in both languages would eliminate disagreements on the subject of religion, but he ventured to hope that familiarity with the gospel must have some effect 'in softening the hearts of all men, and leading them to the exercise of great christian virtues, humility, charitable forebearance and forgiveness.'

An English–Irish Dictionary (1814) compiled by Tadhg Ó Coinnialláin (Thaddaeus Connellan) was printed at Stokes's expense.[40]

Population and Resources

When the catalogue of the minerals compiled by the Rev. Walter Stephens (1807) became outdated Stokes was invited to join his friend, Dr Thomas Taylor, in renewing it. *A Descriptive Catalogue of the Minerals in*

---

[38] *Ibid.*, p. 2.
[39] *Ibid.*, p. 9.
[40] Séamus Ó Casaide, *Irish Book Lover*, (1933); 21: 20.

the Museum of Trinity College, Dublin, was published in 1818.[41]

His *Observations of the Population and Resources of Ireland* was first presented in his home in Harcourt Street, as a lecture to a group of friends. They encouraged him to publish it; he did so (1821) to draw attention to some of his native land's vast resources, and with the object of showing how individuals and voluntary associations could eliminate mendicity, employ the poor and relieve the country without demands on the public purse. He had covered some of the ground already in *Projects for Peace.*

The opening chapter takes issue with Malthus, who in his celebrated *Essay on the Principle of Population* contended that population and the means of subsistence tend to increase by geometrical and arithmetical proportions respectively, and held that vice and misery are necessary checks to an expanding population. Stokes wished to show that Malthus, who had applied his theory 'with peculiar severity to Ireland', was in the main mistaken.

Stokes challenged what he called 'rather an abstract theory, than a deduction from facts', and pointed out that Malthus had taken his increase of population from recently occupied areas of North America, the increase of subsistence from Great Britain —'the increase of man from the most rapid example; the increase of the means of subsistence from the slowest'.[42] Had the data been taken from Sweden, where neither emigration nor immigration was significant, and where most women wed at marriagable age, with Malthus's figures corrected accordingly, a very different situation emerges. The subsistence 200 years hence will be nine times as abundant, the people five times as many.

> Here is great news—so the world is safe enough for two hundred years more, and God is not mistaken after all—it was Mr. Malthus was wrong! Before those two hundred years are out, if we live long enough, we will find some other mistake, which will keep us going two hundred years more. Come, come—things are not so bad.[43]

---

[41] The National Library of Ireland has a copy of the syllabus of a course of lectures on metals and metallic mines to be delivered by Stokes in the Philosophy School, commencing on 5 February 1827.

[42] Stokes, *Observations on the Resources and Population of Ireland* (Dublin: 1821), p. 4.

[43] *Ibid.*, p. 7. We do not know which edition of the *Essay on Population* Stokes read, but the second edition (faulted by Coleridge for 'Verbiage and senseless repetition') seems the more probable. Computing the population of Ireland in *Projects for Peace* (1899) he makes no relevant allusion to the anonymous edition of 1798. His own attitude, at the time, is surprisingly 'Malthusian' for he appears to accept infectious fevers as playing a role in population control. 'If the vicious inhabitants of towns [he wrote] were to encrease as fast as the inhabitants of the country, the world would be overrun with crimes, and call for another deluge. Providence, by the unhealthfulness of towns, prevents much of this evil; the poison kills the part, and prevents its own absorption.' (*Projects*, (note 6), p. 32).

Stokes deplored the English tendency to regard Ireland as 'overpeopled' despite the presence in Wicklow, Connemara and near the Mourne Mountains in County Down, of vast unoccupied tracts of land. 'Can a country, with many such districts, be said to be overpeopled?' The repeated misrepresentations were discouraging—'they damp the hopes, and impede the exertions, of the friends of Ireland', and could have more serious results.

Admit, for a moment, that there are more men in Ireland than there ought to be, what is the consequence? Some should leave it. Now, the next question is, who shall? The poor man who labours, or the gentleman who does not? Mr. Malthus should not stir such questions.[44]

The principles of industry which Stokes adumbrated were:
(1) Supply natural rather than artificial wants; everyday needs rather than the demands of luxury. He complained that many were critical of Ireland for its lack of artificial wants—'they would have us grow rich by throwing away our potatoes, and ordering turtle.'[45]
(2) Remove impediments rather than offer rewards.
(3) Impose regulations regarding qualifications.
(4) Reduce the cost of transport.
(5) Cultivate the home trade. 'The home trade is the better school of industry, punctuality, integrity, dispatch, frugality—of all the commercial virtues.'
(6) Develop domestic industries rather than factories—'the collection of ill-sorted multitudes into extensive manufactories, has been found, by experience, too often injurious to innocence and to honesty.'[46]
(7) The revenue laws require regular revision to avoid an excess of regulations.

Contrary to the opinion of most British agricultural writers, Stokes saw smaller farms as a step 'to relieve the peasantry, to secure the landed interest, to multiply all the products of the earth'. The small farmer had many advantages: 'his flocks and herds lose less by accident; he has less labour in laying out manure and drawing home produce; suffers less loss of time and labour in going to and returning from work; suffers less pillage, less waste, and receives more assistance from his family . . .'[47] There are fewer failures among holders of small farms. Nobody occupying even an acre of ground is ever reduced to seeking parish aid.

He accepted, however, that landlords dreaded dealing with a multi-

---

[44] *Ibid.*, p. 15.
[45] *Ibid.*, p. 16.
[46] *Ibid.*, pp. 16–18.
[47] *Ibid.*, p. 29.

tude of lower-class tenants—'it is not every gentleman who is fit for it'. This difficulty had given rise to 'the middleman' so essential to Irish agriculture. The lower classes in most countries 'are inclined to cunning', a disposition strengthened in Ireland by many irritating circumstances.

Selective breeding and intensive feeding result in more and better sheep and cattle, while human labour is a substitute for productive surface. There should be further cultivation of green crops and of that incomparable root, the potato, which is not to be despised for its cheapness. 'The space that feeds one man with beef, or twelve with wheat, will feed seventy with potatoes.'

Stokes believed the system of leasing could be improved; evils existed, and 'so long as tenants covet land and landlords covet money', would continue to exist unless an ideal form of contract was devised. He cited the relevant authorities, Lord Kames, Dr Anderson, Dr Colquhoun and Bell's *Treatise on Leases*.

He discussed the reclamation of bogs and glens, before turning to fisheries and the manufacture of wool and linen. He dealt with coastal improvements, concluding his observations with a pretty piece of satire in which he exhorts the British to allow the Irish to use their own wool, and grow their potatoes.

> No people are so easily fed; that is what vexes you. Let us have a little clothing of our own; and having food and raiment, we should be content But fear not; we shall not be content. The moment we feel whole clothes on our backs, we will quit burning our shins over the fire; some effort for profit will be made, and then we must be genteel; whatever you say will make us look like gentlemen and ladies, that we buy, name you the price; merely allow us to procure for ourselves absolute necessaries; do not muzzle the ox that treadeth out the corn, the harvest is your own; trust confidently to our inexhaustible folly.[48]

Verses

Stokes was a good judge of painting and music. At the age of twenty, under the pseudonym 'Abednego Squib, Esq', he addressed *The Satanical Remembrancer*, an interview in verse between an apparition and an archbishop, to his friend Thomas C—[o]bbe, Esq. An introductory letter reflects on the reality of ghosts, and the poet reminds Cobbe how the Rev. Eusebius Coming, Vicar of S[words], an able and respected cleric, was popular in his parish—'It is a sensible observation, that a Man is best known within a Mile of his own House'—and conscientious in his min-

---

[48] *Ibid.*, p. 91.

istry.[49] He was, however, subject to severe stomach cramps for which the waters at Bath were the only reliable cure. All went well with him until, at a whim, the bishop ordered him in public 'not to Absent himself from parochial Residence on any Exigency whatever'. Cut off thus from the amenities of Bath he had a bad attack and died.

The events narrated in the poem occurred on the night following the arrival of Coming's successor. The opening stanzas set the scene.

> *When Night the World in Sablest Mantle folds,*
> *And weary Man is sunk to Sleep and Rest;*
> *Save where the Ghost his airy chiding holds,*
> *To wake the Vulture in Guilt's penal Breast:*
>
> *In that dread Hour, around St. Anne's Church-yard,*
> *A sudden Flash shot forth its ghastly Gleam;*
> *And thro' Sepulchre's Chambers straight was heard*
> *A Widow's muttered Curse, a Widow's Scream. —*
>
> *At Bufo's Bed, in Gown and Band array'd,*
> *The Spirit unappeased of Coming's stood,*
> *In his Hand high a Scorpion Whip he sway'd,*
> *In that, a Prospect of a burning Flood.—*

Stokes explains in a footnote that in Latin *Bufo* signifies a toad, an animal well suited by its appearance, 'and a peculiar empty Sufflation of its Body at times', to symbolize pride and malevolence. A suitable nickname, too, for an unkind and mischievous prelate, suspected of wishing to be rid of the Rev. Coming in order to make room for his nephew.

The ghost berates the bishop—'For know, thy Name, thus Execrate on Earth,/Enroll'd already darkens Hell's black Book'—until its disappearance, accompanied by a clap of thunder, leaves his victim quaking.

> *But what Remorse, what Horror seiz'd his Grace!*
> *What Curses on his Counsellors he cast!*
> *Till, thro' a Crevice he the Morn could trace,*
> *He thought each tardy Moment was his last.*

Stokes argues in his introduction that there was sufficient cause to raise a ghost:

> If, therefore, extreme constitutional Delicacy of Nerves wounded by Brutality—if the Dignity conscious Worth and Knowledge insulted by Meanness and Ignorance—if Life rendered unhappy, nay essentially cut off

---

[49] [Stokes] *The Satanical Remembrancer* (Dublin, 1783). See D. J. O'Donoghue, *The Poets of Ireland*, (Dublin: Hodges Figgis, nd) for attribution.

by Oppression, be Provocations sufficient to create, what is emphatically called a perturbed Spirit, to ope the ponderous and marble Jaws of the Sepulchre, we are furnished with an adequate Cause for the Phaenomenon before us:[50]

A black spot, 'the Satanical Mark', is commonly left by ghosts to confirm their visitations. The recorded findings of physicians who examined the bodies of girls infected by Michele Chaudron, a famous Genevan witch, confirmed that 'the Father of Temptation chiefly delighted to Impress with his own Token, the Breasts and Thighs of Women; but in Man, his favourite Parts may be different'[51]; this was so, indeed, with the unfortunate bishop. 'Deep on his Breech the Ghost impresse'd three Blows', the black mark left on the buttocks an unquestionable indication that though the ghost of the late Vicar of Swords was virtuous, it was executing 'a Commission appropriated to his grim Majesty' and deservedly tormenting the wicked.

The poet concludes this curious compilation, which no doubt echoes ecclesiastical gossip he must have heard daily in the rectories of his youth, with a final warning stanza:

> Let each high Prelate, in whose crosier'd Hand,
> The State has left the Power to Vex and Kill,
> Take Warning hence, how he his Flock Command,
> Or use the Scourge or arbitrary Will.

An example of his occasional verses has also survived, an address to the shamrock, celebrating George IV's visit to Dublin in 1821:

> Lov'd, honor'd plant, too long oppressed,
> Beneath the foot of pride;
> At length unfold thy beaming breast,
> And cast the dust aside.
>
> Belov'd! revive—your king appears,
> To wipe your tears away;
> The sorrows of a thousand years
> Are vanishing to-day.
>
> His aged head thy grateful breast
> Shall soothe to safe repose;
> Free from the thorns that still infest
> The Thistle and the Rose.

---

[50] *Ibid.*, p. 22.
[51] *Ibid.*, p. 29.

Stokes's plan for a *herbarium* is said to have influenced the founders of the botanical gardens at Glasnevin, and he also worked towards the provision of a zoo in Dublin.

King's Professor 1798–1812

In November 1803 the governors of the Meath Hospital accepted that Whitley Stokes and Francis Barker, MD, might give clinical lectures on medicine in the hospital, while Richard Dease and Philip Crampton should lecture on surgery. The board of Trinity College agreed to recognise the course if the College of Physicians approved; the latter, noting that of the group only Stokes was its licentiate, withheld its sanction at first, but on reconsideration gave the lecturers the go-ahead, though it caused no little surprise among Dublin doctors that two physicians should associate themselves with a couple of young, and undistinguished surgeons.

In the sphere of religion the 'Walkerites', a Calvinistic sect founded in 1804 by a classics don, John Walker, attracted Stokes who joined them. Their inclination was to follow the advice of St Paul and 'salute one another with a holy kiss', but the custom caused embarrasment in public assemblies, leading to a division into the 'Osculists' and the 'Anti-Osculists'. It is not known whether Stokes favoured one or the other of the sub-sects. He lived at 16 Harcourt Street, and his wife bore him ten children of whom two, William and Gabriel, were to join their father's profession. He had a country-house at Ballinteer where, in view of his interest in agriculture, it seems likely that he farmed.

Stokes received permission on 21 June 1806 to give a course on natural history, provided that he did not disturb his students' routine duties. The lectures were delivered in the law school at two p.m., and were continued for several years. He was commissioned by the board in 1810 to superintend the mines discovered on the college estates. This undertaking was to last for seven years, and Stokes would share the profits arising during the period. He also accepted the post of curator of the museum and, as we have seen, catalogued the minerals.

It is perhaps understandable that however anxious the authorities had been, given the political climate of the times, to expel revolutionaries in 1798, they were prepared tacitly to tolerate the chronic infringment of a university statute imposing celibacy on fellows. Those who ventured to be ruled by their hearts, adopted the convention of passing off their spouses as their sisters. All went well until an eccentric and belligerent barrister, Theophilus Swift, offended by the college's failure to recognise the intellectual merits of his son ('the cleverest lad in Ireland'), decided to expose their equivocation. Embroiled in a legal action, following the publication of a pamphlet entitled *Animadversions on the Fellows of Trin-*

ity College, Swift asked had they not sworn to obey the statutes, and had they not broken them? 'What have they done with their oaths [he wished to know], and with their wives? Have they made no breach in either?'

Swift's revelations did not secure compliance with the unaccommodating statute, nor was it finally removed until 1840. Meanwhile, in 1811, a king's letter enabled the board to reimpose celibacy, but to free from censure those fellows who within two months declared themselves to be married. Stokes petitioned against college money being spent on procuring the letter, and 'because the restraints on marriage contained in this statute appear to me likely to injure the morals of this College and to give countenance to the formation of convents in Ireland'. His protest being unavailing, he gave notice to the provost on 4 January 1812 that he had married Mary Anne Picknell.

Professor and Mrs Stokes respected the traditions of Dublin hospitality, and on one memorable evening in the Harcourt Street residence the dinner guests included such remarkable orators as Charles Kendal Bushe; William Plunket, a future lord chancellor of Ireland; William Magee, Trinity College's professor of mathematics; John Philpot Curran; and Peter Burrowes, an eloquent lawyer. When the question was posed as to the essential qualification of a delightful friend, it was agreed that each person should give his opinion in succession. One said wit, another favoured humour, a third preferred readily accessible learn-ing, and so on until Burrowes cried out: 'Are you all done?' Then with all eyes upon him he struck the table with his fist, saying 'It is honesty, by God!'[52]

Stokes's tenure of the King's Professorship of the Practice of Medicine ended, for some unknown reason, on 6 February 1812. He was surprised and offended when another was appointed to the chair, and considered taking legal action against the electors, but the College of Physicians opposed him with counsel's assurance that three lunar months', rather than three calendar months' notice was sufficient. Thereafter though lacking a chair, Stokes was still permitted to lecture on medicine in a college lecture-room.

He had been admitted to a senior fellowship in TCD on 10 June 1805, holding it until his appointment to a well-paid chair of natural history in 1814 necessitated his resignation. He became an honorary fellow of the KQCPI in 1816, and joined the staff at the Meath Hospital, still in the Coombe, on 14 December 1818 filling the position of the late Dr Thomas Egan; his private practice, if any, was small, and in this regard he was a remarkable contrast to Cheyne. His services were readily available to the sick poor, and he worked valiantly during two typhus epidemics.

---

[52] Sir William Stokes, *William Stokes* (London: Unwin, 1898), pp. 25–6.

Medical writings

The principal medical works of Whitley Stokes are: 'On an Eruptive Disease of Children', published in the *Dublin Medical and Physical Essays* (1808); and *Observations on Contagion* (1818). In the former, Stokes described a disease affecting children that had baffled him for years. Soon after starting practice it was his misfortune to have two cases of the disorder directed to him, both of whom died. One was the child of a close relative whom the young physician warned of the dire prognosis, wisely insisting on having a second opinion.

It was characterised by vesicles behind the ears 'followed by ulcers and copious discharge, loss of substance, rapid tendency to mortification'. Referred to in Dublin and Wicklow as 'the white blisters', in northern counties as 'the eating hive', and in Waterford and Tipperary as 'the burnt holes', Stokes proposed to call it *Pemphigus gangrenosus*.[53]

> One or more vesicles appear mostly larger than the best distinct small pox; these increase for two or three days, burst, and discharge a thin fluid, having a disagreeable smell, limpid in most cases, sometimes whitish and sometimes yellowish, the latter less dangerous; usually the weaker the child's constitution is, the thinner is the matter. Before or after breaking, the vesicles run together, the sore becomes painful, with loss of substance and a thin foetid ichorous discharge, the edges of the ulcer are undermined, and it spreads quickly.
>
> The more usual seats of the disease are, behind the ears, sometimes on the hands or feet, on the private parts, (seldom on the arm-pit,) the breast, folds of the thighs, lower belly, on the inside of the mouth or lips. The disease, however, it is said, seldom passes from the inside to the outside of the mouth.
>
> In the progress of the disorder, the ulcers enlarge rapidly, with remarkable foetor, very great discharge, and livid edges.
>
> If the sores are behind the ears, they destroy the connection of the posterior cartilage with the cranium; they spread to the meatus auditorius; to the eyes, the sight of which seemed, in a few cases to have been destroyed one or two days before death; and they sometimes extend to the vertex.[54]

Death, preceded by convulsions, may take place about the tenth or twelfth day.

Having consulted the available textbooks in vain, Stokes was told by Thomas Cleghorn in Edinburgh in 1792, that Dr James M'Donnell of Belfast was something of an authority on the condition, and had seen several cases. On his return to Ireland, Stokes established communication

---

[53] Stokes, 'On an Eruptive Disease of Children', *The Dublin Med. and Physical Essays*, (1808), 1: 145–53.
[54] *Ibid.*, p. 147.

with M'Donnell, well known for his zeal in studying the natural history of obscure medical disorders. M'Donnell confirmed the gravity of the disease—'that it is very fatal', and poorly understood.[55]

As quinine had not helped, Stokes enquired about the remedies of folk medicine. He discovered a woman named Murray, reputed to have succeeded with several bad cases, and was impresssed by her methods which, *faute de mieux*, he adopted. Using Mrs Murray's ointment, he had some successes.

He mentioned the problem to his students annually, and in 1802 a Mr Quin affirmed that he had seen cases under the care of Dr Spear of Glasslough, County Monaghan. Stokes communicated with the latter who confirmed the efficacy of traditional cures. Stokes collected the recipes for several green vegetable ointments and decided that the active ingredient was *scrophularia nodosa*, the green figwort. He gave detailed instructions for its application.

> I do not pretend to have proved, that the scrophularia has a specific effect on this disease; possibly it is only useful, by supplying the green vegetable matter; but as I and some of my friends have had a success more uniform, by means of this ointment, in a disease in which our failure was almost uniform before, I shall continue to prefer it to other vegetable matters until the subject is better understood.[56]

The typhus epidemic which commenced in 1817 prompted Whitley Stokes to write *Observations on Contagion*.[57] For Stokes the term contagion denoted 'a substance produced on the body of an animal diseased, which will, if applied in considerable quantity to the body of a healthy animal of the same species, give rise to a similar disease'. Smallpox, measles, 'the Venereal Disease', itch and cowpox were spread thus. The contagiousness of certain diseases was disputed 'as in Typhus Fever and the Yellow Fever; in some others doubts naturally rise, as in Dysentery and Catarrh'.[58]

The infectiousness of the plague, Stokes held to be illustrated by the fact 'that those who are carefully secluded escape the disease'. During a severe epidemic at Marseilles, early in the eighteenth century, the monks who shut themselves up in their convents remained well. By closing their houses 'on the first appearance of the Plague', and receiving provisions

---

[55] James M'Donnell has been called the 'father of Belfast medicine'; his son, John, was the first in Ireland to perform an operation under ether anaesthesia, amputating an arm in the Richmond Hospital, Dublin, on 1 January 1847; his grandson, Robert, administered a blood transfusion successfully in 1870 to a woman dying from post-partum haemorrhage.
[56] Stokes, 'Eruptive Disease', (note 53), 152.
[57] Stokes, *Observations on Contagion*, 2nd ed., (Dublin: Hodges and M'Arthur, 1818).
[58] *Ibid.*, p. 2.

only after taking precautions Europeans in the Levant avoided infection.

Certain laws can be formulated, he believed, governing the operation of contagion:

> (1) Contagion could be conveyed directly or indirectly. Dry air does not convey infection to a distance of more than a few feet.
> (2) It seldom produces its effects immediately—there is a latent period.
> (3) A sufficient dose is required to achieve infection.
> (4) Some persons are exempt.
> (5) Some persons achieve immunity.
> (6) Most diseases have animal specificity; others, e.g. the mange, affect animals of different species.

The following measures will help to control an epidemic:

> (1) The destruction of contagious matter. This may involve the destruction of clothes, bedding and houses (especially if the latter are made of wood), but it may be sufficient to apply heat—'such heat as is usually considered sufficient for the baking of bread'—or immersing the substance in boiling water. Acid-gases may also be used. Infected goods should not be handled 'but lifted up by iron-hooks or tongs'.[59] Compensation must be made.
> (2) Separate infected from uninfected persons.
> (3) Avoid exciting causes, e.g. cold, wettings and sitting in wet clothes.
> (4) Inoculation.

Cork Street Fever Hospital, and the fever wards in Steevens Hospital and the House of Industry, are to be used to separate the infected from the uninfected, but as these are soon filled in an epidemic it would be helpful to encircle the city with twelve fever hospitals on the smallest scale. Introduction of further fever cases from the country could be thus prevented—'this circuit of twelve or sixteen houses might be got ready for the purpose of washing the bodies and clothes of such beggars as wish to come into town.' Those refusing to comply 'may fairly be desired to seek their fortune elsewhere'. Those who co-operate should get a dinner, a warm bed and be sent on their way in the morning 'their old clothes cleaned and dried'.

Mendicity [Stokes realised] is a great cause of disseminating Contagion. This has been an observation only too well established in various epidemics. The subject should be speedily attended to. It seems inconsistent to lay vessels from Charlestown under quarantine, and keep the avenues of the city open to beggars, who flock from all the infected districts of our own country.

---

[59] *Ibid.*, p. 40.

We should, however, enter on this difficult question with a firm determination to let no inconvenience, no danger, drive us from the sacred principles of justice and mercy. If we desert these, God and man will desert us. I cannot see on what principle mendicity is treated as a crime: I admit it is a great inconvenience, at present the source of great dangers; still these do not make it a crime. On the contrary, I am of opinion, it may be a man's sacred, bounden duty, if he cannot otherwise support his children, to beg for them.[60]

Stokes adduces reasons for suspecting that the disease formerly known as the plague 'has been softened down into the disease which we now call typhus'. Cases of plague in which buboes do not appear closely resemble typhus. Plague and typhus scarcely differ more than do some varieties of scarlatina and smallpox. 'Perhaps we are wrong in flattering ourselves that the circumstances of society are so altered that we can never again be visited by the Plague; the truth may be, that we have become inured to a mild state of its Contagion.'[61]

Stokes based his belief on the contagiousness of typhoid on the way it ran through families. He had seen as many as eleven individuals affected in a family of twelve and calculated that the chances of this happening in the absence of a contagious factor was 189,600,000 to one. He accepted that the disease rarely selected a second victim in the families of the well-to-do, but attributed this to the fact that the families of the poor 'are more exposed to the exciting causes of the disease, such as filth, damp, cold, and famine, and often sleep in the same bed with the sick'.[62] James M'Donnell of Belfast dealt with the question of the contagiousness of typhus by saying he regarded this 'as a matter quite settled among all thinking men'.[63]

It was clear that while the common people were more disposed to typhus, because of their environment, the mortality rate was higher among the gentry when affected, causing Stokes to point out that if the gentleman while preserving the advantages of cleanliness and dryness in his house can in other respects adapt his life to that of the peasant 'he will probably enjoy a share of the peasant's security'.

Should true plague visit Ireland, Stokes recommended that the uninfected population of Dublin be removed 'in parties of from one thousand to two thousand to the mountain glens', where they should be supported. He calculated that 137,500 lives would be lost if the epidemic were not checked. This figure would not dismay Malthusiasts who hold that the population of Ireland is too high already—'but no man who happens to have four tried friends, will be content to lose one to please Mr. Malthus

---

[60] *Ibid.*, p. 56.
[61] *Ibid.*, p. 17.
[62] *Ibid.*, p. 26.
[63] *Ibid.*, p. 59.

or his disciples'.[64]

Writing to William Saurin, the attorney-general ('the only gentleman in this dismal nation to which I have access') on 26 September 1818 Stokes pleaded for further aid, and urged the government to face its full responsibility.

> Why is an Hospital endowed with funds for the purpose of preventing the extension of the Venereal Disease [?] Is it meritorious to restrain the extension of a disease which is communicated to the guilty [?] Is it less so to restrain fever which affects the most virtuous & affectionate for here
> '—Too oft doe goodness wound itself
> 'And sweet affection prove the source of woe—'
> Why are surgeons paid by Government for attending the health of soldiers and sailors [?] If all other classes of the community are to be left to providence it will be admitted that these at least should be protected [.] How is it possible to have a healthy army & navy while the whole community from which they are supplied are affected with contagion [?][65]

His strongest arguments were the economic ones. How were 'the coffers of their States' to be replenished if the labour force were decimated? 'Can the dead labour? Can the dying labour?'[66]

Chair of medicine

Stokes was elected to the chair of medicine at the RCSI on 15 June 1819, so it was quite natural that his son should enrol at the college in 1822. William Stokes did not remain there very long, however, proceeding instead to Scotland to complete his education.

Whitley Stokes was exceptional among Irish physicians in escaping the bitterness of 'Erinensis', *The Lancet*'s caustic Dublin correspondent, who customarily pilloried the leaders of the profession but detected in Stokes 'none of the trickery, none of the artifice of would-be philosophy about him—he is what he would pass for, "An honest man, the noblest work of God", and a living satire upon the majority of the medical profession in Ireland.'

Stokes was sixty-one when he came under the scrutiny of Erinensis:

> Already beginning to stoop to the influence of time, like a sear leaf bent upon its stem in autumn, we approach him with a deferential feeling inspired alike by his virtues and his years. A blue roquelaire, hanging carelessly from his shoulders, conceals beneath its classic folds, a form of slender pro-

---

[64] *Ibid.*, p. 54.
[65] Nat. Arch. O.P. 474/62. I am grateful to Joseph Robins for drawing my attention to this letter from Stokes to William Saurin.
[66] Ibid.

portions, unincumbered by *sartorial* embellishment. But under this unstudied simplicity of appearance so conformable to the habits of studious old age, we may say with the poet: *'ingenium ingens latet hoc sub corpore'*. And as he now hurries on before us in imagination from the Lecture room to bury himself once more in the beloved solitude of the library, he seems as if unconscious of all around him, and that his thoughts were fixed upon something ulterior to the earth on which he treads. The patriachal repose of his aspect and the unaffected dignity of his demeanour are enlivened by those finer tints of feeling contracted from a long communion with the spiritualities of Creation.[67]

Stokes was regarded with respect, too, by another satirist, Dr Brenan, who praised his charity but commented adversely on his costume, which would have fetched little from the second-hand dealers in Plunket Street:

> *If asked for his coat, he gave with it his waistcoat,*
> *Tho' no Plunket-street man would give much for his vest-coat.*

The Meath Hospital

Whitley Stokes's colleagues at the Meath Hospital included Dr Robert J. Graves, a 'lithe, dark-haired, eagle-eyed, and energetic mannered gentleman' who introduced the stethoscope to the Meath, where Laënnec's recent invention reminded the sceptical students of a 'pop-gun'.[68] The co-relation of clinical and post-mortem findings caused them to have second thoughts, The young innovator's appointment to the staff in 1821 had followed the resignation of Dr Harkans, an event which was not, it appears, purely fortuitous.[69]

Noting the unexpected vacancy, the standing committee on 2 July 1821 ordered: 'That a communication be made to the Medical Board on the subject—'. Two weeks later the committee resolved that the following observation be inserted in the medical communications book: 'The Standing Committee having heard a report that a bargain had been made between two Medical Gentlemen whereby a consideration in money was to be paid on the appointment of a Physician to fill the present Vacancy, and as the Committe are of the opinion that any proceeding of such a nature would be injurious to the welfare of the Hospital and that should the measure be pursued it would become their duty to resist it . . .'

The medical board's response appeared unsatisfactory: postponement of the appointment was requested, pending the availability of counsel's opinion. The medical board ignored this request, correctly holding that it

---

[67] Fallon, *Erinensis*, (note 2), p. 37.
[68] Lambert H. Ormsby, *History of the Meath Hospital* (Dublin: Fannin, 1888); passim.
[69] Ms RCSI: Meath Hospital minute books.

had the right to make the appointment, and on 31 July 1821, at a meeting attended by seven board members, and presided over by Philip Crampton, Robert Graves was elected. The board assured the standing committee 'that in electing a Gentleman of Doct^r Graves Character and qualifications they conceive they have considered the best interests of the Hospital'. They denied that there had been any pecuniary transactions between 'the Candidate and the Electors'. They agreed to meet the committee in conference to guard against possible future irregularities. Three dissentients—Whitley Stokes, Cusack and Thomas Roney—objected to the election, believing that 'practices alluded to, should have been checked in the present instance'.

An appropriate by-law was introduced. Graves took up his duties without further debate and on Monday 3 September the standing committee accepted the list of medicines signed by Dr Graves and Surgeon C. Roney. Meanwhile the erection of the new Meath Hospital was proceeding on a two-acre site at Heytesbury Street and Long Lane. It was completed and occupied on Christmas Eve 1822; the transfer of patients, wrapped in blankets, and carried from the Coombe to the new building in long baskets specially made for the occasion, was supervised by Maurice Collis and William Henry Porter, future presidents of the RCSI. The difficulties were increased by a storm which sent slates flying from the rooftops.

The plaudits showered on a hospital extension are generally charged with superlatives, redolent of old favours and fresh expectations. The picture drawn by 'Erinensis' may have been nearer to reality. He beckoned his readers to the shining new out-patients department 'to observe the practice and study the physiognomy of the nosological benchers assembled, behind a range of desks, in judgement on the ravages of disease, with a crowd of pupils collected round each prescriber, and all seemingly intent on treasuring up in their memories the fortuitous combinations of calomel and treacle and water called "mistura pro tussi"'. He promises that their ears will be assailed 'by a violent objurgation, in which the slender tremor of Mr. Hewson's voice and the screaming soprano of some old inveterate tea-drinker from the cellars of the Liberty mingle into a hideous concert which generally terminates by sending the withered amateur of Bohea to hell, with an asafoetid pill in her stomach to cure her dyspepsia!'

Extracts from the hospital's records, though more prosaic, have the merit of authenticity: 'Damp straw was used for filling the bed of one of my patients, named Hasting—Had not the nurse supplied him with additional blankets, he might have suffered severely, his complaint being rheumatism.' The complainant was Dr Graves; his observations are

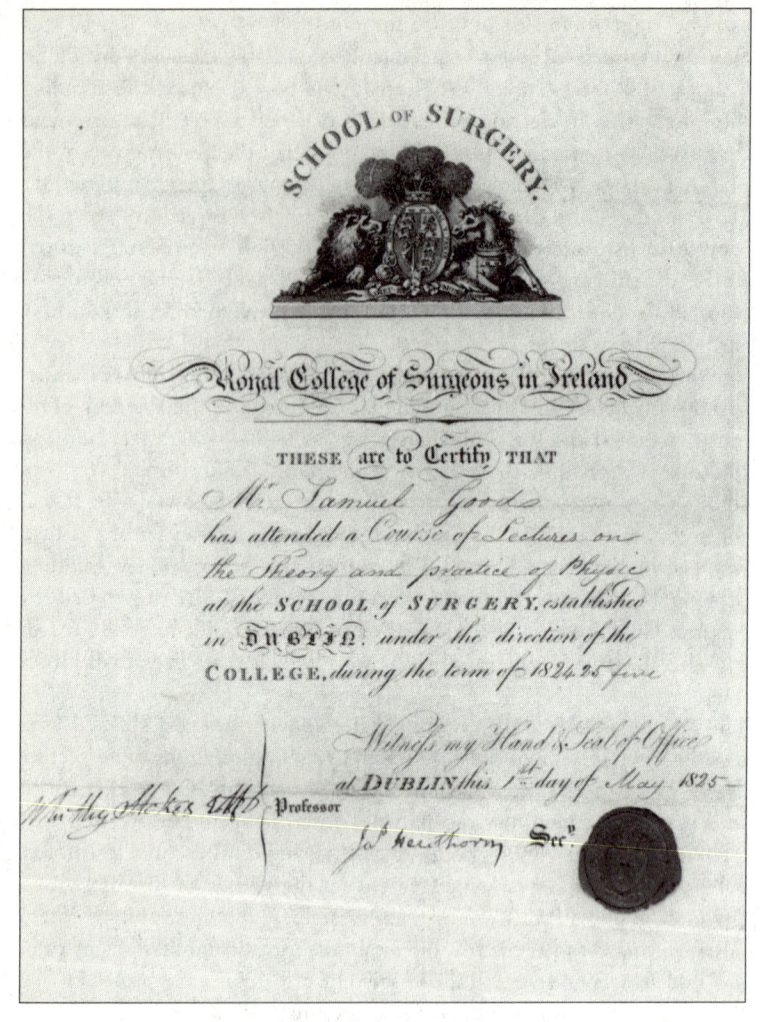

Certificate of attendance signed by Whitley Stokes in 1825

marked 'inquired into'. Surgeon Rawdon Macnamara on 9 October 1825 requested that Nurse Lavelle be fined one shilling and eight pence 'for permitting a patient to sing in her ward at 9 o'clock at night'. The fine was duly imposed. Another disciplinarian reported that on visiting the wards at 10 p.m. he 'found Male Patients sitting at the fire—this occurred several times.'

Andrew Young, a disciple of Graves at the Meath, believed that the amused smiles with which his seniors greeted the stethoscope, must have made the exasperated physician wish for a sympathetic colleague. We learn from Young that Graves soon put out feelers to ascertain whether in the event of Whitley Stokes resigning, his son William could be appointed. And so it came about that the irregularity of Graves's own appointment was paralleled by a singularly felicitous example of nepotism, when Whitley Stokes was replaced by William Stokes at the Meath Hospital in 1826.

Empty benches

Before long the lack of a hospital appointment was to affect the career of Stokes *père* adversely, as became evident when due to the vigilance of Mr John T. Kirby a committee was appointed to enquire into the state of the schools of surgery, and the manner in which professors were fulfilling their duties. Kirby's motion proposed that if any professor fails 'in the punctual discharge of his duty' the authorities shall remonstrate with him, or if necessary impose a pecuniary penalty, or remove him from his office.[70]

At a quarterly meeting of the college in February 1826 a letter from Whitley Stokes requested 'to know their pleasure as to the propriety of giving a Summer Course of Lectures'.[71] The matter was referred to the court of examiners and the necesary permission was granted, but in the following month Stokes explained his problem more fully to Richard Carmichael, PRCSI, and offered a possible solution.

> DEAR SIR:
>
> I understand there is to be a Meeting of the College of Surgeons today, I will be much obliged to you to call attention to the course on the practice of Medicine which I am employed to give.
> Last winter in consequence of some arrangements in other schools I had no class. In February your body gave me permission to commence a course of Lectures in this ensuing Summer if I should deem it advisable. I find my getting a class will depend on my procuring admission to an Hospital for the

---

[70] RCSI minutes, 17 March 1826.
[71] *Ibid.*, 6 February 1826.

pupils who may subscribe.

My Son is now one of the Physicians of the Meath Hospital where he is giving Lectures on pectoral diseases which are well received.

If the College could so far indulge me as to permit him to give part of this course with me he could procure for the pupils admission into the Meath Hospital.

>Believe me Dear Sir
>Yours Sincerely
>WHITLEY STOKES
>Monday April 17th 1826
>R. Carmichael, Esq.

It was resolved that the professor 'be respectfully informed that his request cannot be complied with being contrary to one of the Byelaws'.[72] The decision was entirely without malice, but a door was closed against the young man who by the mid-century would be Dublin's most celebrated physician, and his father remained confronted by a dilemma. The court of examiners reported on 5 May 1828 that 'the Professor of the Practice of Medicine has delivered two or three lectures only' and had responded as follows to their enquiry:

>SIR
>
>In reply to your letter of Yesterday I am to state that having attended at the appointed time at the commencement of the last session and having delivered several lectures I found the number of the attending pupils reduced to three or four of whom only one had subscribed. I therefore thought it best to discontinue the course.
>
>I trust you will find on enquiry that the failure of my class was not owing to the deficiency of the lectures or of my industry but rather to the circumstances in which the pupils were placed which left them with no sufficient motive to enforce attendance.
>
>Please give my thanks to the College for their repeated favours,
>
>>I have the honor to be Sir
>>Your obedient Servant
>>W. STOKES
>>James Henthorn, Esq.,
>>Secretary to the Royal College of Surgeons,
>>Harcourt St., April 30th 1828.[73]

Having considered the professor's explanation it was resolved 'that it

---

[72] *Ibid.*, 17 April 1826.
[73] *Ibid*, 5 May 1828.

is the opinion of the College that the Court of Examiners should not re-elect any Professor who has for Two Years from any cause failed to deliver his course of Lectures'. This edict brought Whitley Stokes's connection with the RCSI to a close; he was replaced in the chair of medicine by Dr Henry Marsh on 4 August 1828. The multiplicity of private medical schools had increased competition; the established influence of Kirby's school in Peter Street, and the growing popularity of the more-recently founded Park Street and Richmond Hospital Schools may explain the empty benches in Stokes's lecture theatre. He was at an age when men become aware of the sprightliness of junior colleagues, who seem to seize on new ideas with surprising alacrity.

Regius Professor

Evidently the strictures of Lord Clare were forgotten, and Stokes was still in favour at TCD where he succeeded the redoubtable Edward Hill[74] as Regius Professor of Physic on 13 November 1830, to resign ten years later well pleased that his own successor was to be his son, William. The latter's *Diagnosis and Treatment of Diseases of the Chest* was published in 1837 and in association with Robert Graves he had enhanced the Meath Hospital's reputation as an important teaching centre.

Early in 1840, increasingly concerned by his father's declining health, William Stokes commissioned Charles Grey to paint the old physician secretly, drawing him first while at prayer in the chapel of his nonconformist sect. The prognosis was unduly pessimistic, for Whitley Stokes lived into his eighty-third year, predeceased in 1844 by his wife. He died at 16 Harcourt Street on 13 April 1845, and was interred in a family tomb at Taney Church, Dundrum, County Dublin.

The intellectual dynasty

Whitley Stokes deserves to be seen today as a salient figure in a great Irish academic and intellectual dynasty, a family accomplished in science, archaeology and letters, with a medical tradition extending from the eighteenth century to the present-day.[75] His grand-nephew, George Gabriel Stokes (1819–1903), FRS, discovered the respiratory function of haemoglobin which he reported in a paper, 'On the reduction and oxidation of the coloured matter of the blood', presented to the Royal Society on 16 June 1864.[76] The term haemoglobin was later substituted for what

---

[74] For an account of the quirky Professor Hill (1741–1830), 'Milton's Dublin editor', see Lyons, *'What Did I Die Of?'* (Dublin: Lilliput Press, 1991), pp. 40–63.
[75] See Lyons, 'A Great Dublin Medical Family', *Proceedings of the XXIII Congress of the History of Medicine* (London: Wellcome, 1972), pp. 1010–16.
[76] C. S. Breathnach, 'George Gabriel Stokes on the Function of Haemoglobin', *Irish J. Med. Sc.*, (1966); 121–25.

Stokes called *crurorine* : 'in its two states of oxidation it may be conveniently named *scarlet crurorine* and *purple crurorine*'.

Gabriel Stokes (1806–81) contributed to Robert Bentley Todd's *Cyclopaedia of Anatomy and Physiology*; he practised in Mullingar, County Westmeath. William Stokes (1804–78), the most celebrated of Whitley's sons, married Mary Black of Glasgow in 1828; for a time they lived at his father's Harcourt Street house, moving later to York Street, and finally to 5 Merrion Square. They had nine children of whom the younger Whitley (1830–1909) became a distinguished Celtic scholar,[77] Margaret (1832–1909) an authority on archaeology and author of *Notes on the Cross of Cong, Three Months in the Forests of France* and other books. Sir William Stokes (1839–1900), FRCSI, a pillar of the establishment, was surgeon-in-ordinary to Queen Victoria in Ireland and PRCSI in 1886; he died of enteric fever at Pietermaritzburg during the Boer War.

Henry John Stokes, another of William and Mary Stokes's sons, joined the Indian Civil Service, and gains entry to this chronicle as father of Henry and Adrian Stokes, surgeon and pathologist respectively. Henry Stokes (1879–1967), FRCSI (surgeon to the Meath Hospital and PRCSI in 1940–41) was a man of rare candour. A former secretary of the Dublin Biological Club recalled that Stokes, when it was his turn to address his club, spoke on 'Some mistakes of Henry Stokes'; when his turn came round again he spoke on 'More mistakes of Henry Stokes'. He was the first surgeon at the Meath, and possibly the first in Dublin, to remove a parathyroid tumour; a pioneer in the techniques of blood transfusion, he acquired the requisite knowledge at the Western Front during the First Great War.[78] Dogs and children are good judges of character, an instinct which the Dublin 'shawlies' also possessed. 'Ah, Mister Stokes!' an old woman from the Coombe exclaimed, 'there's no rhyme or reason in him. He's like the love of God'.

Adrian Stokes was born in Lausanne on 9 February 1887, and educated in Dublin. At Trinity College his interests apart from sport were exclusively scientific. He qualified MB, BCh in 1910 taking the FRCSI and MRCP, London, later. After post-graduate work in St Mary's Hospital, London, and the Rockfeller Institute, New York, he was appointed

---

[77] The publications of Whitley Stokes, LL D, are numerous. They include *Irish Glosses*, 1860; *Three Irish Glossaries*, 1862; *The Middle-Breton irregular verbs*, 1866; *Beunans Meriaseh: The life of Saint Meriasah, bishop and confessor*, (1872); *Goidelica. Old and early middle Irish glosses*, 1872; *Some remarks on the Celtic additions to Curtius' Greek etymology*, 1874; *On the calandar of Oengus* (1880); *The old-Irish glosses at Würzburgh and Carlsruhe*, (1887); *The Anglo-Indian Codes, Vols I and II* (1887–8) with supplements (1889–91); *Lives of saints from the Book of Lismore*, 1890; *A criticism of Dr. Atkinson's glossary to vols I–IV of the ancient laws of Ireland*, 1903; etc. His library was presented to University College, London, by his daughters in 1910.

[78] Lyons, *An Assembly of Irish Surgeons* (Dublin: Glendale Press, 1984), pp. 101–6.

assistant in the department of pathology at TCD. When war was declared in August 1914 he volunteered immediately for service.

A contemporary has recalled him at that time:

> One can see him still on the first day he wore khaki—happy, almost boisterous, striding off down the quays with a sergeant-major and a posse of twenty men to unload stores, and then later, hot, begrimed and tired after hours of work in a blazing sun, but still cheery, coming out of the nearest public house with a huge pile of ham sandwiches and pints of foaming beer for the hungry men, for whom the sergeant informed him there had been 'no instructions' as to rations.[79]

Adrian Stokes took his motor-bicycle and sidecar with him to France and provided the BEF's first mobile laboratory. His research projects included typhoid and spirochaetal jaundice, and he introduced the nasal catheter to administer oxygen.

He returned briefly to Dublin but in 1922, disapproving of the Irish Free State, he accepted a chair of pathology at Guy's Hospital and settled in London. A clinical colleague described him as 'full of strange oaths and native wit', always ready to turn from his own tasks to those of others, and remembered the tea and chat in the laboratory—'heterogenous and inconsequent talk of green days in forests and blue days at sea'. A brilliant career lay before Adrian Stokes but he was fated to fall victim to yellow fever when he was forty.

---

[79] N. P. Hudson, 'Adrian Stokes and Yellow Fever Research.', *Trans. Roy. Soc. Trop. Med. Hyg.* (1966); 60: 170–74.

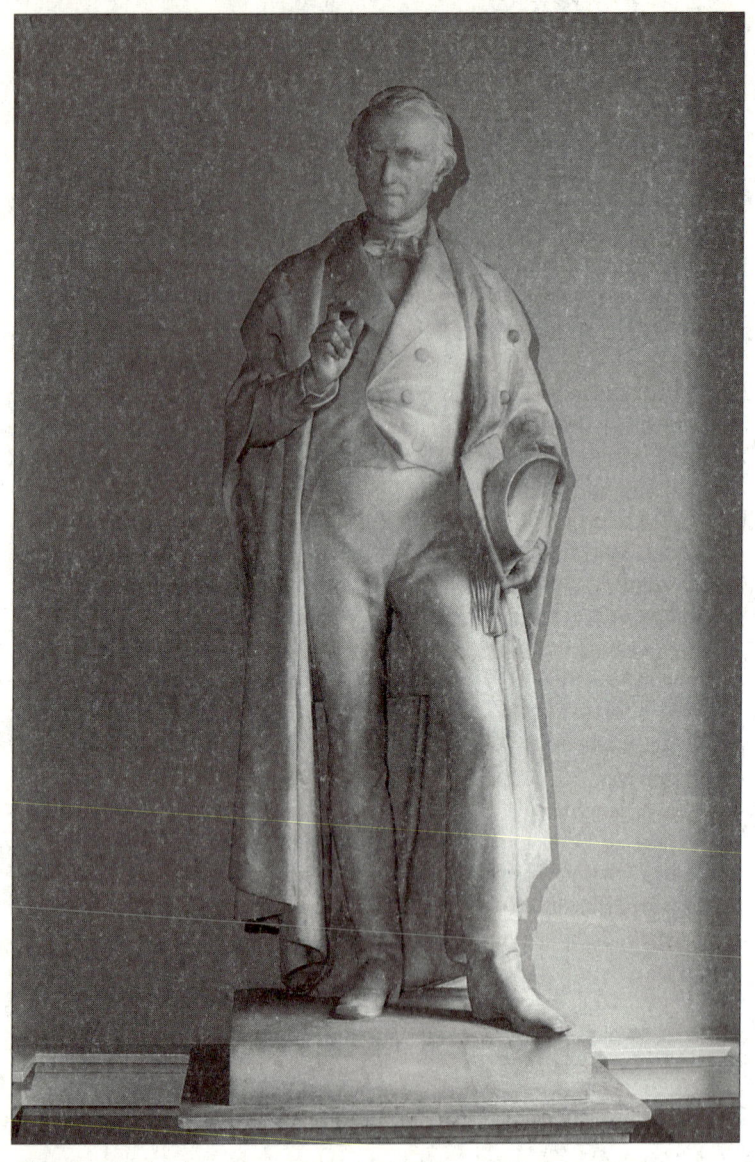

Sir Henry Marsh, 1790–1860 Professor of Medicine 1828–32

Chapter 3: Sir Henry Marsh, Bart., 1790–1860

On a summer evening in 1806, Henry Marsh, a Galway clergyman's sixteen-year-old son, rode one of his father's plough-horses to water. Coming to a crossroads where four roads met, he stopped to speak to a gentleman in a gig. Having directed the affable stranger, he fell into conversation with him and to his surprise found the traveller had been acquainted with his uncle, the Rev. Digby Marsh, fellow of Trinity College, who at the time of his early death in 1791 was professor of modern history in Dublin University.

When the boy explained that his father had encouraged him to farm the glebe, his interrogator placed before him the range of alternative, and preferable opportunities that would follow a university education. The result of this chance meeting was Henry Marsh's decision to leave farming behind him.[1] That a brilliant career should come about almost fortuitously is hardly unprecedented, but the Rev. Robert Marsh's apparently scant interest in his son's education may have been related to the death of the boy's mother within the first year of his life.

Ancestry

Henry Marsh was the scion of a family with roots in Gloucestershire, the first to settle in Ireland being the Rev. Francis Marsh (b.1627) who married Mary, daughter of Jeremy Taylor, chaplain to Charles I, and became Archbishop of Dublin in 1681. Their grandson, the Rev. Jeremy Marsh, rector of Athenry, was Sir Henry Marsh's grandfather. Henry's parents were Robert Marsh, rector of Killinane, and his wife Sophia (née Wolseley), a granddaughter of Sir Thomas Molyneux, the first Irish medical baronet.

Henry Marsh was born at Loughrea in 1790. At the age of nine, he was sent to a classical school in his native town, a school 'as famous at that time for the severity of its discipline as for the number of celebrated scholars it produced'. His father was friendly with the Marquis of Clanricarde, to whom he owed the living of Killinane. Beyond this nothing is known of the Rev. Robert Marsh, but evidently he made no attempt to obstruct his son's change of plans in 1806, hoping now that Henry would take Holy Orders.

---

[1] [William Wilde], 'Sir Henry Marsh, Bart.', *The Dublin University Magazine* (1841); 18: 688–92. See also P. Finnegan 'Sir Henry Marsh, Bart. (1790–1860)', *J. Ir. Coll. Phys. & Surgs.* (1990); 19: 298–300; Norman Morgan, *Sir Henry Marsh, Bart.* (Loughrea: Printing Works, 1995).

The boy entered TCD on 23 November 1807, but coming under the influence of the 'Walkerites', who have been referred to above, he realized that he could not conscientiously become a minister of the Established Church. He took the BA degree in 1812, and being strongly attracted by the adventure of the Peninsular War he attended Kirby's school in Peter Street with the intention of qualifying as an army surgeon, not a difficult task at a time when surgeons were in such demand. The risks of the colourful career he aspired to were pointed out to him by a responsible family member, who prevailed upon Marsh to become indentured to his first cousin, Mr (later Sir Philip) Crampton.[2] This entailed study at the College of Surgeons and the Meath Hospital, but in 1818 towards the end of his apprenticeship, the loss of the right index finger, the result of a dissecting-room wound, effectively ruled out a career in surgery.[3]

He had worked at the House of Industry Hospitals under another cousin, Dr John Crampton, and he now turned contentedly to medicine, becoming LKQCPI in 1818. Most of the next two years was spent in Paris at *La Charité*, and he returned to Dublin expert in the new art of auscultation. His immediate success in medical practice owed at least something to influential relatives. He was appointed assistant physician to Dr Steevens' Hospital on 27 October 1820, being deputed to assist Dr John Crampton whom he was eventually to succeed as physician in 1840.[4] Long before that, his personal qualities had ensured his acceptance as one of Dublin's leading doctors and this, according to a contemporary, resulted from the 'unyielding determination' with which his decisions were made, and the 'undeviating determination and invincible energy' with which any course of action was pursued.

His resourcefulness can be seen from his intervention in the management of a case of severe Sydenham's chorea reported in Graves' *Clinical Lectures*. The fifteen-year-old girl was becoming worse daily, her limbs disturbed incessantly by involuntary movements, her speech and swallowing hampered, her emaciation extreme. The child's parents had summoned in turn Graves, Sir Philip Crampton, Mr Colles and Dr Marsh. The doctors' ineffectuality contributed to the drama, and it was Marsh who suggested tepid salt-water shower baths three times a day, and pre-

---

[2] The Rev. Robert Marsh's sister, Nicola Mary, married the Rev. Cecil Crampton and was the mother of Philip and John Crampton.
[3] The fact that he escaped with his life may have closed his mind to the potential seriousness of the most trivial dissecting-room wound: 'I am certain, from repeated observation, that much more depends upon the state of the constitution and health at the time, than upon the effects of the poison.' *Dublin Hosp. Reps.* (1827); 4: fn. p. 521.
[4] John Crampton (MD Edinb. 1793) was physician to the House of Industry Hospitals, to Steevens' Hospital, and King's Professor of Materia Medica. According to Erinensis: 'He goes through the business of lecturing like one who is bound to the performance of a heavy task ... With chemical experiments he would seem to have nothing whatever to do.'

scribed quinine sulphate with extract of stramonium.

As the modern shower had not yet been invented, Marsh's plan presented difficulties. The patient was placed on a large mattress covered with a sheet, and she was held there by an assistant ('destined unavoidably to enjoy the bath along with her'). Other servants stood on chairs and poured water from large watering-cans, held as high as possible. The unfortunate girl was then taken into another room to be dried, and to the astonishment of Graves her recovery was rapid. The situation may have been aggravated by a hysterical element.

Diabetes

Finding himself with a twenty-year-old diabetic shoemaker under his care in the early 1820s, Marsh was uncertain as to the best manage-ment. Looking into the literature, he found that until Willis discovered sugar in diabetic urine, treatises on the complaint were characteristically vague and uncertain. Opium in large doses was the sovereign remedy, but Dr John Rollo's meat diet (excluding vegetable material) though welcomed initially (1797), had proved disappointing and was loathed by patients.[5]

Marsh was impressed by the fact that many diabetic case histories indicated that the disease was ushered in by 'some cause acting upon the skin, and producing derangement of its function'. Furthermore, sooner or later *every* case of diabetes is likely to show cutaneous involvement. This led him to adopt the diaphoretic action of vapour baths as the basis of his therapy.

Carried away by his enthusiasm and his reading, Marsh began to see the dry skin in a causative light. 'Suppressed perspiration, especially if connected with distress of mind, fear and apprehension, does more frequently than any other cause, give rise to this complaint.' And if diabetes is ('as I suspect') a rare disease in hot climates, where sweating is habitual, this observation could be beneficial to those who could travel. 'It may be [Marsh continued], that a residence of a few years in a warm climate would completely eradicate the disease. This is an important consideration, and well worthy of the attention of medical men.'[6]

The regime proposed by Marsh utilized the vapour bath, daily or twice daily, to produce sweating and reduce urinary output; this could be achieved also by physical exercise—'Active exercise on horseback will excite perspiration without producing fatigue.' Supportive measures in-

---

[5] H. Marsh, 'Observations on the Treatment of Diabetes Mellitus', *Dublin Hosp. Reps.* (1822); 3: 430–465. See also John Rollo, *Diabetes*, (London: Dilly, 1797).

[6] *Ibid*, p. 460. In a later article, Marsh mentioned a diabetic patient who spent autumn in the South of France—'during the whole of the time he was there he perspired profusely, and while in that state of perspiration he could, without the least suffering from it, eat every variety of food'—*Dublin Q. J. Med. Sc.*,(1854); 17: 1–19.

cluded diet, blood-letting, leeches and a daily bowel evacuation. He also recognised the symptomatic value of carbonated limewater.

Fever

Marsh published his views on fever in 1827. Like Whitley Stokes, he accepted contagion and infection as synonymous terms, and his paper, 'Observations upon the Origin and Latent Period of Fever', draws on his experience of infectious diseases since his student days, including a personal illness. Most fevers, he believed, resulted from 'a volatile poison, whose invisible particles, mixed with the air, are, during the act of inspiration, brought into contact with the mucous surface of the nose, fauces, or air tubes'.[7] The subject constantly gave rise to 'keen dispute and intemperate controversy'; there was an associated obscurity which Marsh realised could not be dispelled by reasoning alone—'Nature must be interrogated.'

He wished to consider 'the manner in which febrile disease is produced . . . the symptoms which manifest themseslves during the latent period . . . the treatment adapted to this stage of the disease'. Ten years earlier, a typhus patient in one of Dr Crampton's fever wards in the Whitworth Hospital had told Marsh that her initial symptoms followed the perception of a disgusting smell, arising from a person convalescing from fever who sat close to her. A similar onset was experienced by a nurse in the Richmond Penitentiary who was taken ill on 17 June 1818, after giving an enema to a man dying from typhus—'the smell issuing from the feces produced immediate and most intense headache, and her strength at the same time was so completely exhausted, that she had neither power to move nor to support herself on her limbs'.[8]

Marsh collected sixteen similar examples of fever preceded by a nasty smell or stench, and described how at six p.m. on Friday 4 February, 1825, feeling in the best of health, he had gone to the fever ward in Dr Steevens' Hospital at the end of a long day's work, and turned down the bed clothes of one of the patients. Immediately he perceived a highly disagreeable smell, and straightaway felt oppressed and overwhelmed.

> I hastened home [he wrote], not feeling well, ate a hearty dinner, and made a considerable exertion to go out in the evening. I felt myself however so chilly, that I covered myself with all the coats and cloaks I could procure: but every attempt to excite a sensation of warmth was fruitless; even whilst close to the fire, and wrapped in large cloaks, I still felt chilly and cold. On Saturday night the pediluvium promoted free perspiration, and purgative

---

[7] 'Observations upon the Origin and Latent Period of Fever', *Dublin Hosp. Reps.* (1827); 4: 454–535.
[8] *Ibid.*, p. 457.

medicine operated well. On Sunday, unable to rise; on Monday, went out in a carriage perspiring; yet chilly; severe headache aggravated by the least exertion; expression of countenance remarkably altered. The leading symptoms which succeeded were intense headache, as if a sharp instrument passed from temple to temple, on coughing or moving; great depression of spirits, amounting to absolute and dreadful despair; intolerable mental agony; copious secretion of colourless urine; clammy perspiration, exhaling to my own perception an acid disagreeable smell; a most distressing sensation of contraction or squeezing of the stomach, with occasional vomiting; taste highly disagreeable, yet clean tongue; pulse scarcely accelerated; no increased heat of skin; to a short period of delirium succeeded idiotic manner and gesture; insensibility, spasmodic contraction of limbs, and subsultus tendinum. For several hours my situation appeared hopeless.[9]

On regaining consciouness all the objects in the room seemed black, and beautifully exact and regular in outline. Marsh complimented John Cheyne, who was attending him, 'upon his fine new suit of black clothes'. This surprised Cheyne, whose suit was quite a different colour.

In his paper, Marsh argued that despite the general supposition that 'the febrile miasm' and other poisons, are absorbed and distributed by the circulation before their injurious effects gradually become evident, the extremely rapid action of some poisons indicates a direct effect on 'the sententient extremities of the nerves'. He and Arthur Jacob carried out experiments on rabbits and pigeons and demonstrated to the students that the action of prussic acid was perceptible within five seconds.

'Can it be [he asked], that through the action of the olfactory nerves the effects of the poison are conveyed to the brain? or are the nerves of ordinary sensation those only concerned?' The question remained unanswered, but he believed that the action of cold, too, resulted from the impression made on the nerve endings, and was not due to suppressed perspiration.

He was not prepared to accept the general opinion that the type of fever is always directly related to its cause, believing that atmospheric factors, or a 'constitutional diathesis', had an influence of equal importance to that of the immediate cause of the disease. He was prepared to countenance, too, strong mental emotions as a cause of fever, and refers to 'the slow nervous fever', a non-contagious condition which he had seen in 'delicate and nervous females'.

As most patients with contagious fevers are unaware of the exact circumstances of their initial infection, and pay more attention to any 'exciting' cause, such as cold or fatigue, it may be that many who are exposed to it escape the fever, and only those whose illness is finally determined by the exciting cause become recognised victims. Although

---

[9] *Ibid.*, p. 464.

Marsh thought the smell which accompanied the febrile miasm was actually 'an accidental circumstance' indicative of some coincidental putrescence, he believed that taken in the context of the resulting headache and the subsequent fever, the perception of the offensive odour indicated 'the moment of the impression made upon the system by the febrile effluvia' and the start of a latent period, brief or protracted, which intervenes between that moment and the rigor which makes fever manifest.

> In most diseases [Marsh wrote,] the length of the latent period is extremely variable; in idiopathic fevers it varies from a few hours to as many weeks or months; in exanthematous fevers its duration is more uniform than in other febrile affections; in some diseases it endures to a length of time that is very remarkable; this is strikingly exemplified in cases of hydrophobias, the constitutional symptoms of which are in some instances not manifested for many months after the infliction of the local injury.[10]

A state of perfect health, he points out, does not exist in the latent period, for disturbed sleep, unpleasant dreams, depressed spirits—disturbances primarily of the nervous system—are common. In the acutest fevers the patient may sink and die during the latent period but usually the length of the latent period is variable, influenced by the patients' dispositions to particular affections, and by exciting causes.

Famine, poverty, impure air, cold and wet were important exciting causes. Fatigue should be avoided in those exposed to infection. Avoidance, as far as possible, of the effluvia emanating from the sick, should be arranged by ensuring that bedrooms are well aired.

'The more protracted the latent period, the more formidable is the fever.' Marsh saw the latent period as 'a time during which the judicious application of remedies' could render the ensuing fever less severe and dangerous. Admittedly, the physician was seldom summoned so early; but if he were called he should take the opportunity to impose absolute rest and a light diet. Exposure to cold must be forbidden. An emetic, followed by an opiate might be prescribed and 'the prudent use of purgatives could be singularly beneficial'.

It required nice judgement, however, in such an indefinite situation, to know whether symptoms arose from 'impressions of cold upon the surface', or from contagious effluvia. The former would benefit from tartar emetic or James's powder, which would be undesirable in an early stage of contagion. The subject, Marsh believed, was one of 'great extent and much interest'.

His views attracted wide attention, but Charles Murchison could not accept that 'the facts recorded by Sir Henry Marsh and others' amounted

---

[10] *Ibid.*, p. 493.

to proof of a direct action of 'the poison' on the nerves, without prior absorption into the blood.[11]

Chair of medicine

With Charles Johnson, ex-master of the Rotunda Hospital, and Philip Crampton as co-founders, Marsh established at the rere of his Molesworth Street residence the Institute for Sick Children. This was moved to Pitt Street (now Balfe Street) off Grafton Street, and in 1821 was the first hospital of its kind in the United Kingdom. Treatment was provided free to sick children, clinical instruction was offered to medical students and mothers and nurses were educated in the proper management of children both in health and disease. The Pitt Street Institution was a busy place, treating some 7,000 children in 1826, and in excess of 21,000 in 1831. Eventually it merged with the National Orthopaedic and Children's Hospital (established by L. H. Ormsby in 1875) to form the National Children's Hospital in Harcourt Street.

In association with Arthur Jacob, Robert Graves and others, Henry Marsh established the Park Street School of Medicine in 1824. When a teaching staff was appointed in January 1825, Marsh was lecturer in the practice of medicine, a post he continued to hold in what was regarded as a kind of 'chapel-of-ease' to the RCSI, until 1828 when, as we have seen, he replaced the unfortunate Whitley Stokes in the chair of medicine.[12]

The college minutes for 4 August 1828, the date appointed for the election of a new professor, describe the event. 'The Secretary read the Memorial Syllabus, Certificates and other documents of Doctor H. Marsh a candidate for this chair . . .' The court of examiners and the censors retired to their chamber 'and after some time spent therein' rejoined the main meeting, and Dr Marsh was declared unanimously elected.

Marsh's lectures in the college, unlike those of his predecessor, invariably attracted a large class. His former pupil, William Wilde, has described how the students felt in his addresses, 'that force and felicity of description, which nothing can inspire but a practical acquaintance with the thing described'.

> The closing scene of his career in the College of Surgeons [Wilde continued], afforded the strongest possible indication of his popularity as a teacher. We shall not readily forget the excitement that pervaded all classes of students in medicine, at the announcement that Sir Henry—at that time Dr. Marsh—was about to deliver a series of lectures upon the all-absorbing topic

---

[11] C. Murchison, *The Continued Fevers of Great Britain* (London: Parker, 1862), p. 15.
[12] Sir C. Cameron, *History of the Royal College of Surgeons in Ireland*, 2nd ed. (Dublin: Fannin, 1916), p. 521.

of the day—the swiftly approaching, and justly-dreaded cholera. On each evening, long before the usual lecture hour, crowds of pupils, from every class and school in Dublin—members of the bar—and even judges on the bench, thronged the spacious theatre; and ere the learned professor took the chair, every avenue to the doors was blocked up by masses of eager, but disappointed candidates for admission.[13]

The ease of his spoken addresses has been contrasted with the quality of his writings to the disadvantage of the latter, which were said to display 'lack of lucidity'. Norman Moore's slur in the *Dictionary of National Biography* has been repeated by others, who may not have troubled themselves personally to read Marsh's papers. These, to the present author's mind are not at all wanting in clarity; from a literary viewpoint they err only in their wordiness. Marsh has been criticised, too, for 'the small amount of his contributions to medical literature as compared with the vast amount of his medical experience'. This is equally unconvincing, for he has several substantial papers to his credit.[14] An obituarist in the *Dublin Quarterly Journal of Medical Science* actually referred to him as 'a prolific author'.

Professor Marsh submitted his resignation in 1832:

[24] Molesworth Street, June 5th 1832

GENTLEMEN,

Having been informed that on this day the Censors of the Royal College of Surgeons meet to elect Professors for the ensuing year, I shall take advantage of the opportunity thus afforded of stating that I am come to the resolution of resigning my Professorship, and I shall beg leave further to mention in a few words my reason for adopting (most reluctantly I must say) this Resolution . . .

I feel the undertaking, occupied as I am with daily work, to be too laborious for me, I cannot longer devote to my lectures the time and attention which they ought to have—I think it better to resign the Professorship than discharge its duties imperfectly—

Presumably this was the formal notification of a decision long since conveyed verbally to the authorities. That they had already given thought to his successor is suggested by that fact that following Marsh's resignation, a proposal at a college meeting that the chair of the practice of medicine should be filled by a member or licentiate of the college, was

---

[13] Wilde, 'Sir Henry Marsh', (note 1), p. 692.
[14] Anon., 'Sir Henry Marsh, Bart., M.D., T.C.D., F.K. &.C.P.', *Dublin University Magazine* (1861); 57: 222–8. Sir William Wilde, whose own output was prodigious, may have been the author of this comment.

passed by 27 votes for the motion and 7 votes against it.

On 14 June 1832 an amendment to the fourth section of the by-laws was proposed and accepted by thirty votes to five: 'That no person who is not a Member or Licentiate of the College, shall be elected Professor of the Practice of Medicine.' A further alteration, moved by Arthur Jacob and seconded by Mr O'Beirne, was accepted—the final version reading as follows:

> That no Person shall be elected a Professor of the Theory and practice of Physic, unless he shall have received a regular Surgical education as required by the Bye Laws of this College, and be a Member Fellow or Licentiate of some of the legally constituted Colleges of Surgeons.

A letter in *The Lancet* from an anonymous correspondent ('Observator') drew attention to this illiberal by-law which rendered none but surgeons eligible: '—yes, none but surgeons—to teach the "Theory and Practice of Physic!!!" There is a piece of barefaced corporate monopoly for you!'[15] A barrier had been erected against a fair, open and honourable competition and the question which now presented, 'Observator' pointed out, was 'Who will be the successful candidate?' A possible reason for altering the by-law is discussed in the next chapter.

Phosphorescence

Marsh was appointed consulting physician to the City of Dublin Hospital and also to St Vincent's Hospital, a new Catholic institution on St Stephen's Green, under the auspices of the Irish Sisters of Charity, which was officially opened on 16 August 1836.[16] He was created baronet in 1839; a further honour was his election as one of the six presidents appointed to the newly-founded Pathological Society of Dublin which held its first meeting on 18 November 1838 with Graves in the chair.[17]

Sir Henry's paper 'On Phosphorescence, or Luminous Appearances' was presented to the Royal Irish Academy, of which he was a member, on 10 June 1839, with the purpose of drawing attention to instances of the evolution of light in the living human subject. Certain bodies, such as the sun and fixed stars, he pointed out, are always luminous; others are luminous occasionally, and some are rendered so by friction.

> In recently dead *animal* matter the phenomena of phosphorescence is [sic] most strikingly exhibited. Soon after death fishes become exceedingly luminous. In burial grounds luminous appearances have often been seen.

---

[15] *The Lancet* (1832); 1: 492.
[16] F. O. C. Meenan, *St Vincent's Hospital 1834–1994* (Dublin: Gill & Macmillan, 1995), p. 22.
[17] Davis Coakley, *Masters of Irish Medicine*, (Dublin: Town House, 1992), p. 144.

and fearful and awful are they to the eye of superstition. These corpse-lights, as they are called... take place during the earlier stages of disintegration. A very curious, though not very pleasing appearance of the same kind... has been observed in many dissecting rooms.[18]

Many insects are luminous and light is known to develop in living animals, particularly marine creatures, the presence of which in the water is indicated by phosphorescence in the wake of ships.

Sir Henry proceeded to describe luminous phenomena exhibited by a young lady dying from consumption—'a very extraordinary light which seemed darting about the face, and illuminating all around her head, flashing like an aurora borealis'—and mistaken by her attendant for candle light. The candle was actually removed in case it should disturb her, but the peculiar, silvery light continued for more than an hour.

Similar manifestations, Marsh recalled, were observed near a man dying of 'a lingering disease' in the south-west of Ireland; a light was emitted from a discharging, cancerous ulcer of the breast, and could be seen at a distance of twenty feet from an unfortunate woman in the old Meath Hospital. The physician then drew a comparison between 'a diseased part emitting light', and an occurrence involving the whole body—'spontaneous combustion'. He said that in a case of spontaneous combustion, 'a lambent flame was distinctly seen to issue from the burning body.'[19]

Exophthalmic goitre

Sir Henry Marsh was in the chair when the Dublin Pathological Society met on 25 April 1840, and Dr Law discussed two examples of pathology of the vermiform appendix causing death from peritonitis. Marsh, too, had seen fatal peritonitis from this cause, but neither of them recognised the full significance of what came to be called 'appendicitis', a common and important clinical entity.

Marsh then discoursed on another unusual case. 'The disease under which she laboured', he said, 'merits a distinct notice... Its characteristics are—inordinate action of the heart; habitually quick pulse; enlargement of the thyroid gland; *and in every case... a remarkable prominence and protrusion of the eye-balls*, giving to the eyes a peculiar stare'

---

[18] Marsh, *Proc. RIA* (1839); 1: 317–21. A programme (16 July 1995) on Radio Éireann mentioned that luminous barn-owls had been recently reported, and that cormorants and other birds have been seen to glow in the dark with a reddish-yellow light. The phenomenon is attributed to algae attached to feathers.

[19] *Ibid.*, p. 321. So named by Charles Dickens in *Bleak House*, spontaneous combustion defies belief, but the late Professor P. J. Bofin, sometime city coroner, cited an instance in his own experience in Dublin—during the night of 27 March 1970 an elderly woman burst into flames without apparent cause, and her body was reduced to ashes.

[emphasis added].[20]

Marsh had seen several similar cases; all were female and all presented 'unequivocal marks of the strumous diathesis'. They were thin or emaciated; the pulse 'habitually and permanently quick', and sometimes 'singularly rapid'. Violent palpitations and breathlessness followed exercise or emotion.

> The heart's impulse [he continued] gives to the integuments a considerably increased perceptible motion. The sounds sharp, loud, and short, like those which characterize nervous palpitations. They are heard loudly throughout the chest on both sides; but unmixed with any bellows or other abnormal sound. When the cardiac action is much agitated the venous system is gorged; the veins of the neck prominent and distended. The thyroid gland permanently enlarged, palpably swells and subsides, as the heart's action increases and diminishes. *The protrusion of the eyes likewise keeps pace with the degrees of the heart's action* [emphasis added]. Of the patients thus affected the countenances were pallid, and as the disease advanced the lips and cheeks presented, in various degrees, a purple shade.[21]

Two, of six cases observed, had slight spinal tenderness. Symptoms were aggravated by catarrhal or digestive upsets; the menses were normal in the early phase. If not far advanced the disease responded to treatment by small bleedings, using leeches or cupping, and medication with tonics and sedatives. Small doses of belladonna, prussic acid or digitalis reduced the heart-rate. Iron was needed because of the 'deficiency in the red globules.'

Diet should be nourishing, but not stimulating, and peace of mind and body must be strictly enjoined.

> Nothing in treatment appeared so effectual as prolonged quiet journeying; changing air and place for a long continued period of time. All those affected with this disease were benefitted by this treatment; three apparently were perfectly cured. When the disease, either from neglect of proper treatment, or from other causes, increases, all the essential symptoms are materially aggravated. The heart beats more violently and rapidly; the breathing becomes more hurried and distressing; the veins more swollen; lividity more marked; the thyroid gland increases in size; the eyes assume a more staring and prominent aspect; emaciation advances; and lastly, the patient becomes universally anasarcous.[22]

Despite anasarca, one young patient was twice restored to what her

---

[20] Marsh, *Dublin J. Med. Sc.*, (1841); 18: 335–41.
[21] *Ibid.*, p. 339.
[22] *Ibid.*, p. 340.

friends deemed 'perfect health'; another deteriorated slowly over seven years and died, her sufferings 'prolonged and most painful to witness'.

> Often during that time, she appeared comparatively reinstated in health; but on each occasion, severe catarrhal affections, caused by exposure to cold, sometimes anxiety of mind, or excessive fatigue or exertion, from which she would not be restrained, reproduced, in an aggravated form, all the most urgent symptoms of the disease. [23]

Marsh concluded by saying that the cardiac disturbance seemed 'purely functional' at first, but the 'long continued altered function produces ultimately organic disease'. He was not aware of any previous description of the disease, taking, as he did, exopthalmos to be the cardinal sign.

On 2 January 1841, in the same venue, Marsh showed a specimen illustrative of 'a very curious and interesting affection of the heart', and recalled his earlier presentation. The disorder was characterised by 'remarkable engorgement of the veins, particularly of those of the neck; rapid, violent, and irregular action of the heart, and these, in every instance, co-existing with enlargement and swelling of the thyroid gland'.[24]

He reiterated that he had seen a number of cases of this kind, and said he had 'had more than one opportunity of verifying the condition of the heart' by dissection. The majority displayed 'a remarkable prominence and protrusion of the eyeballs' which gave the group a striking unifying feature. The case he wished to place before the society had all those signs. The prominence of the eyes 'was not so strongly marked as in other cases'; the thyroid gland was enlarged and seemed to swell and increase in size 'whenever there was any inordinate action of the heart'.

Marsh gave a detailed description of the thyroid, which during life 'projected so as to form a very large and prominent tumour', but was now shrunken. 'When first removed its surface was irregularly lobulated, and the lobes or cysts contained a considerable quantity of clear fluid.' The heart was enlarged, its chambers dilated. The margins of the auriculo-ventricular valves were thickened by depositions beneath the lining membranes; this interfered with 'the free discharge of their function'. There had been palpitations and dyspnoea.

He read the notes of another case, a forty-year-old woman, recently under his care. Her illness began with nervous palpitation, and had followed 'nervous excitement and apprehension' caused by her responsibility for the supervision of a relative with epilepsy.

---

[23] *Ibid.*, p. 341.
[24] Marsh, 'Dilatation of the Cavities of the Heart—Enlargement of the Thyroid Gland', *Dublin J. Med. Sc.* (1841); 20: 471.

Her face was pale and somewhat tumid, eyes prominent, lips purplish, the veins of the neck considerably distended, and the thyroid body much enlarged. The impulses of the heart gave motion to the integuments over a space exceeding far the ordinary limits of the cardiac region; and there was a considerable extent of dullness on percussion. The first sound of the heart was short, quick, and loud; the second faint and scarcely audible, in consequence of being masked by the first, but there was no bruit de soufflet or any other abnormal sound. She complained of being subject to attacks of dyspnoea in the morning, accompanied with a sensation of fluttering in the heart; she sometimes had similar attacks during the day, but not so severe. Any unusual exertion, or sudden mental emotion was sufficient to bring on distressing palpitations. Her pulse was quick and jerking, never below 90, her respiration clear and puerile. The bruit in the carotid artery, where it was pressed on by the thyroid gland, was actually perceived by the patient, and caused a great deal of annoyance; she stated that she felt a whizzing sound in her neck, of which she never could get rid, and that it was one of the most distressing sensations she felt.[25]

He had enjoined 'the strictest avoidance of everything calculated to agitate the mind or fatigue the body', and prescribed iron carbonate and hyocyamus. He believed 'that if the affection had been unchecked' damage to the heart valves would have ensued. This statement lacks aetiological specificity, but appears to indicate that Marsh postulated an unknown factor that threatened the valves. It seems unlikely, however, that he suspected primary involvement of the thyroid, for, as we have seen, he attributed variations in the size of the gland of his first patient to 'inordinate action of the heart'.

According to the late M. I. Drury, Marsh's paper was the first to describe an autopsy in what we now call Graves' disease.[26] Marsh does not mention Robert Graves's 1835 publication, 'Newly Observed Affection of the Thyroid Gland in Females', which is surprising as one of Graves's cases (the only case with ocular involvement) was reported to him by Marsh. It is possible, of course, that for Marsh exophthalmos was the essential feature of the new disease, being present in all his cases. Be that as it may, he makes no claim for priority. The eponym 'Marsh's disease' was briefly used, but at least one medical dictionary refers to it as 'the same as Graves's disease'.[27]

Famine fevers

Marsh's little monograph *On the Preparation of Food for the Labourer* took the form of a letter to Joshua Harvey, MD, and contained a num-

---

[25] *Ibid,.* p. 473.
[26] M. I. Drury, 'Graves' Disease, 1861–1961', *J. Irish Med. Assn.* (1961); 49: 115.
[27] Liam Ó Sé, 'Sir Henry Marsh: the Neglected Luminary', *Irish Medical Times*, (December 1989).

ber of sensible observations.[28] Bakeries, he insisted, are as necessary as soup kitchens; food should have bulk and solidity, so as not to be quickly digested. When famine occurred on the borders of Lapland in 1832, 'earth mixed with flour, and with bark of trees, and baked so as to form bread, became a useful article of diet.'

Fish 'should be sought for and provided, whenever possible'; it will be a nutritive adjunct to all soups. Brown bread should be made from the unrefined flour of wheat. 'When famine prevails, everything eatable is earnestly laid hold of—principles are forgotten—the only thought which occupies and pervades the mind, is to arrest and ward off the dreadful cravings of hunger, and to preserve human life.'[29] But when plans are devised, principles should be recalled.

Marsh was a member of a board of health for the city of Dublin which was appointed in anticipation of the cholera epidemic. He was not an original member of the temporary central board of health (CBH) established in 1846 to deal with the famine fevers. The three medical members were Sir Philip Crampton, Dr Robert Kane and Dr Dominic Corrigan who was the dominating figure. The CBH was severely criticised by Robert Graves, but Marsh who joined it after Kane's resignation escaped his strictures.[30]

Clinical lectures

When Dr James Stannus Hughes was a clinical clerk at Steevens' Hospital (1839–42), he took shorthand notes of Marsh's lectures, and towards the end of the latter's life it was agreed that they should be published.[31]

Empyema The examination of the chest carried out by Marsh and his contemporaries included inspection, palpation, percussion and auscultation. Empyema was diagnosed by considering 'the symptoms, age, former state of health, and length of time the disease existed previous to the distension of the affected side'.[32] It was confirmed by the 'explorator' (a very fine trochar and cannula) and when necessary drained by a lancet-shaped trochar. He advocated early surgical drainage as a curative method and by reviewing published cases found that twenty-eight drained cases re-

---

[28] Marsh, *On the Preparation of Food for the Labourer* (Dublin: McGlashan, 1847).
[29] *Ibid.*, p. 10.
[30] R. J. Graves, 'A Letter Relative to the Proceedings of the CBH', *Dublin Quart. J. Med. Sc.* (1847); 4: 513–30. See also Joseph Robins, *The Miasma*, (Dublin: Institute of Public Administration, 1995), p. 123.
[31] Marsh, *Clinical Lectures Delivered in Steevens' Hospital, with Observations on Practical Medicine* (Dublin: Fannin, 1867).
[32] *Ibid.*, p. 2.

covered and eight died whereas conservative treatment almost always ended in death.³³

The medical treatment of empyema consisted then of bleeding, mercury, and in a more chronic phase, cuppings and blisters. The operation of paracentesis thoracis lay within the province of the surgeons and should not be done, Marsh urged, merely as a *dernier ressort*. As late as 1844, the procedure had not gained favour with William Stokes and others, but in 1859 Mr Smyly reported a successful outcome in five out of seven cases operated on at the Meath Hospital. Marsh had found that in cases complicated by pneumothorax (probably tuberculous) the operation was only palliative.

Emphysema Marsh was familiar with John Forbes's translation of Laennec's *On Diseases of the Chest and Mediate Auscultation* (1827) and credited its author with the recognition of emphysema resulting from 'simple dilatation of the air-cells of the lungs'.³⁴ When fully developed it was easily recognised: 'You have on percussion a morbid clearness, no vesicular respiration can be heard with the stethoscope, little or no expansion of the chest during respiration, the breathing appearing to be carried on by the diaphragm, abdominal, and thyroid muscles chiefly.'³⁵

He favoured the management recommended by a Dublin colleague, Jonathan Osborne, whose *On the Nature and Treatment of Dropsical Effusions* he praised warmly. An emphysematous patient of Osborne's happened to visit a London doctor who mistakenly attributed the symptoms to a gastric cause, and imposed a dry, sparing diet, with restricted fluids and large doses of carbonate of iron. Weight reduction amounting to three stone followed, accompanied by great symptomatic improvement. Osborne proclaimed the excellence of the regime; Marsh, too, found it helpful.

Marsh was keenly interested in the pathology of emphysema. He hoped to learn more from a study of the lungs of a large animal, and proposed to do a postmortem examination of an old broken-winded horse which was dying in his stables.

Jaundice 'No age is exempt from Jaundice', Marsh told his students, dividing the many causes into 'the curable and the incurable'.³⁶ A stone in the common bile duct was placed in the latter group, as was pressure caused by the head of the pancreas or by enlarged and swollen glands. Anything that led to congestion or inflammation of the liver could cause jaundice, and it was to be met with occasionally in fevers.

---

³³ Finnegan 'Sir Henry Marsh', (note 1), p. 300.
³⁴ *Ibid.*, p. 60. (A Chichester physician, Sir John Forbes, edited *The Cyclopaedia of Practical Medicine* [London: Sherwood, Gilbert and Piper, 1834] to which a number of Dublin doctors contributed.)
³⁵ *Ibid.*, p. 64.
³⁶ *Ibid.*, 129.

There is a very rare form of jaundice in which there is no obstruction of the biliary secretion, but an over-secretion of it, and this form I have only met two or three times in practice: in such cases the evacuations, instead of being devoid of bile, as in other forms of the disease, are loaded with dark-brown or bottle-green bile, and yet all not getting exit through the ducts, some is driven back on the constitution.[37]

The sheet anchor in the treatment of biliary colic was opium in large doses, with hot stupes applied to the abdomen. Emetics helped in chronic hepatitis by stimulating the liver to healthy action—'hence it is that short rough sea voyages (as to Holyhead from Dublin, for instance) are so often in such cases properly recommended by physicians'.[38]

Death

Henry Marsh was appointed physician in ordinary to the queen in Ireland in 1837 and was created baronet two years later. He was not elected to the fellowship of the King and Queen's College of Physicians until 1839, but he occupied the presidential office in 1841–2 and 1845–6, and contributed £200 towards the building of the college hall in Kildare Street.

He moved from Molesworth Street in the 1840s to 9 Merrion Square North, and at one time or other had country residences, De Maresco at Knockmaroon, and Kirrakill Castle, County Kilkenny. 'His moral was his incentive to action.'[39] He remained free from 'any undue elation on account of his prosperity'; he had a pleasant easy manner and though accustomed to move in the highest levels of society never affected an air of superiority. From time to time he entertained some of his colleagues, and it was customary that a medical paper would be read by one of his guests.

He married twice, and by a curious coincidence both wives were widows. Mrs Mary Henrietta Arthur, the widowed daughter of Thomas Crowe of Ennis, County Clare, whom he married in 1820, was the mother of his son, Colonel Marsh of the 3rd Dragoon Guards who died without issue. The first Lady Marsh died in 1846; ten years later he married a Mrs Mary Henrietta Kemmis (née Jelly), relict of Thomas Kemmis of Shaen, Queen's County, who survived him. Their union was childless.

The first section of Marsh's *Observations on Transmitted Affections of the Stomach* was printed in March 1860 for distribution among his friends. Taking origin in a paper intended for presentation to a mixed audience in the college hall it was written in the author's carriage while on his daily rounds. A second section, *On Disturbances of the Brain which give rise to Somnambulism, Ecstacism,*

---

[37] *Ibid.*, 131.
[38] *Ibid.*, p. 136.
[39] Anon., 'In Memoriam', *Dublin Quart. J. Med. Sc.* (1861); 33: 251–52.

Etc., was nearing completion when fate intervened.[40]

As he was leaving home shortly after 9 a.m on 1 December 1860 Sir Henry was seized with vertigo; he fell heavily fracturing a fibula. He was carried indoors but died in the early afternoon. R. T. Evanson, his former colleague at the Park Medical School and a successor in the chair of medicine, marked his passing with an elegiac verse:

> *Thou'rt gone: but such is life! How strange the lot*
> *Of mortal man upon the Earth! To-day*
> *All absolute: to morrow he is not,—*

Some days after his burial at Mount Jerome Cemetery, a meeting of his friends was called to arrange for a permanent memorial. Mr J. W. Cusack presided and the following resolution was adopted: 'That the high position which Sir Henry Marsh so long held in the estimation of his professional brethren and of the public should be marked by some lasting testimonial of his eminent abilities.' Eventually it was agreed that a marble statue, to be placed in the hall of the College of Physicians, would be the most suitable testimonial.[41]

The statue by Mr John H. Foley, RA, was agreed to be a 'marvellous likeness'. When it was handed over to the College authorities in November 1866, Dr Banks spoke on behalf of the subscribers and praised Marsh's contributions to the *Dublin Hospital Reports*—'The Origin of Fever', 'Jaundice' and 'Spasm of the Glottis'.

Accepting the memorial on behalf of the college, William Stokes recalled the statue of Dr Charles Lucas in the corporation hall, 'the figures on the porticos of the Bank, and the admirable symbolic heads of the river deities of Ireland, which adorn the arches and windows of the Custom House'. Stokes believed that the hall in which they were assembled would become 'the Irish medical Walhalla where will be preserved memorials, which, though dead yet speak of those true soldiers of medicine whose works live after them and whose days were worthy.' This prediction has been amply fulfilled.

---

[40] By request of Major Sir Henry Marsh, his father's book was edited by Dr H. Freke, physician to Steevens' Hospital, and printed for private circulation in 1861.
[41] *The Dublin Builder* (1866); 8: 271.

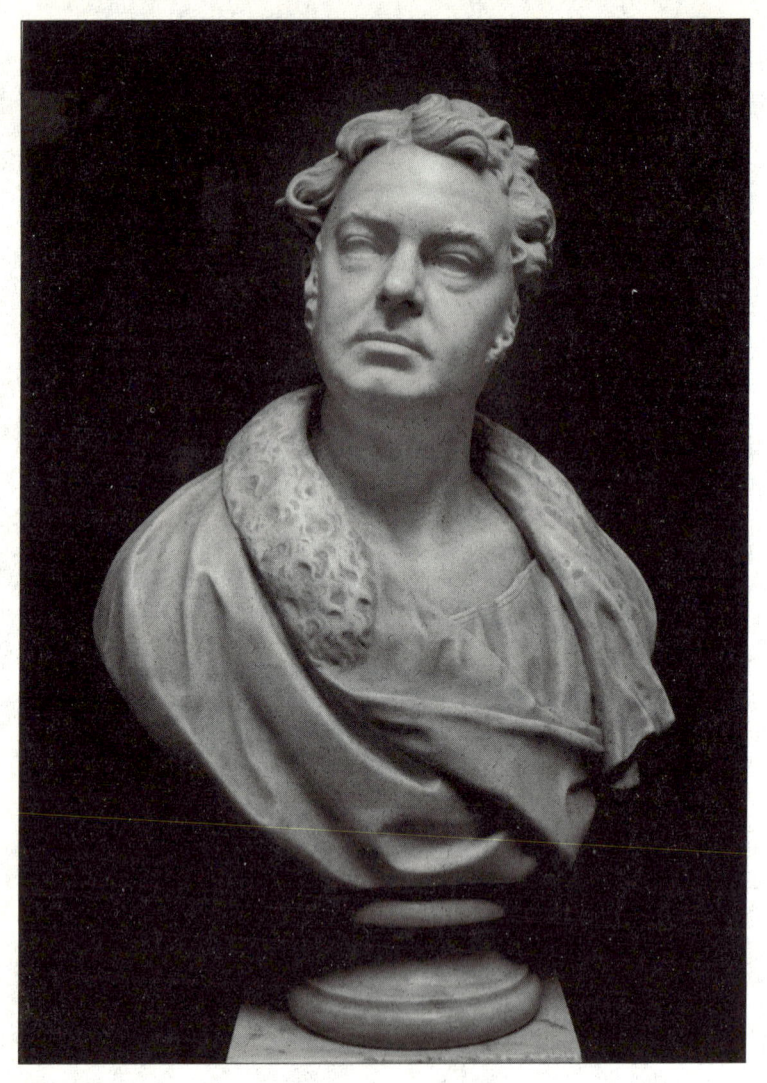

John Timothy Kirby, 1781–1853 Professor of Medicine 1832–6 (bust by Thos. Kirk, courtesy RCSI)

Chapter 4: John Timothy Kirby, 1781–1853

Erinensis, as we have seen, found much to praise in Whitley Stokes, but Kirby cannot have been pleased to read an equivocal description of himself in *The Lancet* five weeks later—'There are few names in the Medical world better known than that of John Timothy Kirby . . . for in every habitable clime, from the Equator to the Pole, where the genius of Irish emigration could find a resting place, there are thousands dying of his precepts, or daily restored to health by the judicious re-application of his skill.'[1] A more factual chapter based on Kirby's unpublished autobiography, preserved by his son, a retired naval chaplain, is provided in Sir Charles Cameron's *History of the Royal College of Surgeons in Ireland*.[2]

Born in 1781, Kirby's father and grandfather were prominent physicians in the South of Ireland; his maternal grandfather, a native of Lochaber, supported Bonnie Prince Charlie in 1745. When Kirby *père* died unexpectedly in 1788 from haemorrhage complicating consump-tion, the family had to exist on limited means supplied by an uncle who had gained control of lands leased by the deceased from the Duke of Devonshire at Lismore, County Waterford.

A case in Chancery to recover John's patrimony was initiated, and he was sent to school in Lismore. Unfortunately, this institution was run by a wayward man of the cloth, the Rev. Mr Crawford, a curate at the cathedral, an inebriate who came into class in his cups and spent the hour chanting drinking songs in an undertone.

> We never had morning or evening prayer. No prayerbook in the school composed of 35 boys. We were allowed to lie, to steal, and to commit even the most obscene abomination. We were washed once a week, only think how filthy, and then what a business; the same water, the same cloth—never called to prayer. *Pro pudor!* I spent seven years at this school. I rejoiced when I left it, which I did in the summer of 1795.[3]

The lack of discipline may have fostered a degree of independence and impetuousness, for having left school in the summer of 1795 young Kirby was engrossed in 'country amusements', until becoming 'military mad' in 1798 he determined to seek an army commission. Setting out on horseback for Dublin, he was accompanied by a servant who had been employed by his father. They rode on through a troubled countryside,

---

[1] Martin Fallon, *The Sketches of Erinensis*, (London: Skilton & Shaw, 1979), pp. 43–53.
[2] Sir C. Cameron, *History of the Royal College of Surgeons in Ireland*, (1916), pp. 440–46.
[3] *Ibid.*, p. 441.

and when the opportunity came to travel by coach guarded by six dragoons, Kirby was glad to do so as an inside passenger.

Putting up at Macken's Hotel in Dublin, he went to the Parliament House to meet his guardian, who being told of his purpose was not at all pleased to see him. Relenting, however, he gave the lad a pass for the theatre, and an entry, as it were, into a different world.

> In a few months [Kirby wrote] I had a commission. I now for the first time began to reflect on the step I was taking, and resolved to return the commission to Sir Robert Musgrave. I did so, and on the 4th November, '98, I was Mr. Halahan's apprentice. This was an eventful time. I was about sixteen years old or seventeen. I here met with a young lady, his niece, to whom in three years I was married. She was a Miss Rose; her father was paymaster of the 59th Regiment.[4]

At TCD, which he entered in 1802, his tutor was John Walker, the redoubtable founder of 'the Walkerites'. He commenced BA in 1805, taking his surgical diploma, LRCSI, in the same year, proceeding MRCSI (equivalent to the present fellowship) in 1808, and obtaining the degrees LL.B and LL.D in 1832.

Demonstratorship

Kirby was a candidate for a post as surgeon to the Armagh Hospital, and in this connection an interview was arranged with the primate. 'He kept me waiting a long time; I grew impatient, left him all my credentials, and retired, believing myself to be badly treated.' The disgruntled doctor turned hopefully to Bartholomew Mosse's Lying-in Hospital, then under the mastership of Thomas Kelly, but disgusted by what he saw there he did not bother to seek a certificate—'This gave me enough of midwifery.' Dr Kelly, it may be added, was soon forced to submit his resignation and sued the governors unavailingly for wrongful dismissal. They accused him of discharging sick patients prematurely to die in their own homes.[5]

Appointed demonstrator of anatomy at the College of Surgeons under the direction of Abraham Colles and Richard Dease, Kirby worked there for two years but then he fell out with his superiors, whom he believed were jealous when the students, to express their gratitude, presented him with a piece of plate worth a hundred guineas. This seems an unlikely story and an interchange of letters indicates that Kirby was planning to enter a rival situation.

---

[4] *Ibid.*, p. 442.
[5] For Thomas Kelly see O'Donel T. D. Browne, *The Rotunda Hospital 1745–1945* (Edinburgh: Livingstone, 1947), p. 264.

JOHN TIMOTHY KIRBY

Dear Doctor,

On meeting Mr. Garnett [vice-president, 1809] yesterday I communicated to him that circumstances had occurred since I last saw him which compel me to retire from the Demonstratorship to which you had appointed me. I conceive it my duty to put you in possession of my reasons. At the period of my former resignation I entered into a partnership, regularly secured by a bond and mutual penalty of £1,000, to conduct a School of Anatomy, &c., for a certain period, and not to hold the Demonstratorship for any part of that time without the full approbation of my partner. With these conditions I in some measure acquainted Mr. Garnett, but, on further conference with his friends, he recalls his indulgence, in opposition to every remonstrance on my part and that of my friend Leahy.[6] These are the motives which *oblige* me to leave you. I resign with reluctance, and fear that you will be put to some temporary inconvenience. Though thus separated I am still sincerely yours,

John Kirby.
Cuffe Street, Sept. 15, 1809.

Colles registered disappointment, and a mild rebuke, in his reply:

I communicated to my colleague, Mr. Dease [PRCSI, 1809] your note of the 15th instant. We regret and are surprised that you should now feel yourself obliged to withdraw from that engagement with us which you entered some weeks ago, when Mr. Garnett waited on you for the purpose of reconciling the differences then existing between you and us. No doubt, we shall be put to some temporary inconvenience by having our arrangements for the season broken up at this late period. These, however, we shall endeavour by suitable exertions, to surmount.[7]

The cause of Kirby's resignation appears to have been directly connected with his plan to start an independent school of anatomy.

Theatre of Anatomy

The case in Chancery had dragged on so long, without any obvious hope of resolution, that Kirby had sold his patrimony for £700, and with Alexander Read as partner he established the 'Theatre of Anatomy' in 1809, at the rear of a laundry in Stephen's Street. The laundress's notice advised 'Mangling Done Here', and the wags inferred that it also applied to the anatomy school.

The first course of lectures opened on 23 October 1809, terminating

---

[6] See note 12 below.
[7] Martin Fallon, *Abraham Colles 1773–1843* (London: Heinemann Medical Books, 1972), p. 139.

> **Royal College of Surgeons in Ireland.**
>
> I, *John Kirby Member* of the ROYAL COLLEGE *of* SURGEONS *in* IRELAND, do solemnly declare upon my Honor, that I have really, and *bona fide*, received the Sum of *One* Hundred & *Fifty Guineas*, with Mr. *Edwd Clarke* who was indented to me as an *Extern* Apprentice, on the 6th Day of *June* 1812.
>
> Given under my Hand, this 6th Day of *June* 1812.
>
> *John Kirby*

Receipt for apprentice fees signed by J. T. Kirby 1812

on 23 March 1810 and was followed by a course extending from late April to September. The school was moved in 1810 to Peter Street and Read resigned about two years later, leaving Kirby sole proprietor of a 'Theatre of Anatomy and School of Surgery'. This flourished until its closure in 1832 when Kirby was appointed to the chair of medicine at the RCSI.[8]

So as to provide the mandatory evidence of hospital attendance required by the army authorities from his pupils, Kirby established a small hospital named for St Peter and St Bridget which was opened on 2 August 1811. Its certificates were not accepted by the College of Surgeons until 1831, for Colles and others held that its bed numbers were insufficient. It was Erinensis who spread the unkind rumour that in 'the celebrated *La charité* of Peter-street' there was only one bed—'and we assure our readers that when we visited the place there was no bottom in the same'.[9]

'I gave my first lecture [Kirby recalled] in a small house near Mercer's Hospital, to a class larger than they had at the College of Surgeons. This aroused envy.' He was succeeded in the college as demonstrator by

---

[8] Kirby's school was reopened in 1836 by George Thomas Hayden who called it 'The Original School' to emphasise its previous existence.
[9] Fallon, *Abraham Colles*, (note 7), p. 45.

Charles Hawkes Todd, whom he accused of slanderous reports calculated to impair confidence in him. He came to regard Colles as a 'bitter enemy', who opposed him in the college and refused to meet him in consultation. Be that as it may, these gentlemen eventually patched up their quarrel, and Kirby in due course was to become censor at the RCSI and to hold high office. 'I became in my turn Vice-President and President [the latter office in 1823 and 1834], and was voted, as usual, the thanks of the College, and was chosen one among the seniors.'

He was fond of fine attire, and wore breeches and silk stockings when lecturing. He walked up and down as he spoke, and the style of his discourse was ornate. In the manner of professional men in every age, he used many ruses including showy horses, and a smart carriage to keep his name to the fore.

> The graceful swing of his chaise [wrote Erinensis], as it plays upon the obedient springs would learn to be communicated by his own more versatile movements—in the solemn rumbling of its wheels, imagination conjures up the awe-inspiring pathos of his oratory. And in the varnished stiffness and profusion of its embellishments, fancy cannot fail in finding a similitude for the gaudy tints of his rhetorical tulips. 'All', indeed, 'are but parts of one stupendous whole'. The very horses as they toss their heads on high, seem proud of their subjection to so stately a master, the light azure livery and silver lace of the mortal Phaeton, holding the reins, are but the creation of his fertile invention; and the military shoulder knots of a blooming boy, perched like another Ariel upon the box behind are emblematic of his picturesque taste. The entire equipage looks big with importance, and as it flouts your gaze in its rapid motion over the muttering pavements, you would think fortune herself was dragged into captivity at its wheels.[10]

Despite the sneers of *The Lancet*'s waspish correspondent, Kirby's success depended on Sir William Osler's 'masterword'—*work*. During the early years of his career he rose at five a.m., tutored a private pupil for two hours, breakfasted and proceeded to lecture at Peter Street. Further lectures, demonstrations, consultations and the writing up of case-reports kept him busy until ten p.m. His 'Lectures on Urinary Diseases', edited by A. J. Walsh were published in the *Dublin Hospital Gazette*.

The Peninsular War, as we have seen, had increased the demand for surgeons, and was the ill-wind that blew good fortune into the College of Surgeons and throughout the private schools, including Kirby's, where to keep up with the physiological demonstrations on rabbits introduced by Macartney at TCD the proprietor outstripped his competitors 'by venturing upon the nine lives of a Cat!' He must have employed 'sack 'em up men' to supply 'stiffs' for his dissecting-room, and he may not have

---

[10] *Ibid.*, p. 46.

been above grave-robbing himself, needing a double supply of corpses in order to give a course on gunshot wounds which was ridiculed by Erinensis:

> For the purpose of demonstrating the destructive effects of fire-arms upon the human frame, Bully's Acre gave up its cleverest treasures for the performance of the experiment. The *subjects* being placed with military precision along the wall, the Lecturer entered with his pistol in his hand, and levelling the mortiferous weapon at the enemy, magnanimously discharged several rounds, each followed by repeated bursts of applause. As soon as the smoke and approbation subsided, then came the tug of war. The wounded were examined, arteries were taken up, bullets were extracted, bones were set, and every spectator fancied himself on the field of battle, and looked upon Mr. Kirby as a prodigy of genius and valour *for shooting dead men*.[11]

There were actually twelve surgical beds at St Peter's and St Bridget's Hospital, but the influential Colles thought this number insufficient. He proposed at a college meeting that no hospital with less than twenty-four beds should be 'recognised'. Kirby countered the motion with the extraordinary claim to have performed more operations in the year at his hospital than were performed in all the Dublin hospitals in the same period. He agreed, however, to add ten medical beds under the supervision of Dr James Leahy,[12] and to appoint a board of governors, but he was obliged to use most of his private funds for the upkeep of his private facility. It was his custom to send private reports to the medical and naval boards in London, being extremely discreet with his recommendations. Then to his distress some of his certificates were copied and sold at a high price.

Kirby's assaults on dead bodies may have evoked smiles from Erinensis and later commentators, but he was an astute surgeon and his observations in the *Dublin Hospital Reports* on a case of a gunshot wound of the head are cited in John Hennen's *Principles of Military Surgery*. After the Battle of Waterloo, Kirby visited Colchester, where the wounded had been sent, and was struck by the case of a young man 'within whose head a musket ball had lodged'. The entrance wound had healed and there were no symptoms apart from some giddiness provoked by violent exercise or mental concentration.

---

[11] *Ibid.*, p. 52.
[12] James John Leahy (1780–1832), MD (TCD and Edin.) was FKQCPI and president of the College of Physicians in 1826 in which year he was appointed to the chair of the institutes of medicine in TCD. He gave a morning lecture on chemistry and pharmacy in the Peter Street school and lectured on medicine at 3 p.m. He died in Sligo of Asiatic cholera.

Skilled surgeon

Though not included in the litany of leading Irish surgeons, Kirby appears to have been skilled and resourceful. He was quickly in demand and dealt with unusual emergencies, such as that facing an embarrassed practitioner whose gum elastic cannula had slipped through the trocar into his patient's bladder, to be removed operatively by Kirby using a pointed bistoury to pierce the bladder, and a scissors-handled dressing forceps to extract the misplaced object.

Aneurism was a relatively commonplace problem, but whatever the surgical procedure it was sound policy to divide responsibility by the presence of colleagues.

> Assisted by my colleagues, Messrs Hamilton, Adrien, and by my old master, Mr Halahan I made an incision, nearly four inches long, through the abdominal integuments, directly over the external iliac artery, commencing about an inch above Poupart's ligament. [December 1811]
>
> Assisted by Mr. A. Colles, Mr. M. Daniel, and Mr. Rumley, I tied the brachial artery, about three inches above the tumour . . . [July 1816]

He had been asked to see one of his cases of wry neck by Dr Benjamin Lentaigne (1773–1813), a French royalist émigré who came to Ireland with the 5th Dragoon Guards, and having married Marie Thérèse O'Neill of Athboy, County Meath, settled in Dublin.[13] Lentaigne attained some prominence for his ministrations to the dying Theobald Wolfe Tone.

Robert Graves praises Kirby in his *System of Clinical Medicine*:

> It has been long known that gout may attack the brain, and the existence of gouty paraplegia is well known by practitioners who have studied attentively the progress of arthritic affections. Thus, in a case which I witnessed some time back, in consultation with Mr. Kirby, he prognosed the supervention of paraplegia at a time when the indications of its approach could not have been discovered by any observer of less experience and sagacity.

A National Surgical Hospital

Attending college meetings regularly, Kirby frequently participated in discussions and was quick to propose amendments. He was elected PRCSI in 1823, and having spent an apparently uneventful presidential year was thanked by his colleagues in January 1824: 'Resolved, that the

---

[13] The National Library holds Lentaigne's treatise in Latin verse, *Testamen Causis Morborum*, written in 1812 under the pseudonym 'Medicus Dublinensis'. See Patrick O'Donnell, 'Wolfe Tone's Death: Suicide or Assassination?' *Irish J. Med. Sc.* (1997); 166: 57–9. His son, Sir John Lentaigne (1803–83) presented a fifteenth-century manuscript 'Practica Magistri Johannis Arderne' to the College in 1851; his grandson Sir John Lentaigne (1857–1916), was surgeon to the Mater Hospital and PRCSI 1908–10.

Thanks of the College be Returned to John Kirby late President for the very able and assiduous manner in which he discharged the duties of that Office.'

Early in the following year, when the executives were devoting their attention to the necessity of enlarging the library and museum, Kirby gave notice (7 February 1825) that he would move at the next quarterly meeting: 'that the Establishment of a National Surgical Hospital under the management of the Royal College of Surgeons in Ireland will greatly contribute to the advancement of Surgical Science in Ireland, to the character of the College and to the interests of its Members'. The college had accumulated a capital sum of at least £9,500, and he would recommend that £6,000 be set aside to build a hospital accommodating one hundred patients.

He summarized his arguments in a pamphlet which purported to answer those who wished to expend money on extending the museum.[14] He asked how could funds 'be disposed of most advantageously to the College, and most beneficially to its Members'? A museum was to be 'considered in a two-fold point of view; first, as a monument of contributive zeal of the Members of the College; secondly, as a depository in which may be seen in a state of anatomical preservation the products of the animal kingdom, and preparation of natural or diseased parts as they occur in the human body.'[15] From the first viewpoint 'no real value can be properly said to be stamped on the collection'; from the second viewpoint recent developments in engraving and colouring had reduced the value of such preparations. And besides, the museum should increase slowly, requiring little expenditure. 'We are not to argue from the sums it has cost under the careless management of its Committee, that equal amounts are to be annually drawn from our funds—nor are we to conclude, that under its new management, economy will be disregarded.'[16]

Having thus antagonized a number of his colleagues, he turned to consider the hospital project. At their last meeting it had been said 'there are hospitals enough', which really meant there were *enough* in the opinion 'of those who are so fortunate as to enjoy the great advantages they afford'.

> But the fact, that Hospital opportunities are not sufficiently numerous, is at once asserted by the reference to the large list of Members whose talents are unemployed during the most vigorous periods of their lives—while they have much leisure to cultivate the Science of Surgery.—While they have

---

[14] John T. Kirby, *Observations on the intended Motion for connecting a National Surgical Hospital with the Royal College of Surgeons in Ireland, addressed to the Members and Licentiates* [Dublin, 1825].
[15] *Ibid.*, p. 2.
[16] *Ibid.*, p. 4.

every disposition to try, by the test of practice, the value of the precepts they have learned.

Of SEVENTY ONE Members of the College resident in Dublin, FORTY EIGHT are without any Hospital opportunity; and of THIRTY Licentiates none are connected with any Institution of the kind. Can it be longer maintained that there is no want of Hospitals, as far as the individuals of the College are concerned? Are those individuals careless on the subject? I say they are not.—Their first ambition is to be connected with an Hospital. To this laudable ambition they devote all the interests they can command, and in the pursuit of this desirable object they are content to expend their pecuniary means. They feel the value of an Hospital as an introduction to public notice; they feel the value of an Hospital in acquirement of professional experience, and they duly estimate the claims it affords to patronage in point of Pupils. They well know without an Hospital, no man in this country has ever taken, or perhaps will ever take a high station in the profession.[17]

London and Paris owed their surgical renown to their hospitals. 'Where do we borrow our present taste for pathological research and pathological science?'

Kirby spoke of Dublin's system of 'harsh monopoly', condemned the tendency to ridicule every individual 'who attempts an innovation', and offered a plan of procedure. 'Such are the views I hold of the value of the proposed National Hospital—such are the funds for its establishment—such are the means for its support—and such are the regulations for its control.'[18]

The college minutes are sparing of details; no information is given of the controversy caused by Kirby's pamphlet. It is clear, however, that behind the scenes he found himself in a minority, and on 21 February 1825 an important notice appeared:

> First, that the Curators of the Museum be instructed to adopt such measures as they may deem expedient to procure a plan and estimate of a Museum on an extensive scale, to be submitted to the College with as little delay as possible.—
>
> Second that a notice of Motion lately entered on the Minutes of the College, by which it is intended to be proposed that a large sum of money shall be applied, from the funds of the College to the establishment of a National Surgical Hospital be erased from the order of the proceedings, it being the opinion of the College, that the extension of the Museum and Library ought not be superseded by the introduction of any new speculation, involving an expense to which the resources of the College are wholly inadequate.

An architect, William Murray, was engaged. The provision of the

---

[17] *Ibid.*, p. 7.
[18] *Ibid.*, p. 15.

desired amenities was to require the extension of Parke's 1810 façade towards Glover's Alley, and entail a rearrangement of the elements of the existing composition which was to give the enlarged building rather a Palladian character.[19]

Kirby's resignation from the museum building committee on 20 September 1825 may have been due to pique, or was possibly related to his bereavement. His personal affairs had prospered; he had saved £2,000 and possessed a fine residence at 56 Harcourt Street, in addition to the school and hospital in Peter Street, but he had experienced the misfortune of losing his wife, Lucinda,—'who supported me by her counsel, and with whom I got £250 a year'. She died in childbed in 1825 after the birth of her sixteenth child.

His resignation was accepted without comment, and in January 1826 he was granted permission to have two additional apprentices. Kirby's motion on 13 April 1826 regarding the duties of professors has been mentioned in an earlier chapter. He was interested, too, in compil-ing a pharmacopoea to be entitled 'the Pharmacopoeia of the Royal College of Surgeons in Ireland' but this project was not completed.

The Charitable Infirmary

He had joined the staff of the Charitable Infirmary, Jervis Street, in the early 1820s, and in common with his surgical colleagues (Richard O'Reilly, Robert Adams, James O'Beirne, James Duggan, William Wallace and Samuel Wilmot) he disapproved of the limit placed on the reception of in-patients by the managing committee. On 1 October 1828 the surgeons wrote to the committee deploring that they were limited to 26 beds, 'particularly as the high Character of the Hospital daily attracts a greater number of applicants that can be accommodated'. They recommended that fifty surgical patients should be admitted.

Having given thought to the matter, they believed that the available funds should support forty in-patients, and they had 'created a fund by subscription among ourselves, for the support of ten Patients, and have agreed to pay monthly to the Managing committee the entire additional expenses of that number . . .'[20] They would provide the extra beds, and be responsible for any other expenses incurred. They had, too, formed a medical board which would be auxiliary to the managing committee.

Their proposal was accepted by the committee, but possibly Kirby's ambition remained unsatisfied and at a special college meeting on 5 September 1831 the plan to create a new hospital was revived. The president

---

[19] Colin Brennan, 'Architectural History (1805–1997) of the RCSI', MA thesis UCD; Dublin, November 1997, p. 17.
[20] Proceedings of Management Committee Charitable Infirmary, Jervis Street 1826–35, p. 100.

Rawdon MacNamara was in the chair when Francis White proposed a motion, seconded by Kirby, 'that the Establishment of a Clinical Hospital under the Superintendence of the College, would greatly contribute to the improvement of surgical education in Ireland'.

An amendment was moved by Abraham Colles, and seconded by Mr McDowell: they proposed that legal opinion should be obtained as to the 'practicabilility of applying the College Funds to the maintenance of a Clinical Hospital'. When the blocking amendment had been defeated by 30 votes to 27 the original question was put and agreed to; a committee was appointed—White, Kirby and ten others.

Censor White reported on 23 September 1831 from the clinical hospital committee that they had not completed their deliberations, and they were allowed further time for their discussions. Their final conclusions never reached the minute book. It seems likely that the committee was disbanded, but in the following year a smaller group agreed to purchase a house in Baggot Street where the City of Dublin Hospital was opened.[21] Kirby was not a party to this transaction having already committed himself to the support of patients at the Charitable Infirmary; he also held appointments as consulting surgeon to the National Eye Hospital, Cuffe Street, and to the Coombe Lying-in Hospital.

Coombe Hospital

When the Meath Hospital moved from the Coombe in 1822 it left an empty building which was taken over in 1823 by Kirby, who with Michael Daniel and Richard Gregory opened a fifty bed general hospital in October. A large ward was provided for maternity cases in 1826, and from February 1829 it functioned fully as a lying-in hospital.

It was still a general hospital when it fell to Kirby to address the pupils on the conclusion of the lecture course in 1825, and he ruminated on a variety of themes, ethical rather than scientific. He impressed upon his audience the 'sacred importance' of the medical profession. 'True, without this conviction, you may obtain profit and independence,—but without a right idea of the duties it imposes, unless you are heartless beings, and regardless of everything except the sordidness of emolument, you will lose the enjoyment of those silent and secret whisperings of conscience which mingle with the morning reflections and shed a delicious peace on the pillow of repose.'[22]

---

[21] Possibly the names of F. White and J. T. Kirby should be added to the list of founders—James Apjohn, Thomas Beatty, Charles Benson, Robert Harrison, John Houston, Arthur Jacob. See Davis Coakley, *Baggot Street: A Short History of the Royal City of Dublin Hospital* (Dublin: Board of Governors, 1995).

[22] Kirby, *A Lecture, concluding the Clinical Course Delivered to the Pupils of the Coombe Hospital* (Dublin: Hodges and M'Arthur, 1825), p. 6.

He communicated a biblical fervour:

> If antiquity commands respect and fixes admiration, medical science must exercise a claim above all others to your veneration. Its origin is coeval with man. In the hour of his disobedience, he felt the sentence of his doom. Then came pain and suffering into the world. Then too, those sympathies were awakened, which, while they display the weakness and wants of human nature, may be said to constitute its most ennobling attributes.
>
> From the history of subsequent ages, numberless examples can be adduced, calculated to inspire a warm attachment to medical science. The best and wisest men devoted themselves to its pursuit. Even our Saviour did not disdain to assume the medical character, when he wished to display the beauty of benevolence, and to shew forth the majesty of that power with which he came clothed from his Almighty Father. He taught eyes which were closed in darkness, to open and receive the light, and into limbs, long fixed in palsied helplessness he infused the strength and vigour of former years.[23]

Kirby was determined that his students would become 'more than mere traders' in the medical profession. 'I would have you wise in skill, that you may be useful in practice,—I would have you kind in heart, that you may fill the channels, which solicit your benevolence.' They must learn how to question the sick, and train their senses to diagnostic service: 'By the ear we frequently determine the existence of fractures... From the eye we have many of the external features of disease...'

> Health is a valuable treasure [he concluded]; when society commits it to your care, it confers on you the highest rank of confidence and esteem. This is the greatest reward you can receive; and the inestimable consciousness of having discharged your duty, the dearest recompense of the human heart.[24]

Delivering a similar address in the same year to students in Peter Street, Kirby presented himself as 'the first founder[25] in Ireland of a private Institution for the promotion of Anatomical and Surgical Science', and proceeded to describe the 'excited surprise' caused by the venture, and the difficulties encountered.

> The natural obstacles offered by the celebrated schools of surgical science to the feeble competition of an infant establishment, raised by an individual who had little to recommend him but his zeal—who had no patron but his own industry—and in a country, too, where every scheme was accustomed to wither in neglect, and meritorious efforts to be consumed without reward;—

---

[23] *Ibid.*, p. 9.
[24] *Ibid.*, p. 26.
[25] Here Kirby is incorrect. Cameron, *History of the RCSI* (note 2), lists many eighteenth-century predecessors, p. 647.

these constituted impediments of a formidable magnitude.[26]

The obstacles, as anticipated, had given way to 'the irresistible force of perseverance'. He had surmounted, too, 'the illiberal attacks of combining interests and undermining calumny'.

Were you, gentlemen, aware [he continued] how far the progress of surgical science had been interrupted in this kingdom by a narrow spirit of monopoly, which ever affords resistance to every attempt at improvement, you would, with me lament, that it ever had its fatal existence; you would feel indignant at such principles. Were these principles no longer operative, indignation might subside, and lamentation cease. It is melancholy, however, to be obliged to confess, that this spirit of opposition is still abroad.[27]

When the Peter Street school was first attacked he had remained silent, to avoid pleading his own cause; but nowadays, when the sneers were directed elsewhere, he was free to condemn them. He was glad to find senior students thinking for themselves, and seeking instruction 'at every foundation which promises to produce it'.

The terms imposed at Peter Street were seven guineas for a course of lectures and dissections.[28]

The chair of medicine

Kirby was one of the delegates who represented the college in London in 1831 when bills affecting surgical education were contemplated. In the following summer we find him a candidate for the chair of medicine, and under *The Lancet*'s close scrutiny. The journal's purpose was educational reform, and the destruction of the cliques and coteries that led to an abounding nepotism.

It was suggested by *The Lancet* that the altered by-law referred to in the previous chapter had the purpose of making the chair of medicine 'safe' for Kirby. This is a flimsy assertion. As early as February 1830, when it was unlikely that anybody, including Kirby himself, had the proprietor of the Peter Street school in mind as a candidate for a chair of medicine, Richard Carmichael had given notice 'that he would move, that whenever the chair of the Practice of Physic in this College shall in future become vacant by death or resignation, that such candidates be alone eligible to that situation as are or have been Members of this College'.[29] His purpose, according to Fleetwood, was retaliation against TCD and the College of Physicians which had refused to accept the col-

---

[26] Kirby, *Clinical Course*, (note 22), p. 9.
[27] *Ibid.*, p. 12.
[28] *Theatre of Anatomy—Rules* (Dublin: Hodges and M'Arthur, 1827), p. 10.
[29] College minutes, 1 February 1930.

lege's certificates.[30]

Carmichael took no further action, but following Marsh's resignation on 9 June 1832 a series of proposals and amendments led to the version finally accepted on 23 June 1832 by a 'Committee of the whole College':

> That no person shall be elected a Professor of the Theory and practice of Physic, unless he shall have received a regular surgical education, as required by the Bye Laws of this College, to be a Member, Fellow or Licentiate of some of the legally constituted Colleges of Surgeons[31]

The candidates were Kirby, Orpen, Hargrave, Benson, Greene, Alcock and Evanson. John T. Kirby was unanimously elected. By whatever means this was achieved, fair or otherwise, Kirby's chair was secure and one learns with surprise that hardly had he embarked on the new academic venture than he found it necessary, ostensibly for health reasons, to tender his resignation. This was 'accepted with regret' on 5 November 1832; then either he had second thoughts or a welcome return of health, for the following letter was read at the next meeting:

> GENTLEMEN,
> When I resigned the Professorship of the Practice of Medicine, I was influenced by the severity of my late Attack, and by the Advice of my Medical friends.
> The Office not being filled up, and my health, improving, so far as to encourage me to undertake a Professor's duty, I beg leave to express a hope that you will permit me to resume the Chair—
>
> I have the honor to be
> Gentlemen
> Your faithful Servant
> J. KIRBY

He was permitted to withdraw his letter of resignation, and not many days later he wrote again to the college secretary.

---

[30] John F. Fleetwood, *The History of Medicine in Ireland*, 2nd ed. (Dublin: Skellig, 1983), p. 74. Relations between Dublin's medical schools were disturbed from time to time for trivial reasons. On 19 June 1818, Macartney complained 'that some of the Members of the Royal College of Surgeons have represented my Apprentices as not being admissable to an Examination for a Surgical Diploma in that College'. He believed that no by-laws existed to explain the decision; if such did exist there they could be set aside legally.

Charles Hawkes Todd replied that he was unaware that any decisions had been taken in regard to Professor Macartney's apprentices. No relevant by-law existed, but 'as documents relative to the professional Education of your Apprentices have not been submitted to the Consideration of the Court, their qualifications for Admission to such Examinations cannot now be decided on'.

[31] College minutes, 23 June 1832.

JOHN TIMOTHY KIRBY

Harcourt Street
21: November 1832

SIR

Having always intended to present my Museum to the College, whenever I retired from the duties of Lecturer on anatomy and surgery, I now beg leave to offer it for acceptance, and I trust the Collection will be found not unworthy of a place in our National establishment.

I have the honor to be
Your faithful Servant
J. KIRBY

The professor received the college's appropriate thanks and as a mark of gratitude it was agreed that his bust should be sculpt.

Resignation

Kirby held the chair of medicine for less than four years, and his resignation (like his appointment) created a controversy. A regulation notice was issued by the college on 19 November 1835: 'The Royal College of Surgeons in Ireland will hold a special meeting on Monday next, at two o'clock, to receive Mr. Kirby's resignation of the Professorship of the Theory and Practice of Physic. By order, C. O'Keefe, Dr.' Naturally this attracted the attention of *The Lancet*, quick to read between the lines, and to hazard a hidden and damaging interpretation: 'Thus terminates in disgrace and disappointment, a job that was conceived in the worst spirit of corruption, and carried into effect by means which cannot be safely described.'[32]

Few indisputable facts are available, but the college minutes confirm that Kirby's letter was read at a special meeting of the college on 23 November 1835:

SIR,

I beg you to communicate to the proper Authorities of the College that I resign the Professorship of the Practice of Medicine, to which I have been four times annually elected.

Circumstances connected with my health reluctantly compel me to such a measure—I confess I regret the necessity, however I am consoled by the reflexion that my place can be adequately filled by many of our distinguished Members and Licentiates.

I delayed this Communication in the hope that I should be able to pro-

---

[32] *The Lancet* (1835–36); 1: 418.

ceed, I cannot at present go forward, and I think it better not to commence a duty, which I may be obliged to interrupt with much inconvenience, and which could not be performed with the regularity required in a public Institution without unjustifiable neglect of my health.

When Kirby's letter had been read, and his resignation accepted, a resolution proposed by Professor Harrison, and seconded by Mr Tagert, was put from the chair and carried unanimously. This thanked Kirby, and commended him in conventional terms. It was then agreed that two professors, instead of one, should be appointed, and it was reaffirmed 'That all future professors of the Theory and Practice of Physic, shall be bona fide practising surgeons, being Members, or Licentiates, of the Royal College of Surgeons in Ireland.' Kirby, regular in his attendance at college meetings, was absent for a short time but returned to the college on 14 December.

The Lancet alleged that Kirby was obliged to retire because his class had fallen to 'ten or a dozen pupils this season', and not on account of a 'fit of the gout', as he would have his colleagues and the public believe. 'It was, in fact, the class of the College School which took the gout; and if we are not very wrong in our conjecture, the disease will, in a short time, become general in other departments of the same establish-ment.'[33] The journal insisted that sympathy for Kirby was hardly to be expected. Had he not walked 'into the house of sin' with his eyes open? 'His commerce with its leprous occupants was an act of free-will and deliberate consideration.' The best that could be said for him was 'that he was the least criminal, though the most injured party, in this dis-graceful transaction'.

What truth was there in the radical periodical's innuendoes? Kirby did suffer from gout, and as we have seen it almost prevented his taking up the chair. Even if the malady was used as a convenient excuse, and his class had fallen to negligible numbers this was not necessarily the professor's fault. Such things happen. Whitley Stokes, too, had found himself without a class. And the decision that Kirby should be succeeded by two professors may have been an acceptable attempt to draw students from two flourishing hospitals.

The fact that in January 1835 Kirby completed his second term as PRCSI, and was thanked in the usual way, must be some assurance that he was unlikely to have been compelled to resign. He was a member of the finance committee, and an influential person in the college. His successors, R. T. Evanson and Charles Benson, were appointed on 7 March 1836.

---

[33] *Ibid.*, p. 419.

Publications

Kirby's *Cases in Surgery*,[34] price six shillings, was published in 1819, its full title sufficing for a table of contents: *Cases with Observations on Wry Neck; on the reduction of Luxations of the Shoulder Joint; on the Operation For Hare Lip; on Cartilaginous Substances of the Knee Joint; on Aneurism; on the Use of the Extract of Stramonium, and on the Extraction of a Gum Elastic Catheter from the Bladder, By an Incision above the Pubis, Under singular Circumstances.* His 'easy laudatory' on the virtues of Stramonium for tic douloureux, ardor urinae, chordee and other nervous disorders elicited a rhymed comment from the pen of Erinensis:

> *Stramonium's still an emptier sound,*
> *Not worth a pinch of snuff!*
> *By all despised or only found,*
> *In Kirby's modest 'puff.'*

His contributions to the *Dublin Journal of Medical Science* give no hint of any interest in the revelations of morbid anatomy, highly valued by Cheyne, and so very fruitful in the hands of Addison, Bright, Osborne and other nineteenth-century investigators, but they do indicate an admirably critical attitude towards medical therapy. The advocacy by an army surgeon, Dr Lehman, of hot water applied to the region of the larynx as a cure for croup led to Kirby's observation that the simplicity of a remedy may delay its acceptance. He reported a device he had found effective, if applied early in croup:

> My first advice is, that the neck shall be invested with a bolster of hot salt, sufficiently long to surround it thoroughly, and sufficiently full to fill the whole of the cervical hollow; a flannel case is to be preferred to linen. When the former cannot be procured, a large woollen stocking will be found to answer as a convenient substitute. Care must be taken that it be not too tightly stuffed, as then it would force the head into a constrained position, and interfere with the action of the laryngeal muscles; besides it cannot be so conveniently accommodated to the form of those parts with which it is designed to lie in contact.[35]

It acted quickly as a rubefacient, causing 'a sudden general and copious perspiration'. He had little faith in mercury and saw leeches and blisters, which he found useless, as 'the resource of men who are in the habit of pursuing a practice of routine'.

He disagreed with 'R. J. G.' (presumably Robert James Graves) who advised 'instant' bleeding for croup from one or both arms, or from the

---

[34] Kirby, *Cases in Surgery* (London: Burgess and Hill, 1819).
[35] 'On the Treatment of Croup', *Dublin J. Med. Sc.*, (1836); 8: 332–38.

jugular vein. 'Now, I am perfectly convinced [Kirby wrote] the rule which is thus delivered is expressed with too general an application.'[36] He favoured the immediate stimulation of sweating, and described how when passing through the hall of the hospital he was approached by a young woman carrying an extremely distressed two-year-old. Kirby had taken the opportunity of demonstrating the clinical features of croup to his students, expressing the most gloomy prognosis: 'I said I had no hope and yet I would try an experiment. I procured a piece of lapis infernal, and applied it extensively to the back of the neck, as if I designed to establish a large issue; I shall only add that the boy was quickly relieved, and rapidly recovered from the extreme danger in which I perceived him to be placed.'[37]

Like so many Irish doctors, Kirby became familiar with the ravages of cholera in the 1832 epidemic, but in reporting 'a case of genuine Asiatic Cholera' in September 1839 he seems not to have reflected that an isolated case of diarrhoea, however profuse, in a temperate climate, is unlikely to be due to cholera.[38] The clinical problem represented by his well-to-do female patient was that of what today might be tentatively called severe gastro-enteritis with dehydration and shock. Called in by a Dr Price, Kirby prescribed lead acetate which he had found helpful in 1832—'I administered it in doses of two grains, with two minims of Battley's sedative liquor; at first every half hour, and subsequently every hour.' Starch-and-opium enemas with 'a scruple of the acetated cerussa' were also given. 'It is more than pleasing to be able to state, that the subject of this case recovered, convalescence having been established on the eighth day.' The 'Notice' sent to the *Dublin Journal of Medical Science* 'Concerning a Case of Cholera' was somewhat self-congratulatory.

He was less fortunate when called by Dr Churchill on 13 October 1839, to see Mrs Wall of Mill Street. A few days previously, she was 'favourably delivered of a healthy child' but now she was in what today might be called 'bacteraemic shock'. The lochial discharge had ceased, and questioning his patient Kirby was told of a 'trifling scratch' on the right thumb where on inspection he found a small vesicle 'moderately distended with an opake, milk-coloured fluid'. Was this the wound through which the fatal poison seeped, or was it puerperal fever?

> The treatment during the short period of our attendance, was stimulant: from the first we despaired; and although we ordered ammonia, turpentine, opium, brandy, &c., yet we felt the distressing conviction that we prescribed

---

[36] *Ibid.*, p. 335.
[37] *Ibid.*, p. 338.
[38] 'Notice Concerning a Case of Cholera, and a Case of Diffuse Inflammation', *Ibid.* (1840); 16: 285–88.

with painful hopefulness. It did not seem to our judgement, that there was any thing in the local appearance to indicate any particular topical operative management, or remedial application.[39]

Death

After an arduous life, John T. Kirby died at Newtown House, Rathfarnham, on 26 May 1853 and was buried at St Kevin's Graveyard. Of those children who survived to adult life the son named for him, John Timothy Kirby, a surgeon in the 74th Regiment, predeceased him; Hickman Rose Kirby served with the 4th Native Infantry, Madras; the Rev. James Kirby was rector of Kiltegan; Lieutenant-General George William Kirby died on 28 June 1890; another son was the naval chaplain who preserved the autobiography. His daughter, Jane Rose, married Surgeon George Foster West of County Leitrim, sometime demonstrator at Kirby's school.

---

[39] *Ibid.*, p. 287.

The title page of Richard Evanson's treatise on diseases of children (1840)

Chapter 5: Richard Tonson Evanson, 1806–1871

Comparatively little is known of Professor Evanson, who for seven years shared the chair of medicine with Charles Benson. Illness compelled him to resign in 1843, and he eventually settled at Torquay, Devonshire. He was co-author with Henry Maunsell of *A Practical Treatise on the Management of Diseases of Children* (1836), and also published *Nature and Art. A Poem.* (1868).

A native of County Clare (b. 1806), and the son of a soldier, Richard Tonson Evanson was indentured to Mr (later Sir) Philip Crampton. He attended the schools of surgery of the RCSI, and the Meath Hospital, taking the letters testimonial of the college in December 1827 and proceeding MRCSI (equivalent to the present FRCSI) on 3 May 1830. Having obtained the MD of Glasgow in 1832, he embarked on private practice in the Irish capital.

Chair of medicine

In 1830, Evanson became lecturer in materia medica at the Park Street Medical School, of which Erinensis wrote: 'of all the bad schools in Dublin, we think this will be the best'.[1] His colleagues there included Marsh, Arthur Jacob, William Stokes and others, and, as we have seen, he applied successfully for the position of professor of medicine in the RCSI in 1836.

The election did not pass without attention from the watchful *Lancet* which on 19 March 1836 published a letter from 'Amator Collegii'. This inferred that the election was dictated by vested interests: 'one [Evanson] vacates a share in the Park-street School, and the other [Benson] leaves a piece of patronage (that of demonstrator) in the hands of our *College*-school professors—advantages which would not result from the promotion of Dr. Orpen [a third candidate], or any other reformer.'[2] These advantages, according to the pseudonymous letter-writer, were so apparent that 'we all knew what *must* be the result long before the election took place'.[3]

A week earlier, another correspondent (who inappropriately signed himself 'Silens') complained that owing to unabated corruption the appointment 'of the favourite of corruption' could be predicted 'especially if he come from the manufactury in Park-street, whence have been drafted in latter times no less than six professorial pedagogues'.[4]

---

[1] Martin Fallon, *The Sketches of Erinensis*, (London: Skilton & Shaw, 1979), p. 80.
[2] Charles Orpen, FRCSI, became a missionary in South Africa, where he died *c.* 1857.
[3] Amator Collegii, 'Election of Professors at the Dublin College of Surgeons', *The Lancet*, (1835–36); 1: 982.
[4] Silens, 'Continued Corruption in the Dublin College', *The Lancet*, (1835–6); 1: 909–12.

Paediatrics

Meanwhile, Evanson's interest in what is now called paediatrics had gained for him an attachment to the Pitt Street Institute for Diseases of Children, where in August 1832 Mary Brown brought her distressed, thirteen-month infant whose illness furnished material for a dramatic paper in the *Dublin Journal of Medical and Chemical Science*.[5]

The stridulous infant was hot, restless and uneasy; the pulse and breathing were rapid. Its throat seemed swollen, and it 'had one of the hands applied to the throat as if to indicate the seat of distress'. Croup was unlikely, but the history suggested to Evanson that a foreign body, a herring bone, had stuck in the trachea a few days earlier.

Surgeon Crampton was consulted. As the infant did not then appear to be in any immediate danger leeches were applied to the throat, and calomel and jalap given as a purgative. Next day, in view of the lack of improvement, Crampton advised operation. Some hours elapsed before the parents reluctantly consented. They brought the child to the Meath Hospital, and by the time of its arrival it seemed on the brink of death.

A tracheotomy was performed without further delay, but no foreign body was located. 'On the morning after the operation, however, some amendment was manifest.' Mrs Brown was allowed to take the child home a week later leaving Evanson still puzzled.

> That the child had been rescued from impending death, by the operation of bronchotomy, no doubt could be entertained, and this may be deemed a sufficient corroboration of the correctness of the opinion which led to the performance of the operation; for had a different course been adopted, it is but reasonable to suppose that a different result would have taken place. Still it was unsatisfactory that no foreign body had been found, and that neither during the operation, nor at any time subsequently, was the bone detected, though anxiously looked for by the medical attendants.[6]

He called on the Browns, in due course, to see the infant. When he mentioned his surprise that no bone had been found, he thought he saw the parents exchanging covert glances. He pressed Mrs Brown on the matter and she produced a portion of fish bone, explaining that on the fourth post-operative day, when attending to the wound, she felt something hard sticking in the sponge. She had managed to extract the bone. She said nothing about it, in case the surgeon should decide to perform another operation.

John Cheyne, as we have seen, was the author of *Essays on the Diseases of Children*; Whitley Stokes published 'On an Eruptive Disease of Children'; Marsh with others founded the Pitt Street Institute; Evanson's main contribu-

---

[5] Richard T. Evanson, 'Report of a Case in which a Foreign Body was supposed to be present in the Trachea', *Dublin Journal of Medical and Chemical Science* (1834); 5: 19–29.
[6] *Ibid.*, p. 25.

tion to paediatrics was the textbook he wrote with Maunsell. This was well received, going through five editions; it was reprinted in America and translated into German. *The Dublin Journal of Medical Science*'s anonymous reviewer commented on the absence hitherto of 'a commodious treatise on the diseases of childhood, suited to the present advanced state of medical science'; he felt that 'this want the work before us has abundantly supplied'; he said he had 'derived unmingled gratification' from its perusal. He discussed the contents in some detail.[7]

Evanson wrote six, and Maunsell seven of the book's thirteen chapters. The physiological introduction appears singularly slow to recognise a difference between the sexes:

> Beyond the eighth year, we would not employ the term child—though applied by some until the age of puberty: but before then the peculiarities characteristic of childhood have been merging into the attributes of adult age; while the influence of sex begins to be discernible, and the individual may thenceforward be designated boy or girl.[8]

Prominence is accorded to the antiphlogistic plan of treatment, and Evanson relied on bleeding in the first stage of inflammation. 'In the infant, or young child, we can seldom draw blood from the brachial veins . . . We can generally, however, procure as much as we require from a vein on the dorsum of the foot, or back of the hand.'[9] Or leeches may be preferred. Blisters also are recommended. The common occurrence of jaundice within a few days of birth is recognised—'it can scarcely be called a disease, commonly disappearing spontaneously, and requiring no medical treatment.'[10]

Evanson accepts Cheyne's definition of acute hydrocephalus as consisting of 'a diseased action of a peculiar kind, but of which we can as little explain, as we can the nature of scrofulous action'. He is, however, familiar with W. W. Gerhard's papers in the *American Journal of Medical Science* (vols. 13 and 14), and accepts the condition as frequently tubercular. In several cases in which tubercles were reported in the brain by Ruz, white semi-transparent granules were detected in the arachnoid membrane, while tubercles were also present in the lungs. He endeavours to equate the classic stages described by Whytt with Cheyne's three stages—the quick pulse of Whytt corresponds with Cheyne's period of increased sensibility; the slow pulse with the diminished sensibility; the rising pulse with the convulsions or palsy.

Maunsell regarded syphilis as an infection, but accepted scrofula as the out-

---

[7] [Anon], *Dublin J. Med. Sc.* (1837); 11: 113.
[8] Evanson and Henry Maunsell, *A Practical Treatise on the Management and Diseases of Children*, 3rd ed. (Dublin: Fannin, 1840), p. 2.
[9] *Ibid.*, p. 127.
[10] *Ibid.*, p. 186.

come of a strumous diathesis, rather than 'the product of any peculiar virus'.[11] He credits 'Stokes the elder' with the first accurate description of the 'Burnt Holes'. An official preparation of the only available remedy, *scrofularia nodosa*, had recently been added to the *Dublin Pharmacopia*.

Preventive medicine

Henry Maunsell,[12] Evanson's co-author (and co-editor with Arthur Jacob of the *Dublin Medical Press*) held a chair of midwifery in the RCSI from 1835 until 1841 when he resigned in order to take a newly-founded chair of hygiene or political medicine. This was the first chair in the United Kingdom devoted to preventive medicine. Widdess[13] traces its origin to a lecture given by Maunsell himself in 1839, and subsequently published as a pamphlet, entitled *Political Medicine; being the substance of a discourse . . . on Medicine, considered in its relations to Government and Legislation*. Maunsell castigated the leaders of the profession for 'having abandoned the higher and more honorable walks of their profession, to pursue, exclusively, the less exalted, though more profitable trade of the empirical curing of disease'. He pictured the doctors 'employed in driving with ostentatious hurry through the streets, and in courting the favour of nurses, apothecaries, and other menial attendants of the sick'.[14]

He focused on larger measures to benefit communities rather than individuals; improvements in the health of seamen; amelioration of the deplorable conditions in the prisons; vaccination which, since its introduction to Dublin in 1800, had made the mortality rate for smallpox plummet. These were matters for political medicine (a term, as mentioned above, replaced later by public health, or community medicine) to control, but there also were endemic fevers traceable to dirty dwellings, uncovered drains, heaps of rubbish at the bottom of close courts and in corners.

---

[11] *Ibid.*, p. 462.

[12] Henry Maunsell (1806–79) lacks the full biography he merits. The eldest son of the general manager of the Grand Canal Company, he was by birth a Dubliner, educated at a school in Stephen's Green and (after apprenticeship to Charles Johnson) in the RCSI. He took the letters testimonial in 1827, becoming MD Glasgow in 1831 and proceeding MRCSI on 7 May 1832.

He held the post of MO to Letterkenny dispensary briefly. Returning to Dublin he was elected (for a fee) lecturer on midwifery at the Park Street School, and assistant accoucheur to the Wellesley Lying-in Institution. He published *The Dublin Practice of Midwifery* (1834).

Maunsell was elected secretary to the council of the RCSI from 1844 to 1860; in that year (possibly influenced by the example and success of his friend Charles Lever as a literary figure) he purchased *The Dublin Evening Mail* and retired from medicine. He died in Greystones on 27 September 1879, and was buried in Stillorgan Cemetery. Twice married, he had several children, many of whom predeceased him. His surviving son succeeded him as editor of the *Evening Mail*.

[13] J. D. H. Widdess, *The Royal College of Surgeons in Ireland and its Medical School 1784–1984*, 3rd ed., (Dublin: RCSI, 1984), pp. 76–7.

[14] Maunsell, *Political Medicine* (Dublin: Fannin, 1839), pp. 2–3.

> And why [Maunsell asked] is such a state of things allowed to continue? Simply because, in latter days, those who should have assumed the useful and honorable position of leaders of the medical profession, have too often failed to use the opportunities which their success in life has opened to them, of raising their profession and themselves in public estimation, by engaging in the performance of public duties. Simply, because such gentlemen have been fighting with their juniors for the paltry gains of their trade, instead of employing in the service of the community and of their own reputation, and, as a natural consequence, that of their profession, that leisure which their early success would have allowed them to enjoy....[15]

Unwholesome trades should be regulated, and the treatment of lunatics controlled by political medicine; medical aid should be supplied 'for the public generally, and especially for the poorer classes'.[16]

Verses

The illness that led to Richard Evanson's resignation, and from which he never recovered fully, has been described as 'an affection of the intestinal mucous membrane'.[17] He was obliged to seek a milder climate, and leaving Ireland he became something of a wanderer on the continent, practising here and there and attracting English travellers as patients. In the late 1850s, he settled at Holme Hurst, Torquay, being elected FRCP, London, in 1859. He was consulting physician to Erith House Institute for Diseases of the Chest, and sometime president of the Torquay Natural History Society.

Evanson's second book was published in 1868. Its cumbersome title was *Nature and Art, or, Reminiscences of the International Exhibition, Opened in London on May the first, 1862. A Poem; with Occasional Verses, and Elegiac Stanzas.* He admitted to a 'life long dalliance with the Muse', but was inconsistent in this relationship. A year might pass without a line being written, but if stirred by some public event or private incident the impulse to commemorate it would strike him, 'and rhymes would flow in upon me, unsought and uncalled for'. He could retain the verses in his mind, and even correct them, and when an opportunity presented he wrote them down. 'Composed as a divertisement to thoughts, as a solace in care, or as a mental recreation to relax the mind when wrought by sterner studies or over burdened with the weight of professional responsibility,—the heart was relieved and the mind refreshed by a diversity of even mental toil.'

His ambition was to write 'a large Poem' and he devoted some 3,5000 lines to the exhibition, with the aim of leaving a record 'of the greatest of all International Exhibitions', in the hope that 'the very novelty of such an attempt in Rhyme' might succeed in its being read when other records were forgotten. He

---

[15] *Ibid.*, p. 26.
[16] *Ibid.* p. 34.
[17] *The Lancet* (1871); 1: 696.

looks at what nature, art and science have provided—'The lightning now Man's messages must take', is an allusion to the electric telegraph—and considers the functions of commerce. Inventions have their advantages, and their drawbacks:

> *By steam man sows and reaps and works the plough*
> *Nay, by a new Machine, can milk the cow!*
> *Whatever aim your innovations dare,*
> *In England's homesteads England's milkmaids spare!*
> *Think of the wrath in each fair damsel's heart*
> *To find her hands supplanted thus by art.*

He describes a sculptor's triumph:

> *But marble may be jubilant with joy;*
> *See Ino leaning o'er that wayward boy,*
> *The infant Bacchus, who lies laughing there,*
> *With feet upturned and hands outspread in air . . .*

He marvels at attempts to invade the heavens:

> *Does man desire above the earth to rise,*
> *And be a traveller in yon far skies?*
> *In vain the huge Balloon is seen to soar—*
> *In vain its lessening bulk, mounts more and more.*

He arrives finally at a conclusion almost inevitable to the Victorian mind:

> *What is the greatest wonder Man beholds?*
> *Himself! In his own Maker's Image made,*
> *In him God's mightiest work has been displayed;*
> *Accountable and placed above the whole,*
> *Entrusted with that awful gift, a soul . . .*

The elegiac poems, twenty-five in number, include verses commemorating the deaths of Sir Henry Marsh (cited in a previous chapter) and of James William Cusack, MD: 'Adieu! Loved friend, adieu! Can time replace/The friends whom we have lost: among them, thee?' The occasional poems, of which there are ninety-five, commemorate events as diverse as an ode to mark the opening of the international exhibition in Dublin by the Prince of Wales on 9 May 1865, and verses to announce the arrival of the mayfly. The former opens thus:

> *The Emerald Isle, the Emerald Isle!*
> *What Island of Ocean can lovlier be*
> *Than Erin's green Isle, ever fresh as the smile*
> *Of Venus herself when she rose from the sea?*
> *The famed land of Erin, our own native home,*
> *The birthplace of all that's brilliant and fair;*
> *O'er the Isles of the Ocean full far may we roam,*

> *But the beauties of Erin we find not elsewhere.*

The Mayfly is greeted with a fisherman's ditty:

> *The May-fly comes dropping*
> *Like dew from the skies;*
> *The angler is stopping*
> *To mark where trout rise;*
> *His hooks, strong but slender,*
> *Two May-flies now bear,*
> *With a cast light and tender*
> *Blow out on the air.*

Evolution

Darwin's *Origin of Species* appeared in November 1859, selling out on the day of publication. On 10 October 1862, Evanson wrote 'Man and Monkey', in which a man addresses ('but not respectfully') his remarkable forefather, the gorilla.

> *Most uncouth monster! tell us do we see*
> *A veritable ancestor in thee?—*
> *In thee, with thy flat forehead, hideous face,*
> *Huge, awkward arms, bare teeth, and broad grimace*

Has Man, Evanson asks, grown gradually from 'some primaeval germ, unnamed, unknown'? Has he passed through varying races 'to so high a lot that to Gorilla he ascends at last'.

> *And now, the great Gorilla-period past,*
> *Having attained to be a tailless brute*
> *(Although still senseless, and although still mute),*
> *The rising race progressing on the whole,*
> *At length achieves a language and a soul.*

Natural selection—'nature's plan'—has enabled herbs to become trees, 'and monkey becomes man!' All we see, 'however old or young', derives from a single line and creation is nothing but development.

Philosophy, Evanson concedes, is entitled to spectacular flights. Man, too, has his rights and he may claim the right 'To read his Bible, and believe it true.'

> *The famed Gorilla or most able Ape*
> *Shows but a parody on human shape;*
> *So write or argue as you may or can,*

Man is not monkey nor is Monkey Man.[18]

The outcry against Darwin in England, together with the defence by T. H. Huxley and others, has been amply documented. But what of *The Origin*'s reception in Ireland? Pens other than Evanson's had been active in protest.

No notice appeared in either the *Dublin Journal of Medical Science* or the *Dublin Medical Press*, other than a brief mention in the former (in a review of another book): 'Mr. Darwin's work . . . pretends to account for how the present races of animals and plants have established themselves'. Cudgels had, however, been already taken up by the Rev. Samuel Haughton, who in an address to the Geological Society of Dublin on 9 February 1859 referred to papers laid before the Linnaean Society in the previous year by Charles Darwin and Alfred Russell Wallace, and sponsored by Sir Charles Lyell and Dr Joseph D. Hooker. These were 'supposed by a certain class of geologists to prove more than they intended, and to lead to conclusions which are rather hinted at than asserted'.[19] Their speculation, he insisted would not be worthy of notice were it not for 'the weight of authority of the names under whose auspices it has been brought forward. If it means what it says, it is a truism; if it means anything more, it is contrary to fact.'

In the *Proceedings of the Natural History Society of Dublin* (1860) Haughton places Lamarck in contrast with Darwin:

> The Frenchman, with the vivacity and perception of the ridiculous belonging to his nation, seizes upon the quality most likely to elevate a monkey into a man, selects the faculty of imitation, and, with a bitter satire, endows his monkey with the human desire to better his condition, and lift himself above his brother chatterers. He thus magnifies the monkey power of imitation,—which is truly wonderful, and extends to the most wonderful actions,—into the position of a law of nature, sufficient to create man! The Englishman, on the other hand, firmly believes his theory, and, with a confident faith in the power of food and comfort, equally characteristic of his country, elevates the desire to supply the stomach into a law of sufficient force to convert an eel into an elephant, or an oyster into an orang-outan.[20]

Writing in the following year in the *Dublin University Magazine*, Haughton posed a rhetorical question:

> [Are we to believe] that the Crustaceans, Fishes, Reptiles, and Mammals, because they have lived and tyrannised in succession on the earth, followed from each other by a law of descent? that the Crustaceans produced the Fishes; that the Fishes gave birth to the Reptiles; that the Reptiles were developed into the Mammals. No—the Rep-

---

[18] Evanson, *Nature and Art. A Poem* (London: William Hunt, 1868), pp. 237–9.
[19] Samuel Haughton, 'Address to Anniversary Meeting', *J. Geological Soc. of Dublin* (1859); 8: 137–56.
[20] Haughton, 'On the form of the cells made by various wasps' *Proc. nat. hist. soc. Dublin* (1862); 3: 128–140.

tiles are not born of the Fishes; the Mammals are not sprung from the Reptiles; and God forbid that Man should be born of an Ape. Base, degraded, and cruel as he is, he was once made in the 'image of God,' and carried with him in his degradation the ineffacable lineaments of his parentage.[21]

'Who, then, are we?' Haughton asks. As the 'vicegerents of God' we govern the globe. But we rule 'not by dint of numbers, not by virtue of superior size or strength, but by the power of intelligence.'

Haughton, who held the chair of geology in Dublin University, re-turned to the subject of evolution in his lectures:

> My apology [he said in his opening remarks] for taking the Anthropomorphic, instead of the Pithecomorphic view of nature, is that I am a Man, and not an Ape, and therefore cannot help doing so; and I admit that my idea of the Creator is perhaps as clumsy as the illustration supposes, and that I can no more imagine an abstract Creator, à la Lamarck or à la Darwin, than Martinus Scriblerus could imagine an Universal Lord Mayor, without his Horse, Gown, and Gold Chain.[22]

Continuing another day:

> ... I believe the simplest and the most truthful hypothesis that we can make on this subject is the oldfashioned one derived from final causes, that, according as the Creator arranged conditions of life on the globe physically suited to various creatures, He placed in succession on the globe by His own will, creatures suitable to those conditions to enjoy them.[23]

In his concluding lecture, the Rev. Haughton regretted that he should feel ashamed ('in the lecture halls of such an institution') to be obliged 'to offer an apology for the existence of a Creator'. It was, however, difficult to believe in the natural origin of man while retaining a Christian's conviction of an immortal feature. 'Surely the animal that grew from a monkey, which monkey had its origin in a lower type of life, that again proceeded from still lower forms, cannot hope to live beyond the time when his perishable body shall return to the elements from whence it came.' A belief in the resurrection of the body, Haughton held to be 'inconsistent with these natural theories of life upon the globe'.[24]

'Darwinism' was frequently discussed in *The Irish Ecclesiastical Record*. When 'JBC' consults 'the Naturalist's College of Heraldry, he is at a loss to decide, 'so much do pursuivants differ—whether we descend from a chimpanzee or a gorilla, from a jelly or from a seaweed, or derive from a collection of gases electro-

---

[21] Haughton, 'The History of the Earth and its Inhabitants', *Dublin Univ. Mag.* (1861); 58: 105–13.
[22] Haughton, *Manual of Geology*, 3rd ed. (London: Longmans, Green, 1871), p. vii.
[23] *Ibid.*, p. 95.
[24] *Ibid.*, p. 360.

chemically combined'. This Catholic clergyman, who accepts the authority of *Genesis*, concludes his article with the verdict of Agassiz: 'The transmutation theory is a scientific mistake, untrue in its facts, unscientific in its methods, and mischievous in its tendency.'[25]

Father J. Murphy complained that Darwin 'has bounded to a con-clusion unscientific, illogical, degrading, which places on the same level the beasts that perish and the soul that never dies'. He rejects 'the dreamings which our scientists offer as a substitute for our faith'.[26]

The apparent incompatibility of Darwinism and *Genesis* was debated for decades, but the judgement of a *Catholic Encyclopaedia* in our more dispassionate age is that the solution of the basic difficulties was found to lie in Biblical research and scholarship, and not in rejection of the new theory. Darwin's sustaining influence on biology was undeniable, and in his encyclical *Humani Generis* Pope Pius XII urged (1950) that evolution 'should be professionally studied by both anthropologist and theologian'.[27]

Marriages

Returning to Evanson after this digression, we find the attractions for him of the opposite sex expressed in 'Woman's Eve', 'The Kiss', 'Woman's Voice' and other poems. The following jingle is from 'The Beautiful Lady':

> *Her beauty, her beauty!*
> *I dreamed of it long:*
> *But oh! it surpasses*
> *All praise and all song!*
> *Her dignified grandeur,*
> *Her exquisite grace,—*
> *A Juno in presence, A Venus in face!*
> *Such beauty, such beauty!*
> *Not often has been;*
> *And 'tis well for man's peace*
> *Such beauty seldom is seen*

Evanson married three times: his first wife was a daughter of Admiral Fortescue; his second was the widow of a son of the Duke of Manchester; his third wife, also a widow, was Mrs Johnston of Torquay.

Despite his recurring ailment, Evanson remained throughout his life bright, cheerful and warm-hearted. When the British Medical Association's annual meeting was held in Plymouth in August 1871 he was an unanimous choice as

---

[25] [J. B. C.] 'Darwinism', *Irish Ecclesiastical Record* (1873); 9: 337–61.
[26] J. Murphy, *Irish Ecclesiastical Record* (1873); 9: p. 594.
[27] *New Catholic Encyclopedia* (New York: McGraw Hill 1967), vol. V, p. 693. See also, William Reville, 'Science Today', *The Irish Times* (20 October 1997).

chairman of the excursion to Torquay. His delight at meeting an old friend, Dr Thomas Beatty[28] of Dublin, was recorded in verse:

> *My Friend and I talk of the old, early times,*
> *When the days passed all merrily as wedding chimes,*
> *While he sang his songs, and while I wrote my rhymes,*
> *In the gay joyous days of our youth.*
> *And then we reflected, and thought of the past,*
> *And our looks o'er a long varied lifetime were cast.*
> *Till we felt how old age stole upon us at last;*
> *For old men are we both, now, in sooth.*[29]

Feeling unwell, Richard Tonson Evanson remained in bed during the morning of 26 October 1871; towards midday he was found to have died in his sleep.

---

[28] Thomas Edward Beatty (1800–72), surgeon, obstetrician and physician, b. at 28 Molesworth Street, Dublin, on New Year's Day 1800, was the son of John Beatty, a medical practitioner, and his wife Mary (née Betagh). Apprenticed to Charles Hawkes Todd at fourteen, and having studied in Dublin and Edinburgh became BA (Dublin, 1818) and LRCSI (1821), proceeding MRCSI (1824).

He held chairs of medical jurisprudence (1830–35) and midwifery (1842–57) in the RCSI and published *Contributions to Midwifery* (1866). He became a licentiate of the King and Queen's College of Physicians in Ireland in 1860, and within a month was elected an honorary fellow of that body. As his surgical fellowship prevented further promotion in the physician's college he withdrew from it in 1862. He was elected FKQCPI in 1864, and succeeded Dominic Corrigan as president, being the only man to have held that office in both Royal Colleges. He had a beautiful tenor voice; his duets with the Rev. Charles Tisdall, chancellor of Christchurch, were regular features of Sir William Wilde's dinner parties. Wilde sought his advice during the ENT surgeon's unexpected involvement in medico-legal aspects of child abuse. (See J. B. Lyons, 'Sir William Wilde's Medico-Legal observations', *Medical History* (1997); 42: 437–54.)

Beatty was twice married: Margaret, his first wife, was a daughter of Judge Mayne; after her death he married her second cousin Maria, eldest daughter of Captain John Mayne. He died on 3 May 1872.

[29] *Brit. Med. J.* (1871); 2: 337.

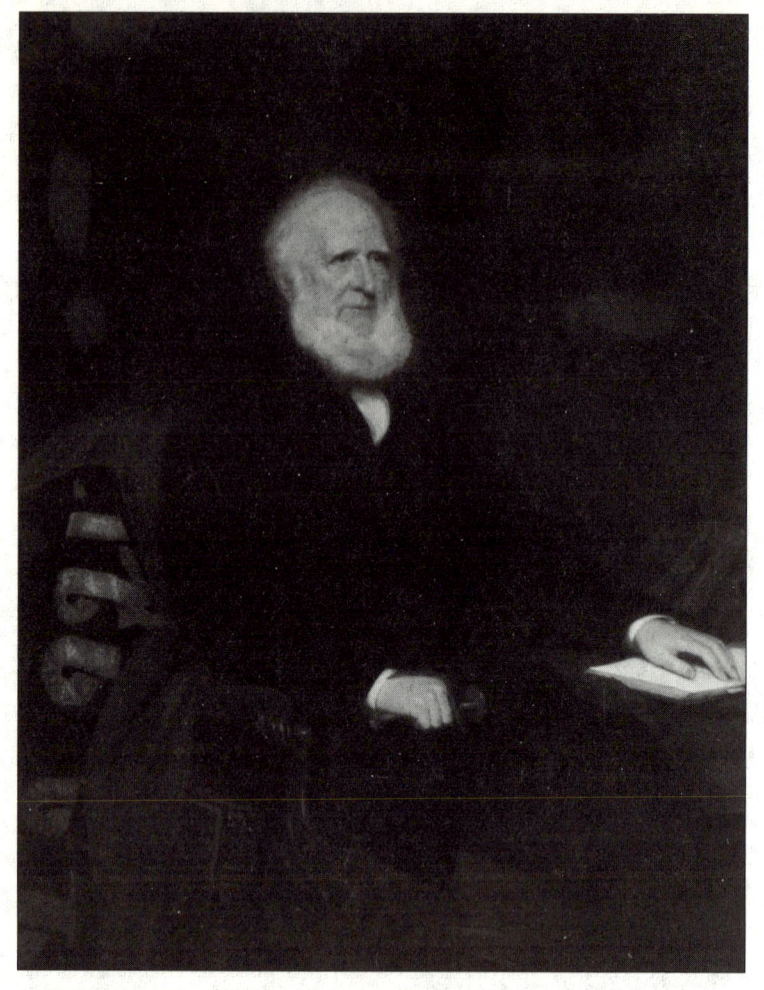

Charles Benson, 1797–1880 Professor of Medicine 1836–72 *(portrait by Stephen Catterson Smith jnr)*

Chapter 6: Charles Benson, 1797–1880

Like Kirby, Charles Benson held both a professorship and the office of president. This was not uncommon in the college's early years: the Deases, Abraham Colles, Arthur Jacob and others held chairs during their presidencies. The present college charter excludes RCSI professors from election to council, in effect barring them from presidency. And besides, a professor of medicine would not nowadays aspire to the highest rank in an institution dominated by surgeons. Things were different in many respects in the early nineteenth century.

Benson was born in Sligo in 1797, the son of a land-agent, Charles Benson, who married Elizabeth Gray, a local beauty.[1] He was educated locally, before being apprenticed in Dublin on 28 January 1815 to Charles Hawkes Todd, surgeon to the Richmond Hospital, under whose tutelage he first learned anatomy in a dissecting-room near the Hardwicke Hospital.[2] He was a pupil at both the RCSI and TCD, and won a scholarship in classics in 1818. He commenced BA in 1819, obtained the letters testimonial of the RCSI in 1821 (proceeding to membership in 1825); he took the MB in 1822, proceeding MD in 1840.

Dissecting-room deaths

For many years, Benson was a demonstrator in the RCSI's anatomy department, and he contributed articles on bone, the axilla and the diaphragm to Robert Bentley Todd's *Cyclopaedia of Anatomy and Physiology*. On Tuesday, 30 December 1834 a student whose brother, a twenty-two-year-old medical student, was laid-up with fever asked him to visit. The sick man had spent the previous Saturday 'dissecting an old half putrid subject', and was taken ill on the following morning.[3]

'I found Mr J— in a very confined room [Benson wrote], complaining of excruciating pain in the head, his eyes suffused, his face flushed ... his skin hot and dry, his pulse above a hundred and somewhat hard.' It was the student's first term as a dissector, and Benson thought he had 'taken the fever so common among students in the first months of their anatomical pursuits'. He bled him and gave a purgative. Next day the student was worse. 'He urged me to bleed him again...' Leeches were ap-

---

[1] Sir C. Cameron, *History of the Royal College of Surgeons in Ireland*, 2nd ed. (Dublin: Fannin, 1916), pp. 470–72.
[2] Apprenticeship to a surgeon, initially compulsory for RCSI students became optional in 1812; it was abolished in 1844.
[3] C. Benson, 'Fatal Effects of a slight Wound received in Dissection', *Dublin J. Med. and Chem. Sc.* (1835); 7: 189–97.

plied to the temple, and a few ounces taken from the arm. 'Thursday. He passed a wretched night, sleepless and unhappy, sometimes delirious.' The brother mentioned a small scratch on one of the fingers, and on close examination Benson was alarmed to find 'a little wound, not more than one-fourth of an inch long, such as a spicule of bone might have occasioned, and was nearly healed'. There was, too, tenderness below the axilla on the pectoral muscles.

The doctor's optimism evaporated. The situation was grave; it looked as if the student would die—as Richard Dease (1819) and John Shekleton (1824) had done, from contaminated dissecting-room wounds. He arranged to have the painful pectoral area stuped with a decoction of poppy heads, prescribed a camphor mixture with ammonia daily and gave calomel at night. He summoned Abraham Colles in consultation, but their ministrations were unavailing in this pre-antibiotic era. The young man died a few days later. The limited post-mortem permitted, disclosed what Benson called 'healthy-looking pus' under the pectoralis major.

He was disappointed that events had not justified his initial optimism. Scratches and slight incisions were common in the dissecting-room, and a useful rule of thumb held that wounds acquired while working on a fresh subject were the most dangerous. The deceased student had dissected a decaying subject; the wound showed no local inflammation; there were no red lines on the forearm and the dominating feature was fever. To explain these anomalies, Benson offered a convoluted argument based on 'the absorption of a peculiar animal poison, generated, in some way, at or about the time [of the subject's] death, and losing its specific virulence when putrefaction occurred'. Such ingenious explanations, as we shall see, were to be replaced within his own lifetime by the acceptance of the germ theory. Meanwhile, he and his colleagues would be guided by plans such as the following:

In all cases of dissecting wound, I advise the part to be well sucked, and then dipped in spirits of turpentine; a generous diet, and good air, from the receipt of the injury; and when a smart inflammation sets in locally, I consider the case will end favourably.[4]

Venous pulsation

Benson was physician to the City of Dublin Hospital in Baggot Street, the foundation of which has been discussed in an earlier chapter.[5] On 14

---

[4] *Ibid.*, p. 197.
[5] The hospital was opened in November 1832. The other founders were James Apjohn, Thomas Beatty, Robert Harrison, John Houston and Arthur Jacob, all of whom held chairs in the RCSI with which for many years the hospital was closely associated. See Davis

August 1835 Mary Oliver, a sixty-year-old fruit-seller was admitted under his care in a restless and confused condition, unable to give any account of herself other than to say 'it was all about her heart'. There was marked cardiac enlargement, and a loud bellows murmur was audible all over the precordium. On the day after her admission she went into a state of coma.[6]

'While feeling her pulse, and reflecting on the symptoms before me [Benson wrote in his subsequent report] I was struck with an appearance of pulsation in a vein on the back of the hand. Further examination showed a distinct pulsation in every superficial vein of the two upper extremities.' The easily visible but impalpable pulsation puzzled Benson intensely. 'My colleagues and the hospital pupils now joined me in observing the pulsations.'

Opinion was divided: some envisaged pulsation derived from the *left* side of the heart, communicated through the capillaries; others interpreted it as regurgitation from the *right* side. Repeated venesections seemed to effect temporary improvement, but the patient died during the night of 20 August. An autopsy was performed next day: 'The right auricle was dilated, and a little hypertrophied . . . The right auriculo-ventricular opening was very large and gaping.' The right ventricle was enlarged, and there was mitral stenosis.

Intent on proving the diagnosis of tricuspid regurgitation beyond doubt, Benson had an arm removed from the body and injected it through the brachial artery. 'Fine wax, largely diluted with oil of turpentine, and coloured with vermilion was used, but not a particle of injection passed into the veins.' A review of the literature convinced him that 'the curious phenomenon of venous pulsation' was most uncommon. 'And yet the *dissection proved*, I think, incontestably, that hypertrophy with dilatation of the right ventricle, was the true cause.'[7]

Chair of medicine

Having been an unsuccessful contestant for the chair of medicine in 1832, Benson was elected professor on 7 March 1836, sharing his responsibilities with R. T. Evanson[8] until the latter's resignation in 1843. Benson continued to hold the chair until 1872, a duration of tenure unequalled in its history. Neither Cameron nor Widdess, the college historians, indicate that he made any significant changes in the curriculum

---

Coakley, *Baggot Street: A Short History of The Royal City of Dublin Hospital* (Dublin: Board of Governors, 1995).

[6] Benson, 'Case of Pulsation in the Veins of the upper Extremities', *Dublin J. Med. and Chem. Sc.* (1836); 8: 324–32.

[7] *Ibid*, p. 331.

[8] On 27 November 1835 the college resolved to appoint two professors of medicine.

during that long period, but fortunately the *Dublin Medical Press* carried his lectures on the theory and practice of medicine in 1840–42, enabling us to view his performance during those sessions.

He lectured on Mondays, Wednesdays and Fridays at three p.m. He did not speak from a prepared script but gave careful thought to each lecture, using notes. He welcomed questions, and believed he benefitted from them himself, suggesting new subjects for enquiry. 'We are all learners, and must be so in medicine, perhaps in every thing, as long as we live.'

In his introductory lecture at the college in November 1840, Professor Benson explained to the students that it was introductory in the proper sense of that word, 'but not in the sense now so often attached to it—not abstract declamation—not a set speech—not a panygeric on myself, or my school, or my subject—but an account of what I have to do, and how I propose to do it, and with what instruments'.[9]

> In this College [he continued] we are sparing of 'Introductories,' seldom using them except when some important subject calls for special notice; but I dare say you have had an ample store of them brought before you in other places. I did not go to hear any this season—but a couple of years ago I went in search of them and was not disappointed. Their variety was amusing: one man gave a history of medicine from Aesculapius, through Machaon and Podalirius, Paracelsus, and Van Helmont, down to himself. Another lauded his school and himself—promised wonders—and acted the showman to life. A third gave an excellent lecture on the numeric method of accumulating facts; and a fourth gave us a discussion *de omnibus rebus et quibusdam aliis.*[10]

Having listened to them he was reminded of the last chapter of Dr Johnson's *Rasselas:* 'The conclusion in which nothing is concluded.' Those were 'introductories in which nothing was introduced'. The object of his own course on the principles and practice of medicine was to describe 'all the medical diseases to which the body is liable'; and he hoped to direct the students 'in the discovery of their first stealthy approaches', going on to their full development, means of prevention and cure.

He warned them that it was impossible to learn medicine from textbooks alone: they must also attend lectures.

> The lecturer leads you through a systematic course—he brings before you, in regular order all the important subjects—he points out the most important and dwells on them —he compares the opinions of the various writers—he tells you what to believe, and assigns his reasons. He gives you the

---

[9] Benson, 'Lectures on the Theory and Practice of Medicine', *Dublin Med. Press*, (1840); 4: 321–4.
[10] *Ibid.*, p. 321.

latest information, the received notions of the day, and the results of his own experience. Just fancy a student wading through the big books that come out in thick battalion; or galloping over the 365 volumes on medical subjects that are published every year.'[11]

A lecturer uses drawings, plates, casts and recent specimens to illustrate his talks, and fix his words indelibly on his hearers' minds. 'Lectures, books and hospitals are all indispensably necessary, if you would acquire a competent knowledge of your profession.'

Defining *disease* as 'any departure from health', Benson reminded his audience of the complexity of the human body and its organs, explaining that disease consisted 'in some derangement of the structure or the functions' of organs. Here, no doubt, he was influenced by the work of Bright, Hodgkin, Addison and other leading figures of that fruitful period; Virchow's *cellular pathology* (1858) would add a further dimension.[12]

The term *aetiology*, the lecturer said, denotes the study of the varied causes of disease many of which are avoidable or controllable. Some are born with disease, or possess a hereditary tendency; old age brings its inevitable woes, to describe which Benson invoked Dr Johnson's lines: 'From Marlborough's eyes the tears of dotage flow,/And Swift expires a driveller and a show.'

Causes are divisible into *remote* and *proximate*. The former may be subdivided into the *predisposing* and the *exciting* and Benson gave phthisis as an example: 'The remote predisposing cause was hereditary delicacy of lung, the exciting cause, also remote, was exposure to cold, and the proximate cause is tubercle in the lung.'

No disease is perfectly alike in any two persons—'The age, sex, habit, diathesis, the mental and physical peculiarities individualize the disease'—which is also influenced by temperament.

> *Temperament* or *crasis* [Benson explained] meant a mixture or tempering of elements or principles. The ancients thought that there were four elements, air, earth, fire and water, which entered into the composition of all bodies; and Hippocrates thought that the fluids of animals consisted of four secondary elements composed of these, *viz.*, blood, phlegm, yellow bile, and black bile. Bodies were named according to these as these compound elements predominated in their systems—if blood, they were called sanguineous; if phlegm, phlegmatic; if yellow bile, choleric; and if black bile, atrabil-

---

[11] *Ibid.*, (note 9), p. 321.
[12] Rudolf Virchow (1821–1902), saw the body as 'a cell-state in which every cell is a citizen'; disease was 'a conflict of citizens . . . brought about by the action of external forces'. See F. H. Garrison, *An Introduction to the History of Medicine*, 4th ed., (Philadelphia: Saunders, 1929), p. 370.

ous or melancholic.[13]

What Benson and his contemporaries (who no longer supported a belief in the four elements, or the humours), understood by temperaments was 'certain combinations or groups of peculiarities of mind and body'. Though inborn they could be modified by circumstances and rendered their possessors more liable to some diseases than to others. They included the *sanguine* (thoracic), the *lymphatic* (abdominal), the *bilious* (hepatic), and the *nervous* (cerebral).

Preliminary appraisal

In his second lecture Benson discussed the meaning of terms such as *idiosyncracy, diagnosis, symptoms, pathognomic* etc., and he indicated how much a physician learned from an initial inspection.

> The organs may all be reviewed more quickly than I could describe to you the process. You judge of the feelings from the countenance—of the lungs by the respiration and the colour of the face—of the heart and arteries by touching the pulse at the wrist—of the skin by the same touch. You see the excretions and the tongue by which you form an opinion of the digestive organs. You hear the patient speak and thus learn the state of the larynx. The eye and voice give you information of the brain. A few questions serve still further to direct you. If possible you look at the chest—you lay your hand on the region of the heart and feel the abdomen all over.[14]

This preliminary appraisal is followed by the closer examination that leads to diagnosis, prognosis etc. Treatment may be rational or empirical, and nature's tendency to resume its healthy function is known by the name of *vis medicatrix naturae*. Sydenham[15] was one of Benson's favourite guides to treatment—'you see I am fond of this fine sensible old writer, though his language is quaint, and his theories are not always orthodox.'

He discussed *nosology* and classifications adding, predictably, that an ideal classification is lacking. Cullen's was the best-known, and they should be familiar with it.

> Cullen arranges all diseases under four heads, which he calls classes viz;— *Pyrexiae, neuroses, chachexiae, locales*, and each of these he divides into ORDERS which are each sub-divided into GENERA and SPECIES. His classes are very faulty—no one principle of anatomy, physiology, or pathology is

---

[13] Benson, 'Theory and Practice of Medicine', (note 9), p. 323.
[14] *Ibid.*, p.354.
[15] Taking Hippocrates as his exemplar, Thomas Sydenham (1624–89) based his practice on observation and experience. *Processus integri* (1692) containing his views on treatment was read by generations of British practitioners.

followed in them. The first class is dominated from the temperature. The second from the nervous system which is chiefly deranged. The third from the depraved state of the fluids—and the fourth from the local character.[16]

His own nosology, he claimed, was simple, natural and useful in practice. 'I arrange the organs of the body into groups or systems . . . and I consider their diseases of structure and of function—using for the most part, the established names for each disease.'

He wished to make the students think for themselves, and not to rely on the thoughts of others; to see them become wise, rather than merely learned. Cowper, he told them, contrasted these accomplishments:

> *Learning and wisdom, far from being one,*
> *Have oft-times no connexion. Learning dwells*
> *In heads replete with thoughts of other men;*
> *Wisdom in minds attentive to their own.*
> *Learning, a rude unprofitable mass,*
> *The mere materials with which wisdom builds,*
> *'Till smooth'd and squar'd, and fitted to it place,*
> *Does but encumber what it means to enrich.*
> *Learning is proud that it has learned so much;*
> *Wisdom is humble that it knows no more.*

Gastrointestinal tract

Subsequent lectures purported to deal with diseases of the digestive organs, but Benson first embarked on what today would be called the infective conditions of the mouth and throat, including tonsillitis, quinsy and diphtheria.

> Well, then, diphtherite occurs as an epidemic at particular times, and is now and then contagious too; a detached case may also be met with, as you see in our hospitals; and it so often shows itself at Tours, where Bretonneau first met and named it, that it might be called an endemic there. That town is in a rich plain, through which two rivers flow, the Loire and the Cher, and there are rows of trees in some of the streets. These circumstances, by causing damp, are believed to predispose to this malady. It is not common in Ireland, where we have richer plains, and trees, and rivers, and damp enough; but we are not relaxed with any superabundance of heat.[17]

The lecture course continued in 1841 dealing with contagious conditions such as cynanche parotidea, 'very well known as "the mumps"', before proceeding to disorders of the oesophagus, gastric physiology and

---

[16] Benson, 'Theory and Practice of Medicine', (note 9), p. 355.
[17] *Ibid*, p. 389.

intestinal anatomy. He discussed in turn diseases affecting the gastric mucous membrane, the muscular tunic of the alimentary tract and the pathology of the peritoneum, illustrating his talks with pathological specimens: tubercles attached to the peritoneum; intussusception, diaphragmatic hernia and the like.

In May 1841 a lecture was devoted to acute, subacute and chronic gastritis. Treatment of the acute condition consisted of bleeding, enemeta and starvation. From ten to twenty leeches were applied to the epigastrium. 'Leeching has the most beneficial effect—the general bleeding goes for nothing without it . . . and it ought to be repeated again and again, every eight or ten hours.'[18]

Benson's lectures on the gastro-intestinal tract seem to have been fluent, comprehensive and up-to-date, containing many references to contemporary literature and some complimentary asides to Dublin colleagues with relevant publications, for example—'In the third volume of the *Dublin Hospital Reports*, Sir Henry Marsh gives a very nice paper on jaundice and shows that inflammation of the mucous coat of the duodenum is a frequent cause of it.'[19]

Several lectures were devoted to diarrhoea and dysentery. He referred to the late Dr Cheyne who 'with talents scarcely inferior to those of Sydenham, with more correct views of pathology, and with all the advantages of modern science, had found himself, in 1818, in the midst of the dysentery which was then decimating Dublin'. He referred his audience to Cheyne's articles in the third volume of the *Dublin Hospital Reports*, recommending them 'to study the entire of it (it is too short) with the utmost care'.[20]

He also discussed 'colic'.

> When you hear of 'colic', many of you will think of an old woman's belly-ache, which a little ginger cordial has so much potency in removing, or a little castor-oil with Daffy's elixir and peppermint. You are right; I mean such a disease, but I mean much more. The term colic includes not only some of the most painful, but some of the most fatal affections of the intestines. Under that name I place *ileus* or the iliac passion, intussusception, and other rapidly destructive derangements.[21]

Colica Pictonum, a severe disease, had various appellations, lead colic, painter's colic, Devonshire colic—the latter because cider was contaminated by lead used in pipes and cisterns.

He spoke on *ascites* (fluid in the abdominal cavity), a term derived

---

[18] *Ibid.* (1841); 5; 321.
[19] *Ibid.* p. 394.
[20] *Ibid.* (1841); 6: 2
[21] *Ibid.*, p. 289

from the Greek for a leather bag or bottle—'not the glass bottle of the present day, but the large round leather bottle of the olden time, or such wine bags as Don Quixote so valorously cut open at the inn'—not omitting to stress that pregnancy had been mistaken for ascites, and vice versa. He illustrated his lectures on the liver with specimens of hepatic cirrhosis, acute hepatitis, hydatids, scrofulous tubercles, secondary carcinoma, abscess and an organ ruptured by the kick of a horse. He included emotional disturbance as a cause of jaundice: 'It seems strange that mental emotion should give rise to jaundice, and yet nothing is more certain.'

Tiedemann and Gmelin regarded the spleen as an appendage of the lymphatic system; Mr Hargrave,[22] the RCSI's professor of anatomy, believed its chief function was to receive blood 'as a temporary reservoir, or diverticulum' when cardiac, pulmonary or hepatic conditions demanded relief from vascular congestion. Many other functions had been assigned to the spleen and S. T. Soemmering, not altogether seriously, offered a catalogue of these uses, which Benson recapitulated: 'The seat of laughter, the cause of sleep, the seat of venereal excitement, from which the blood was directed to the genital organs . . . That the globules of the blood were formed in it . . . That it was of very little use, that it was of no use at all.'

> Soemmering's own opinion [the professor continued] was that it prepared and fitted the blood for the secretion of bile. And Paley, in his beautiful remarks on the 'Package' of the viscera, suggests that the spleen may be merely a *stuffing*, a soft cushion to fill up a hollow, which unless occupied, would leave the package loose and unsteady. Perhaps Soemmering, Paley, Tiedemann and Hargrave are all, to a certain degree, right, and that the spleen, like the nose, the mouth, the urethra, and many other organs, serves more than one useful purpose in the economy.[23]

Asiatic cholera

Benson was held in high esteem by his students, and on at least one occasion a presentation of plate was made to him. His lecture-course cannot be discussed in its entirety, but the account of the pandemic of Asiatic cholera merits inclusion because of the value of his contemporary evidence. Commencing in the basins of the Ganges and the Brah-

---

[22] William Hargrave (1797–1874), a native of Cork, was Benson's colleague in Baggot Street. As a graduate student of the RCSI he visited London and continental clinics (working with Dupuytren and others in Paris) in the early 1820s. On his return to Dublin he established himself as a private teacher of anatomy and surgery. Elected professor of anatomy in the RCSI in 1837 he moved to the chair of surgery ten years later and was PRCSI in 1853–4. He was the author of *A System of Operative Surgery* (1831).
[23] Benson, *Dublin Med. Press* (1842); 8: 290.

mapootra rivers in 1817, the disease spread throughout India sweeping to reach the Persian Gulf four years later. 'In Basra on the Euphrates, fourteen thousand died of cholera in one fortnight, and in Baghdad, on the Tigris, one-third of the population were swept away.' Russia was affected in 1823 and the disease entered Moscow in 1830. It was in Dublin on 23 March 1832.

> I well remember [Benson told his audience] the fearful anxiety with which its progress on the continent of Europe was watched, and the dismay with which the news of its arrival on the British coast was received. Everyone's heart seemed to fail him as he observed its unrelenting north-western progress; and when it actually touched our shores the most awful results were dreaded. Nor were the gloomiest fears unfounded, as we shall see, for the ravages of this pestilence were tremendous.[24]

Benson described the characteristic features of cholera: copious and violent purging, with vomiting of fluid resembling whey, or rice-water; painful cramps affecting the abdomen and limbs; a feeble pulse and hurried breathing.

> In eight or ten hours the vomiting ceases, or is less frequent, the spasms are less observed, the pulse cannot be felt at the wrist, the extremities are stone cold, and indeed nearly the entire surface, which is also bathed in a cold clammy sweat. The face and hands are generally blue, as if the blood were not arterialized; the hands assuming a peculiar sodden and shrivelled appearance, like those of a washer-woman after her day's work, and the face getting an old, sunk, and cadaverous look. I have seen men of thirty, after a few hours' illness, not to be distinguished from men of seventy—nay, I have seen them look like old men who had died of some wasting disease, and whose bodies had begun to putrify; more like the loathsome *subjects* of a summer dissecting-room, than patients of one day's sickness.[25]

He drew on the accounts of Mr Simon M'Coy and Dr Cranfield, assistants to Dr Lindsay at the Grangegorman Cholera Hospital, and cited Dr John Colvan of Armagh who divided cholera into three types: choleric fever; simple or spasmodic fever; and the blue congestive fever—and referred to 'its proteiform nature.'

Benson had been puzzled when autopsies in Sunderland, the first English town to experience the epidemic, showed only venous congestion and 'nothing to account for death—no lesion of sufficient importance to give rise to the symptoms, or to cause the fatal result'.

---

[24] *Ibid.*, p. 178
[25] *Ibid.*, p. 178.

But you will ask what was the result of dissection in Dublin, where [pathological] anatomy is so thoroughly understood, and where it is studied with so much zeal and success? I believe there was no additional light thrown on the subject by the Dublin anatomists. I was myself a demonstrator of anatomy in this school, and examined a great number of bodies, but in no instance could I say that there was any morbid appearance, except the most extraordinary congestion, in any of those who died during a stage of collapse. Congestion, congestion, some congestion, great congestion—such were the only epithets I had to use, as one organ after another was exposed.[26]

The congestion was so severe that the bones were blue. Their pristine whiteness could not be restored, to the great disappointment of Kit Dixon, the RCSI's dissecting-room attendant, who had planned to sell the skeletons which now were unsaleable.[27]

Many investigators had examined the blood and Benson mentioned Dr William O'Shaughnessy's findings—'cholera blood had less water than healthy, the serum had more albumen than it ought, but was very deficient in salts'.[28] This, had he known it, was the key to the understanding of the disease's most dramatic features, but Claude Bernard's concept of an 'internal milieu' and the vital importance of homoeostasis, lay in the future. Nevertheless, Benson was greatly taken by these changes. 'Was it a primary lesion of that fluid?' he asked. 'Or was the first morbid impression made on the nervous system and then communicated elsewhere?' He inclined to answer the second question in the affirmative.

For my part I am satisfied that the first impression was on the nervous system, which changed the properties of the blood, and then that the altered blood and the depressed nervous influence together, suspended all the secretions, suffered the exhalations to be poured out, as if passively, on the skin and mucous membranes, and occasioned the color, the spasms, and all the

---

[26] *Ibid.*, p. 210.

[27] Christopher Dixon was a 'resurrectionist'; according to J. D. H. Widdess, *A History of the Royal College of Physicians of Ireland* (Edinburgh: Livingstone, 1963), p. 36, his annual takings exceeded £100.

[28] Speaking to the Westminister Medical Society in Saturday 3 December 1831, W. B. O'Shaughnessy proposed the use of 'highly-oxygenated salts' intravenously in the treatment of cholera, 'the nitrate of potash or chlorate of potash', with a view to oxygenating the 'black and thickened blood' and re-establishing the circulation. At the conclusion of his lecture, he remarked that another worker had just published a similar recommendation 'nearly in the words I uttered last Saturday evening when giving notice of my intention to propose the injection of saline substances into the veins'. (*The Lancet* (1831–32); 1: 366–71).

A later issue of *The Lancet* (2 June 1832, p. 284) credits O'Shaughnessy's experiments as having discovered the deficiency of water and salts that can be restored intravenously. See also Davis Coakley, *Masters of Irish Medicine*, (Dublin: Town House, 1992), pp. 149–56, for an account of the career of Limerick-born William Brooke O'Shaughnessy (1809–60) who graduated in medicine at Edinburgh University.

other sensations and actions and appearances.[29]

Severe cholera resembles the action of a poison so closely, that the ignorant of most countries have suspected that in some way a poison had been administered. It is proverbial that 'the multitude is ever in the wrong'; while another adage tells us that 'what everybody says must be true'. And here the multitude was surely half wrong, and half right—'the disease *was* occasioned by a poison, but the poison was *not* administered by man'. It had its generation, Benson believed, in the miasmata or effluvia that rise from marshy places under a tropical sun and spread through every climate. 'The rice-eating Hindoo, the beef-eating Englishman, and our own potato-eating variety of the human species, all fell before it with similar symptoms.' The question of its contagiousness was fiercely contended, and Benson sided with the contagionists.

Cholera mainly affected 'the poor, the debilitated, and the debauched'; bad food and clothing, fear and intemperance were predisposing factors, whereas those with warm clothing, a wholesome way of living and a cheerful state of mind tended to escape. A thousand and one modes of treatment, according to Benson, had their advocates, but the first cases in any place were unlikely to be cured by any therapy. He gave examples of therapeutic measures applied in India, Russia and France. Bleeding, calomel, opium, camphor, stimulants and applications of heat were common to most regimes. Andral of Paris regarded the mercury-containing calomel sceptically, saying, 'I cannot account for the prostrate veneration, which English physicians pay to this metallic drug; I can only compare them to those poor Indians, who, faithful to their ancient creed, persist with words of mystic import, in plunging their sick into the charmed waters of the Ganges.'[30] At the Hôtel Dieu, Dupuytren used acetate of lead, opium, bleeding and vigorous supportive measures.

Sir Matthew Tierney introduced cajeput oil to England. Soon no house 'was considered safe without a little vial of it on the mantel-piece . . . and no prudent old bachelor would think of going out without a dose of it in his waistcoat pocket'. Fortunes were made by its sale, until it was agreed that oils of cinnamon, cloves and peppermint were equally effective.

Non-purgative salts were given to restore the loss of salts in the blood:

> Dr Smart of Cranborne, suggested that the salts sufficiently diluted, might be injected into the veins, as more likely to be efficacious than by the stomach, and Dr O'Shaughnessy, who had analysed the blood with great care, advanced the same opinion, and enforced it with so many arguments,

---

[29] Benson, *Dublin Med. Press* (1841); 6: 212.
[30] *Ibid*, p. 243.

that it was extensively tried, and according to some, with success, but it always failed in Dublin.[31]

According to Benson, claims for priority in the discovery of the saline treatment led to 'much argumentation and skirmishing'. He said it would be difficult to name any item in the pharmacopeia that had not been 'tried and praised and blamed in turn' in Dublin. They included galvanism, mustard emetics, croton oil, Ponsonby's drops, and good brandy. Simon M'Coy 'could not bring himself to use the saline injections of veins', and when the epidemic was at its acme in mid-July 1832 he gave only calomel. Dr Cranfield was influenced by Dupuytren in favouring lead acetate. At the Townsend Street Hospital, Dr Hart used a warm rhubarb-based purgative.

Hart had tried intravenous saline in twelve cases, 'selecting those only in which there appeared to be no reasonable hope of recovery under other treatment'. The pulse returned to the wrist but the vomiting and purging, which had ceased, also returned. He merely succeeded, as he saw it, in 'bringing back the disease from the moribund state and postponing the fatal event for perhaps 12 or even 24 hours'.

Dr Apjohn found the application of heat distressing to patients, and resorted with benefit to friction with camphorated oil. Ice relieved thirst, and was substituted for effervescing draughts and leeching. Calomel with camphor was given hourly, and he lost no patient in whom salivation was produced. He came to regard opium, usually a powerful and valuable medicine, as 'a regular poison' in Asiatic cholera.

Despite the relatively poor showing accorded to intravenous saline in Dublin, it caught the students' imagination and they wished to know the composition of the fluid. Benson's formula was a drachm of the muriate of soda, with ten grains of carbonate of soda to be dissolved in three pints of water.

It is relevant to add that John Snow (b. York 1813) was an apprentice surgeon in the north of England during the cholera epidemic of 1831–32. He moved to the Hunterian medical school in Great Windmill School, London, in 1836 and in due course became MRCS and MD (London). Snow reasoned that cholera was a water-borne infection, and his essay on its mode of communication was awarded a prize by the French Institute. During the 1854 London cholera epidemic he predicted that if the handle of the Broad Street pump were removed the epidemic would end. A pioneer anaesthetist, Snow administered chloroform to Queen Victoria in 1853 and 1857 during the births of Prince Leopold and Princess Beatrice respectively.

---

[31] *Ibid.*, p. 243.

Examination for fellowship

As a member of the court of examiners, Benson took part in the examination for the letters testimonial for many years. He was one of the members of the council who attended the first examination for fellowship, on 27 and 28 May 1845. On that occasion the council and the examiners met at 1.30 p.m and at 2 o'clock the candidates, Messrs Tufnell and Blake were called in and given a series of questions in anatomy and physiology, surgery, medicine, midwifery, chemistry, materia medica and medical jurisprudence. They 'were directed to answer as many under each head as time would permit'. The answers to each numbered question were to be written on separate sheets of paper. One member of council and one examiner remained in the room and the examination concluded at 4 p.m.

On the following day at 2 p.m. the candidates were required 'to perform operations on the dead Body', in the anatomical theatre. Next they were submitted to a viva voce examination in the examination hall. 'The Examiners then deliberated, and decided on reporting to the Council that Mr [T. Joliffe] Tuffnell was qualified to be admitted to the Fellowship, but they could not recommend Mr Blake as duly qualified.'

The germ theory

Cholera caused the panic in Ireland that elsewhere has accompanied epidemic visitations of, say, plague or yellow fever.[32] Individual cases of scarlatina or typhoid, on the other hand, appear to have been accepted with accustomed toleration, despite the significant mortality.

Hans Zinsser tells us in *Rats, lice and history* that infections have been about for millions of years, and the Vienna Museum holds remains of prehistoric bears which display signs of large abscess cavities of teeth and jaws.[33] The validity of the germ theory of disease, discussed intermittently for centuries, was confirmed by Pasteur, Lister, Koch and others. The provenance of its initial enunciation is conjectural but the controversy became clamant in the mid-nineteenth century.[34]

---

[32] William Howison (*The Lancet* (1832–3); 1: 203) has described how cholera broke out with great violence in Sligo. 'Forty, fifty, sixty individuals died every day, and were put into the same pit. Coffins could not be procured for one-half of them; the others were wrapped up in tarred canvas, and carried to their graves. Of 18,000 inhabitants, the population of the town, in a few days 16,000 fled the place, in terror—the wealthiest families paying £40 or £50 for a small room in the country to live in—the poorer classes living with their families under canvas, while others slept in the woods and under hedges. Provisions in a short time became an extravagant price . . . Of thirteen medical practitioners settled in the place, seven or eight died within the first few days.'

[33] Hans Zinsser, *Rats, lice and history* (New York: Bantam Books, 1960), p. 77.

[34] Girolamo Fracastoro published *De Contagione* in 1546; Antoni van Leeuwenhoek saw micro-organisms through his wonderful instrument (1675), and Giovanni Cosimo Bonoma

Cheyne and Whitley Stokes were contagionists. Sir Henry Marsh, as we have seen, held that fevers were caused by invisible particles, mixed with the air. He realized that reasoning alone would never solve the conundrum. 'Nature must be interrogated', or as John Hunter said less ponderously, 'try the experiment'. But Marsh's and Jacob's experiments on pigeons and rabbits were ill-designed to supply constructive information.

'Chance favours the prepared mind' was Louis Pasteur's pregnant aphorism, to which he might have added 'and men with hands trained in a laboratory'. John Tyndall, the Carlow-born physicist, enjoyed that advantage; his experiments supported those of the French industrial chemist.

Pasteur (b. Dôle, France, 1822), had graduated from the École Normale Supérieure of Paris in 1847, moving from the study of isomeric forms of crystals to investigate major problems in the beer, wine and silk industries. He proved that fermentation is a chemical process caused by living germs, and showed that spoilage of wine is prevented by partial heat sterilization at 55° to 60°C (Pasteurization). He discovered the cause of *pébrine* and *flâcherie*, diseases which were destroying silkworms. To his logical mind it seemed highly likely that the contagious diseases of humans were caused by living organisms. Opponents of the germ theory ridiculed the suggestion that infinitesimal living agents could kill vastly larger organisms. They invoked traditional doctrines which attributed epidemics to meteorological conditions, noxious effluvia, chemical poisons, or inanimate particles. But evidence of the role living parasites played in the aetiology of trichinosis, scabies and fungal skin diseases was accumulating. Then Casimir Joseph Davaine, a Frenchman, isolated the rod-like 'bacteridia' that cause anthrax, and in 1876 Robert Koch demonstrated the full life cycle of this organism (Koch's *Bacillus anthracis*), thus revealing the existence of resistant spores.

In due course Pasteur went on to develop preventive innoculation against anthrax and rabies. He had supplied, too, a rationale for the antiseptic regime introduced with obvious benefit at the Glasgow Royal Infirmary by Professor Joseph Lister, whose five-part article 'On a New Method of Treating Compound Fracture, Abscess, etc., with Observations on the Conditions of Suppuration' was published in *The Lancet* in the spring and summer of 1867. Lister spoke 'On the Antiseptic Principle in the Practice of Surgery' at the annual meeting of the British Medi-

---

(d. 1697) proved that scabies is caused by the itch mite; John Crawford, an Irishman (b. 1746) who settled in Baltimore, Maryland, postulated a *contagium vivum* as the cause of fevers; Schönlein, a Zurich professor of medicine, reported (1839) a fungus as the cause of ringworm; Jacob Henle, also of Zurich, published *On Miasmata and Contagia* (1840) and postulated the presence of *contagia animata*.

cal Association which was held in Dublin in August 1867. The 'first object', he said 'was destruction of any septic germs which might have been introduced into the wound' with full strength carbolic acid.[35]

The principle of Lister's method was to exclude germs, but many of his opponents abhorred the carbolic spray which he recommended to destroy air-borne germs; they ridiculed it and other details of his regime. The first sympathetic report published in Ireland (1868) was written by Mr John Machonchy, surgeon to the County Down Hospital, who described an excision of the knee-joint performed by him in 1867, and other applications of antisepsis. Mr (later Sir) William MacCormac, then surgeon to the Belfast General Hospital, visited Glasgow to see Lister working. Professor H.J. Tyrrell introduced antiseptic catgut to the Mater Hospital in 1873. These indications of support, however, were exceptions rather than the rule, and 'Listerism' as it was called became one of the most controversial aspects of the germ theory, to which we shall return in the next chapter.

Introductory address

Benson delivered an introductory address on 8 November 1859 to mark the commencement of the annual course of clinical lectures at the City of Dublin Hospital.[36] His discourse, it must be admitted, was not outstanding; it followed a familiar pattern, exalting the medical practitioner whose position is 'with one exception, the noblest and most useful you could select. I am content to give the study of divinity the first place'.

Stressing the importance of health, he regaled his audience with an incident from the career of Dr John Radcliffe who was consulted by King William III about his dropsied legs. 'I would not have your Majesty's two legs,' said the candid physician, 'for your three kingdoms.'

Benson referred to Jenner's 'beautiful discovery' of vaccination against smallpox, and to Marshall Hall's 'ready method of restoring suspended animation' by artificial respiration. How many lives had been spared? The number was incalculable.

Charles Dickens gave nineteenth-century medical students a bad name, and it is surprising to find how much Benson expected from them:

> I hope you all have had a good preliminary education; that you have a competent knowledge of Greek and Latin; of history, geography and chronology; of arithmetic, algebra, Euclid, and logic; that you write a good hand

---

[35] Isabella Lister married Thomas Pim of Dublin; her brother (the future Lord Lister) had visited the Irish capital and stayed with the Pims. Mr Lister brought his own wife, Agnes, to Dublin in August 1857 when the British Association held its meting there. He discussed 'the Flow of Lacteal Fluid in the Mesentery of the Mouse', a subject remote from the great contribution that lay ahead.

[36] Benson, 'Introductory Address', *Dublin Med. Press* (1859); 62: 305–08.

and spell correctly. I should be glad, too, that you all understood German and French, especially French. Indeed, without a fair acquaintance with all the subjects I have mentioned, you will find it hard to get on in your studies, and will but imperfectly understand what you read or hear; your prescriptions are in Latin; your technical terms are chiefly derived from the Greek; the names of diseases are for the most part Greek or Latin, and so are the names of the medicines.[37]

It was never too late, he told them, to remedy deficiencies in their education. 'Many of you have sisters, and all ladies know French, let them teach you that language; it will only be an amusement and relaxation from severer studies, and it may keep you from less innocent amusements.' They would sink in the estimation of their patients, if they were not well-educated men.

PRCSI

A polite and mild-mannered man of charitable disposition, Benson was one of the founders of the Medical Benevolent Fund, a member of the Royal Irish Academy (in which capacity we find William Wilde writing to him to remind him that the second volume of the *Catalogue of Antiquities* was available), vice-president of the Royal Zoological Society and physician and surgeon to the Four Courts Marshalsea.

He attended the first Anniversary Meeting of the Medical Association of Ireland on 27 May 1840, and seconded G. W. O'Brien's resolution enumerating the objects of the Association:

(1) The protection of medical practitioners' just and legal rights.
(2) To seek legislative enactment directing a competent and uniform standard of medical education throughout the Empire
(3) To secure for the public a scientific apothecary protected in the exercise of his profession and not engaging in the practice of medicine.

Benson said the resolution stated the association's aims so clearly that further discussion was unnecessary. The advantages the association offered were so obvious that he felt astonished that every man in the profession had not joined it immediately. The object of the association was 'to raise every man to the same situation and rank . . . and to protect all from the dangers by which they were attacked'.[38]

He was elected a member of the RCSI's first council under the supplemental charter on 16 January 1844. He held presidential office in 1854–5.

Charles Benson was the 'guiding spirit' of the Junior Surgical Society,

---

[37] *Ibid.*, p. 307.
[38] Benson, *Dublin Med. Press* (1840); 3: 374.

a students' medical society which was established in the college in 1862 and flourished for a decade. Meetings were held in Benson's lecture theatre; he attended its first meeting on 10 December 1862. 'The proceedings were opened at 8.30 p.m. with an address by Professor "eulogising to a great extent the Society".'[39]

Acute rheumatism

Benson's publications included 'Lectures on the Diseases of the Digestive Organs' (*Dublin Medical Press*, 1840–2), and 'Auscultation' in Costello's *Cyclopaedia of Practical Surgery*. He was one of a number of physicians whose opinions were canvassed in 1869, regarding the treatment of acute rheumatism. He was convinced 'that treatment does influence favourably, the duration of the disease, and lessen the percentage of hearts damaged'. His preference was for 'the alkaline' treatment, using potassium bicarbonate with lemon juice in effervescence, sometimes with decoction of cinchona, or with colombo.

Colchicum was given 'to eliminate the *materies morbi*'; digitalis was added to the mixture with the same intention, 'while by its sedative instinct it lessens the danger of cardiac complications'. Cod-liver oil was used freely; a little potassium iodide was sometimes prescribed. Dover's Powder was the selected opiate. Poultices of linseed meal were applied to particularly painful joints and he had recourse to a blister when effusion was present.[40]

Last years

On 26 October 1872, in which year Benson retired from the chair of medicine, the council honoured him by its decision to have his portrait painted, and he was given an honorarium of £250 in view of his long and distinguished services to the college. The artist chosen was Stephen Catterson Smith, RHA. Another portrait of Benson was presented to Baggot Street Hospital by Benson's friends.

During the last decade of his life, Benson's sight had failed. This did not prove calamitous, for he still managed to get about, retaining an interest in professional matters and occasionally attending the lectures on public health given in the college by Professor Cameron. The latter recalled that Benson wrote 'a poem of considerable merit' on the subject of vision.[41] He died peacefully at his home, 42 Fitzwilliam Square, on 21 January 1880.

Charles Benson was twice married. He lost his first wife (née Lamb)

---

[39] See J. D. H. Widdess, *The Royal College of Surgeons in Ireland and its Medical School 1784–1984*, 3rd ed. (Dublin: RCSI, 1984), p. 81.
[40] Benson, 'Treatment of Acute Rheumatism', *Dublin Quart. J. Med. Sc.*, (1869); 47: 433.
[41] Cameron, (note 1) p. 471.

and their daughter, when the child was twelve years of age. His second wife, Maria, was a daughter of Maunsell Andrews, High Sheriff of King's County, and Mary Hawtrey a descendant of the Hawtreys of Chequers, Buckinghamshire, now the country residence of the British prime minister. Three of their sons[42] entered the medical profession: Sir John Hawtrey Benson, the second son, was physician to Baggot Street Hospital and president of the RCPI, 1910–11; George Vere Benson, the third son, a doctor and a barrister, was coroner for East Sussex; the fifth son, Arthur Benson, FRCSI, a widely travelled ophthalmologist, and one of the founders of the Royal Victoria Eye and Ear Hospital, gained a footnote in literary history by prescribing glasses for the little James Joyce.[43]

---

[42] The eldest son, Charles Maunsell Benson, MA, was rector of Lucan; the fourth son, Sir Ralph Sillery Benson, was under-secretary to the Madras government and vice-chancellor of Madras University. There were three daughters, Charlotte (d. 1893), Mary and Sarah, whom Cameron credited with 'considerable artistic ability', producing paintings praised by critics; Cameron, *ibid.*, p. 472.

[43] See J. B. Lyons, *James Joyce and Medicine* (Dublin: Dolmen Press, 1973), p. 185. Arthur Benson organized a bazaar and fête at Ballsbridge in 1893 in aid of Baggot Street Hospital, an occasion reminiscent of the Araby and Mirus Bazaars featured in *Dubliners* and *Ulysses* respectively.

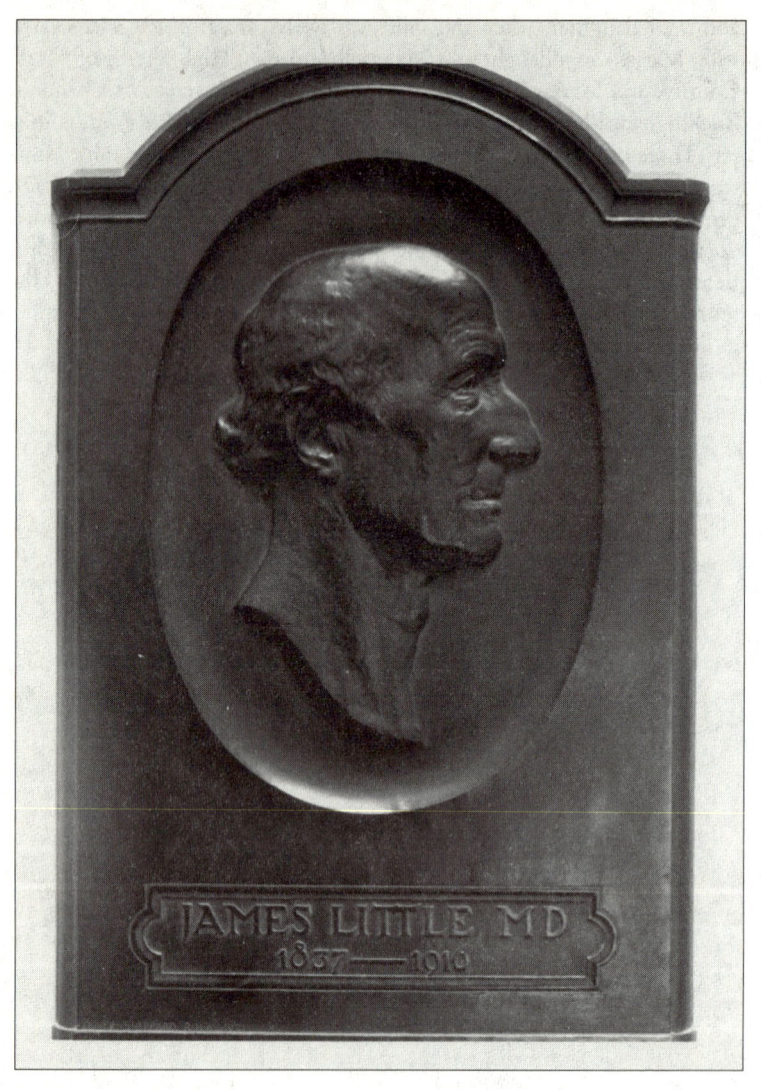

James Little, 1837–1916 Professor of Medicine 1872–83 *(plaque by Oliver Sheppard RHA, courtesy RCPI)*

Chapter 7: James Little, 1837–1916

James Little, son of Archibald Little and his wife Mary Coulter, was born in Newry on 21 January 1837, and educated at Cookstown Academy and the Royal School, Armagh, before his apprenticeship to Dr John Colvan, physician to the Armagh Fever Hospital. He was instructed, too, by Alexander Robinson, surgeon to the County Infirmary.[1]

With the advantage of this clinical experience, he entered the schools of surgery of the RCSI in November 1853, attending clinics at the City of Dublin Hospital and the House of Industry Hospitals. With a view to taking a degree at Edinburgh later, he fulfilled a regulation requiring attendance at two courses of lectures at the University of Dublin. He took the LRCSI on 29 June 1856, then worked for six months at the County Infirmary, Armagh, visiting the County Lunatic Asylum also by permission of Dr Thomas Cuming.

In the spring of 1857, Little was appointed surgeon to the Peninsular & Oriental Steam Navigation Company, and posted to the Calcutta Station where he remained for three years. He returned to the United Kingdom in 1860, and in the following year graduated MD in Edinburgh. He won a prize for psychological medicine awarded by the Commissioners of Lunacy for Scotland. Two years of general practice in Lurgan were followed by twelve months' study at continental clinics.

Settles in Dublin

A major decision had now to be made, and Little resolved to practise in Dublin. Like most newcomers his first year in the capital proved difficult, but Dr Alfred Hudson[2] put work in his way and his election as

---

[1] Sir C. Cameron, *History of the Royal College of Surgeons in Ireland*, 2nd ed. (Dublin: Fannin, 1916), pp. 611–13. See also J. W. Moore, 'In Memoriam: James Little', *Dublin J. Med. Sc.* (1917); 143: 73–9; James A. Lindsay, *ibid.*, 79–80; Walter G. Smith, *Irish J. Med. Sc.* (1922): 1–4; David Mitchell, *A Peculiar Place* (Dublin: Blackwater Press, 1989), p 62.

[2] James Little, 'Life and Work of the late Dr. Alfred Hudson', *Dublin J. Med.Sc.* (1882); 74: 1–9. The son of a Congregational clergyman, Alfred Hudson (1808–80) was born in Staffordshire and apprenticed to a local medical practitioner who did little to further his education. His distant ambition was to become a fellow of the College of Physicians of London, and to this end he required a degree from Oxford, Cambridge, or Dublin. As a nonconformist he was excluded from the English universities and prevailed upon his father to support him in Dublin, where he entered Trinity College in 1830.

Already acquainted with the writings of Cheyne and his contemporaries (whose therapeutic methods he never quite abandoned), Hudson was instructed in later developments by Macartney, Crampton, Graves and Stokes, and completed his education

physician to the Adelaide Hospital (1866) was almost a guarantee of ultimate success. Two years later he was appointed lecturer in medicine in the Ledwich School of Medicine, and took over the editorship of the *Dublin Quarterly Journal of Medical Science* from Dr G. H. Kidd. He held the editorial chair for five years, and having arranged for the journal to revert to a programme of monthly issues in 1872 revived the earlier title, *Dublin Journal of Medical Science*. His friend Dr John William Moore then succeeded him.[3]

Little married Anna Murdoch, the daughter of a leading solicitor, in 1872; they had three children, two sons and a daughter.

Cheyne-Stokes breathing

Little's first publication (1868) discussed the 'ascending and descending breathing' described by Cheyne and Stokes.[4] This was generally regarded as pathognomic of fatty disease of the heart, but in 1860 Dr Seaton Reid of Belfast reported its occurrence in a case of left ventricular hypertrophy associated with aortic and mitral valve incompetence, the myocardium being free of fatty change. Little's own experience, based on three autopsies, indicated 'that breathing of ascending and descending rhythm occurs in fatty degeneration of the heart, and also in cases in which the left ventricle is hypertrophied as a consequence of valvular or arterial disease'. What, he asked, do these two morbid conditions have in common? The answer appeared to be that in both situations the circulation is embarrassed.

> Blood would, therefore, accumulate in the left auricle, in the pulmonary veins, and in the capillaries of the lungs. That blood, having already absorbed as much oxygen as it required, would fail to produce that impression on the ultimate filaments of the penumogastric which black blood does, and which impression is converted by the nervous centres into the motor impulse

---

in Edinburgh.
  While considering a tentative invitation to join the staff of the Birmingham General Hospital in 1836 he felt obliged to take over the practice of his fiancée's father, Dr Gilroy of Navan, who was ill and disabled. He remained in Navan (where he was physician to the Fever Hospital) until his father-in-law's death nineteen years later, and then ventured to take a house in Merrion Square and open a practice in the capital. 'Here is Hudson come to Dublin to starve', Sir William Wilde remarked to a friend. Against the odds he prospered, joining the staff at the newly-established Adelaide Hospital from which he retired when appointed to the Meath in 1861. Hudson became regius professor of physic in the University of Dublin, physician in ordinary to the Queen and a member of the GMC. He was president of the KQCPI (1871–2).
[3] When founded by Robert Kane (1832) the title was *The Dublin Journal of Medical and Chemical Science*.
[4] Little, 'Ascending and Descending Breathing; its Value as a Symptom, and its Mechanism', *Dublin J. Med. Sc.* (1868); 46: 46–52.

which produces breathing. Breathing would, therefore, cease ...'[5]

But when a few cardiac contractions had propelled red blood onwards, the flow of venous blood stimulated deeper respiration.

Dr J. Hawtrey Benson contributed two articles to the *Dublin Journal of Medical Science* on 'Ascending and Descending Respiration'. Not quite satisfied with Ludwig Traube's contention that the cause is 'a diminished excitability of the respiratory centre', Benson postulated a combined aberration of cardiac and nervous factors.[6]

On the eve of his retirement, Little returned to the intriguing problem of Cheyne-Stokes breathing, reviewing recent observations that attributed it to 'an anaesthesia of the vagus or of the medulla itself', or to a lowered percentage of carbonic acid in the alveolar air removing the normal stimulus to the respiratory centre. 'In many points [he wrote] the explanation I offered so many years ago is founded on the same premises.'[7]

Typhoid fever

Enteric or typhoid fever was a common illness in the nineteenth century. Commencing insidiously with a cloudy awareness of ill-health, its course was slow, its toxic victims (commonly young people at the threshold of adult life) displaying mounting pyrexia, rose spots, abdominal distension and diarrhoea. Providing that the Scylla and Charybdis of perforation and intestinal haemorrhage were circumvented, the fever could be expected to decline in the third week, and a week later the devastated patients should reach the happy harbour of convalescence. Quite a number, however, passed into a delirium, a pseudo-wakeful state dubbed coma-vigil, characterised by senseless mutterings and twitchings of the fingers and wrists, a critical phase during which many succumbed.

The cause of the disease was not yet established; its management in the 1870s was largely a matter of husbanding the patient's strength, while placating the relatives. It was a major trial of character for all concerned, and it is paradoxical that the modern doctor who cures typhoid fever speedily with chloramphenicol, is unlikely to gain anything like the credit accorded to predecessors who withstood the prolonged sieges of infectious illness in the past.

When James Little lectured on the treatment of typhoid fever in the Ledwich School early in 1872 he ventured to disagree with the standard text-books regarding diet:

---

[5] *Ibid.*, p. 50
[6] J. Hawtrey Benson, 'Ascending and Descending Respiration', *Dublin J. Med. Sc.* (1869); 48: 127–32; 'A case of "The Cheyne-Stokes Phenomenon"', *ibid.* (1874); 58: 519–22.
[7] Little, 'Cheyne-Stokes Breathing', *Dublin J. Med. Sc.* (1911); 131: 321–8.

Next to early confinement to bed, which perhaps more than anything else lessens the severity and risk of the fever, I rank the rigid exclusion of animal broths and jellies from the food, as tending to keep the disease mild. On this point I find myself quite at variance with the text-books in which such articles as beef-tea and Liebeg's essence of meat are recommended. Dr Hudson in his Lectures on Fever insists on the liability of all kinds of broths to increase the diarrhoea, and I cannot but attach the utmost importance to this matter, as I have repeatedly seen a patient who was passing four to six stools on a milk diet have eighteen to twenty during the day and night after he had taken beef-tea. Milk should be the chief article of diet in enteric fever.[8]

Following the example of Dr Cuming, whose opinion he valued, he advocated cold baths and explained that the Adelaide Hospital had full-sized baths which ran on castors, and were brought to the bedside, half full of water at 75° Fahrenheit. The patient was lifted into the bath and kept there for from five to fifteen minutes, three or at most four baths being given in the twenty-four hours. His recommendations included a full dose of quinine when nervous symptoms were prominent; leeches should be applied to the temple to counteract delirium and insomnia; dry cupping of the loins should be resorted to if the urine was scanty.

Some degree of pulmonary congestion was to be expected; it hardly required medication.

When there are cooing and wheezing rales, and the sleep is broken by fits of coughing a turpentine stupe at bed-time is usually sufficient to relieve. When there is any deficiency of resonance posteriorly I attach most importance to the precaution on which I first heard Dr. [William] Stokes insist, of not allowing the patient to remain on his back, but keeping him alternately on his right and left side, supported if need be by pillows.[9]

Little endeavoured to perform autopsies whenever possible, and brought specimens to the Academy's section of pathology from time to time. The majority of his publications, however, deal with therapy. On 8 January 1873 he addressed the Medical Society of the College of Physicians 'On the Use of Digitalis in the Failing Heart and Delirium of Acute Diseases'.[10] The use of wine as a stimulant in acute diseases was well established, but Little pointed out that there are persons 'whose brains are unusually susceptible to the influence of wine and brandy'. In

---

[8] Little, 'The Treatment of Enteric or Typhoid Fever', *Dublin J. Med. Sc.* (1872); 53: 370–76.
[9] *Ibid.*, p. 376.
[10] Little, *Dublin J. Med. Sc.* (1873); 55: 245–9.

such circumstances he recommended digitalis.

> I have given it [he wrote] with the special object of increasing the force of the cardiac contractions in more than twenty cases of fever (of these, six were typhus, one rheumatic fever with typhoid symptoms, and the remainder cases of enteric fever), and although my experience of it is by no means large enough to justify me in speaking positively, it has produced a strong impression on my own mind . . . I give half a drachm of the tincture every fourth, third, or second hour; in some cases every hour. I have not seen any ill effects produced by it except sickness of the stomach . . .[11]

He discontinued the digitalis when the pulse fell to eighty, not venturing to use it to the complete exclusion of alcohol, either in typhus or enteric fever. He solicited a trial of the drug 'at the hands of those whose observation of fever has been sufficiently extensive and sufficient-ly precise to qualify them for estimating the effect of the remedy'.

Geographical distribution

Little had withdrawn from the Ledwich School in 1872, on succeeding Charles Benson in the chair of medicine in the RCSI. His lectures in the college were well attended, and attracted students from other schools. In terms of professional status he had 'arrived', and he was among those invited to participate in a series of 'Afternoon Scientific Lectures' on public health delivered in the lecture hall of the Royal Dublin Society in the months of April and May 1873.

His choice of subject, 'The Geographical Distribution of Disease', is likely to have been influenced by his employment with the P&O on the Calcutta Station. There, he had seen India's cauldrons of disease, and became familiar with beriberi and cholera in their endemic situation. 'Cholera has in Lower Bengal, and especially in the great towns of Dacca and Calcutta, a home; when its ravages have ceased elsewhere, it still prevails in this region.' He was familiar with the delta of the Ganges, that alluvial plain, 'so flat, that for 200 miles inland it barely rises above the sea level, exuberant vegetation, vast expanses of jungle, a great network of rivers and canals, and a tropical sun; in the habits of the people too we find everything favourable to the spread of an epidemic.' He could see in his mind's eye the busy port of Alexandria, where conditions existed for the rapid diffusion of infection. 'In it you may see every day the flag of almost every European nation. It is the great highway between Europe and the East, and from it are daily starting English, French, Russian, and Austrian steamers.'

The world was free of cholera in January 1864, with the exception of

---

[11] *Ibid*, p. 246.

the insalubrious *bustees* (native villages) of Lower Bengal. It spread first to Central India, and to Bombay reaching the latter in 1865. By the summer of 1866 the pestilence was in Ireland, and Little traced out its dolorous journey.

From Bombay it had followed the trade route to Arabia, and the pilgrims' route to Djeddah, the port for Mecca. There were 30,000 deaths in the Islamic encampments leaving survivors from the north to return to their homes via the Red Sea and Suez. They crossed the isthmus by train to Alexandria. 'The first case of cholera occurred at Alexandria on June 2; on June 11 it was at Marseilles, on June 28 at Constantinople, and on July 7 at Ancona.'

Precautionary measures imposed at English ports were successful, and the disease did not appear at Southampton until 17 September. It was not conveyed to Ireland by the direct route, however, and Little followed other trails of infection which took it from Constantinople via the Black Sea to the Danube, or through the agency of a party that travelled overland. These were Persians who carried cholera to the Persian Gulf and along the valley of the Euphrates to the Caspian Sea, its portal to Russia.

Northern Europe was contaminated in the spring of 1866; Holland was severely affected, and two persons from Rotterdam died of cholera in Liverpool on 2 May. When a girl died of the disease in Dublin on 26 July Edward Mapother, the city MOH, found that she had come from a Liverpool lodging-house patronised by Dutch sailors.

The subsequent epidemic spread to many distant Irish counties, with 4,309 cases and 2,308 deaths, but was at its worst in the capital, where between July and December 1866 there were almost a thousand deaths.[12] It may be added that Robert Koch visited Egypt and India in 1883, leading the German cholera commission, and discovered the *Vibrio cholerae* which colonises the small intestine.[13] Its exotoxin causes secretion of isotonic fluid by all segments of the small bowel. The adult cholera stool is nearly isotonic, with sodium chloride concentrations slightly less than those of plasma, a bicarbonate concentration approximately twice that of plasma, and a potassium concentration three to five times that of plasma.

Germ theory again

The leading proponents of the germ theory in England included Dr (later

---

[12] Joseph Robins, *The Miasma* (Dublin: Institute of Public Administration, 1995) p. 205.
[13] See Sir William Coleman, 'Koch's Comma Bacillus: the First Year', *Bull. Hist. Med.* (1987); 61: 315–42. Koch reported on 2 February 1884 the isolation of a comma-like bacillus. This was invariably present in cholera and absent in all other circumstances. Like so many discoveries it was not entirely new; Koch's comma bacillus is officially known as *Vibrio cholera Pacini* to commemorate a Florentine, Fillipo Pacini, who described it in 1854. 'What Koch and his associates did . . . was to see once again, but then go on to build, via rigorous experimental work . . . a strong case for the causal role of the vibrio.'

Sir) John Burdon Sanderson and John Tyndall.[14] The former (known to his students as 'the Burder') had been MOH for Paddington (1856–67) and a precis of his work was reported to the *Dublin Journal of Medical Science* in 1871 by Dr (later Sir Charles) Cameron: 'Dr. Sanderson defines microzymes as "living particles which in the earliest stage of their existence, are spheroids . . . but subsequently lengthen into rods."' Tyndall's experiments were referred to by Dr T. W. Grimshaw in 'state of the art' lectures delivered at the KQCPI on 4 and 11 March 1878. He accepted that Tyndall and Pasteur had 'pretty well disposed of all the arguments in favour of spontaneous generation'.[15]

Grimshaw used the term zymotic disease as synonymous with infective disease, and wished to call his audience's attention to a process 'strictly homologous to, if not identical with, fermentation', which had an important bearing in relation to infective diseases.

> There are certain little organisms [he continued] whose name, 'bacteria', is now in the mouth of everyone. They are generally talked of as if those who discuss them were intimately acquainted with their appearance and nature. The name, in consequence of sensational lectures, has come to be commonly employed in the same sense as disease germ; so 'bacteria' and germs are now looked upon as almost equivalent to 'plague and pestilence'. Now bacteria in themselves appear for the most part to be harmless little creatures; they or their germs swarm in millions in the air we breathe, the fluids we drink, and the food we eat. They can be collected from our mouths at any time, and when washed clean by distilled water have been injected into the blood without producing any evil result. It is quite clear that if bacteria were possessed of the terrible powers attributed to them they would soon have the world to themselves, having eaten up or decomposed all other organised beings.[16]

Despite the apparent harmlessness of many of these organisms it seemed 'to be almost certain that their existence is necessary' to the production of zymotic or infective diseases, a fact which offered an impor-

---

[14] Like Pasteur, with whom he corresponded from 1871, John Tyndall (1820–93) was not a physician. Born in humble circumstances to Protestant parents at Leighlinbridge, County Carlow, he worked as a surveyor in Ireland and England before gaining an education in science.

Tyndall devised experiments to demonstrate and quantify particles in the atmosphere; he showed that he could remove them by passing air through a flame, or through a tube containing platinum gauze heated to redness. His main opponent, Dr Henry Charlton Bastian, held that bacteria were 'pathological products' created by the diseased body. See *John Tyndall: Essays on a Natural Philosopher*, ed. W. H. Brock, N. D. McMillan and R. C. Mollan (Dublin: RDS, 1981).

[15] T. W. Grimshaw, 'The Intimate Nature of Infection and Contagion', *Dublin J. Med. Sc.* (1878); 66: 1–15.

[16] *Ibid.*, p. 5. The word zymotic was used by W. Farr in 1842.

tant corollary: 'their destruction will either prevent or cure diseases'.[17] At the time of Grimshaw's lectures certain organisms had been found that were constantly related to specific contagious diseases. These included the germs of anthrax, relapsing fever and leprosy. J. W. Bigger has listed the more important discoveries made between 1880 and 1900.[18]

The acceptance of Listerian surgery should have come about more easily, but despite Sir Joseph Lister's personal demonstration of his method in the Richmond Hospital on 26 June 1879, the controversy dragged on in the Surgical Society of Ireland, where on 27 February 1880 Mr (later Sir William) Stokes spoke on 'Ovariotomy and Antiseptics'. Stokes posed a rhetorical question—'Did not antiseptics, or I should say "Listerism" play a chief rôle in bringing about the result?'—and supplied his own answer: 'He would be, I think, a hardened and hopeless sceptic who would answer the query in the negative.' The chairman on that occasion, Mr E. Hamilton, of Steevens' Hospital, told how his enthusiasm was followed by wavering faith, then by a full conversion to Listerism, only to be recently disturbed by results which had given a further check to his belief.

Edward Halloran Bennett said he had seen surgeons use carbolic lotion and the carbolic spray during the operations, but 'the arteries were tied with silk from a roll which the resident pupil took out of his pocket'.

On 12 March, Mr Henry Gray Croly, of the City of Dublin Hospital, reported favourably on Listerism at the Surgical Society and was supported by Mr (later Sir William) Thornley Stoker of the Richmond Hospital. Mr (later Sir Lambert) Ormsby, surgeon to the Meath Hospital, held that it did not matter which antiseptic was used providing complete cleanliness in the dressing was aimed at. He objected to the expense involved in the full Listerian ritual, which involved an outlay of 1s 2d for each dressing.

Mr Robert M'Donnell said Lister had imported into practical surgery 'the modern and received theory . . . that organic fluids were set going and worked through the means of organic germs'. Dr T. Darby, an elderly practitioner from Bray, County Wicklow, objected, saying that for his part he did not believe in the germ theory of disease.

When the debate was resumed on 5 May, opinion was evenly divided but the most trenchant critics of Listerism were Mr Rawdon Macnamara,

---

[17] *Ibid.*, p. 11.
[18] 1880 : the typhoid bacillus—Eberth; 1881: Staphylococci—Ogston; 1882: Tubercle bacillus—Koch; 1883: The cholera vibrio—Koch; 1884: Tetanus bacillus—Nicolaier; 1885: B. coli—Escherich; 1886: Pneumococcus—Fraenkel; 1887: Meningococcus—Weichselbaum, M. Melitensis—Bruce; 1888: B. enteritidis—Gaertner; 1892: B. welchii—Welch and Nuttall; 1894: the plague bacillus—Kitasato and Yersin; 1896: B. botulinis—van Ermengem; 1898: B. dysenteriae—Shiga. Taken from Joseph W. Bigger, *Man Against Microbe* (London: English Universities Press, 1939), p. 165.

and his friend Samuel Haughton, DD, MD, whom we have already encountered in an anti-Darwinist role. Macnamara said it was clear that those who supported the antiseptic plan based their arguments on Pasteur's experiments—experiments which had been disproved by no less an authority than Dr Bastian.

The Rev. Haughton had seen the antiseptic treatment in Edinburgh, Newcastle-on-Tyne and London. He pronounced it to be 'occult, beyond all religious belief . . . the newest fangled notion going'. Listerism was a perfect humbug based on extreme cleanliness. He could not produce statistics for or against the carbolic system but on the question of germs he was more authorised to speak:

> As a scientific man [he said], not merely as a medical man, I believe there never was a more miserable idea brought before the world of science than that expressed in the words *omne vivum ex ovo*. Where did the original ovum come from? We have witnesed at the British Association the contemptible spectacle of Sir William Thompson telling us that the germ came on a meteoric stone from some other planet. He had the audacity to say in my presence that the Papa Beetle brought in the germ with him.
>
> I cannot allow such an absurd physiological statement to pass muster [Haughton continued]. There are a number of ladies present and they well understand perfectly that unless the Mamma Beetle came as well as the Papa there would be no disastrous consequences.
>
> It is nonsense to say we cannot go back for the origin of life beyond some living germ. There must have been a time on this planet when the laws directed by an Almighty Creator of all things, who predestined and created everything in heaven and earth, arranged that from some complex organic chemical compound a living thing should proceed. I am perfectly certain of that.
>
> It is absurd to say that this world cannot produce a living germ. . . . The laws are there that when certain unknown conditions are fulfilled, the germ shall arise. That the germ, the living thing, can come from organic things is as certain as anything in the world. Hence to postulate for any living thing in the world a previous living thing is nonsense.[19]

Accepting the occurrence of spontaneous generation, Haughton believed the germ might arise from the complicated conditions of a festering wound.

Closing the debate, Mr Mapother, PRCSI, approved of a suggestion that a committee should visit the Dublin hospitals where antiseptic surgery was practised, and those where it was ignored. He had never used it in St Vincent's Hospital and never would. The late hour left him insuf-

---

[19] *Med. Press & Circ.*, (5 May 1880); p. 369. Haughton's contribution has been changed from passive to active mood.

ficient time to explain why he was an unbeliever.

In the course of a paper read to the Surgical Society on 21 January 1881 entitled 'A Record of Cases Treated Antiseptically, and of Cases Acording to Lister's Method', Mr William J. Wheeler remarked: 'If I understand Lister's theory, he accepts Pasteur's views, that there are germs in the air which cause putrefaction on their admission to wounds, and that these develop *ad infinitum*, whenever they meet a suitable medium, and that by spraying the air with carbolic of prescribed strength, he washes it of these impurities, and prevents their deleterious effects. This theory I cannot hold to be tenable . . .'[20]

Wheeler was criticised by Thornley Stoker, who said he 'utterly and entirely dissented' from the views expressed. He objected to Wheeler's terming one system 'antisepticism' and the other 'Listerism', implying that Lister's method was not antiseptic at all. 'Antiseptic surgery was associated with Lister's name, and antisepticism and Listerism were used as convertible terms.'[21]

By the early 1890s the germ theory was generally accepted by both physicians and surgeons. Papers for the fellowship examination in January 1890 asked: 'What is septicemia? How would you treat the condition?' A paper set by Sir William Stokes in November 1893 instructed candidates to 'Enumerate the forms of micro-organism met with in acute suppuration, and discuss their connection with the process.'[22]

Practical therapeutics

Little's popularity as a teacher was a source of great satisfaction to him, but by 1883 the demands of his by then enormous practice (it was said to have been larger than Cheyne's) forced him to resign his professorship. Having bidden his class farewell he was emotionally overcome, confiding later to Dr John William Moore that he went home, 'shut himself into his study, and wept like a child'.

He addressed the medical section of the recently-established Academy of Medicine on 19 November 1886, a duty that fell to him as president of the College of Physicians, to which office he had been elected some weeks previously. He spoke on practical therapeutics, dwelling on defects that hindered a just appreciation of the value of remedies. Preconceived notions, for instance, dictated that potassium iodide should be given in tubercular meningitis (where it was useless), while its potential benefits in asthma were neglected. Claret, commonly given to anaemic girls, actually has no power to make blood. He believed that alcohol may be prescribed

---

[20] W. J. Wheeler, 'A Record of Cases Treated Antiseptically, and of Cases According to Lister's Method', *Med. Press & Circ.* (1881); 82: 155–59.
[21] W. Thornley Stoker, *ibid.*, p. 161.
[22] See court of examiners minutes.

with undue liberality as a stimulant in acute diseases, but withheld because of its moral dangers in other situations where it could help.[23]

He complained of the multiplicity of proprietary preparations produced by the 'ingenuity of pharmaceutical chemists'. Few of these were more effective than corresponding pharmacopeial medicines, and were devised solely for commercial reasons. He explained in some detail that 'apparently slight differences in the manner in which [medicines] are administered often make a great difference in their effects'.[24] Iron in effervescence acts more rapidly. Morphine relieves cough more fully when dissolved in a viscid menstruum. The salicylate of sodium acts more effectively when taken in a large dose at night, than if given in smaller doses during the day.

It was the age of mixtures (an age that lingered on well into the middle of the twentieth century) but when prescribing, say, digitalis, nux vomica and belladonna, Little directed the patient to take the required number of minims of each tincture separately in a little water. He also insisted that the ingredients of the celebrated Baillie's Pill (digitalis, squill and mercury) should be prescribed individually. And he continued to favour certain medicines the use of which he had learned from the heroes of his youth, Dr Thomas Cumings's morphine syrup, and Dr Alfred Hudson's white mixture.

Migraine

Little's 'Note on the Relief of Migranous [sic] Headache' was presented to the section of medicine on 20 April 1888:

> Up to October, 1885, I did not know of any treatment which had any distinct power of cutting short the attack when it came, or even mitigating its severity. Most patients found that if they refrained entirely from any attempt to take food, and were able to lie in a darkened room, they did all which was possible to lessen the intensity of their sufferings. Those who had on the previous evening a warning of their impending attack sometimes thought they kept it off by a full dose of bromide taken at bed hour. Others found that a dessertspoonful of the granular citrate of caffein was beneficial, while some told me that lemon juice or vinegar relieved the sickness and headache; but at this time it occurred to me to try salicylate of sodium, and after more than two years experience of its strikingly beneficial effect, I feel justified in commending it to the members of the Medical Section.[25]

Other speakers confirmed that having been advised by Little of the

---

[23] Little, 'Practical Therapeutics', *Dublin J. Med. Sc.* (1886); 82: 438–47.
[24] *Ibid.*, p. 444.
[25] Little, 'Note on the Relief of Migranous [sic] Headache', *Dublin J. Med. Sc.* (1888); 85: 489–92.

efficacy of sodium salicylate, they had prescribed it with benefit. Dr John William Moore believed the relief followed its action on the liver. 'Once the bowels were freed and the tendency to nausea was relieved, the headache disappeared almost like magic.'[26]

Myxoedema

On 11 December 1890 Little was consulted by a thirty-four-year-old unmarried woman who presented the typical appearance of myxoedema. 'Her face seemed swollen and had a mixed pale and livid look. Her fingers had become clumsy; she felt the cold terribly, and she was occasionally hoarse.' He prescribed Turkish baths and tincture of jaborandi. When he saw her again in July 1892, the patient was inclined to say that she was a little better, but her sister disagreed, pointing out that she had just become accustomed to the discomfort.

In the interim, however, George R. Murray of Newcastle-on Tyne had reported to the annual meeting of the BMA in Bournemouth, in July 1891, the striking benefits that followed hypodermic injections of thyroid juice, obtained from a sheep's thyroid, in a single case under his care. He published an account of this patient on 10 October 1891[27] and confirmation of the value of the therapy was supplied by others, including Little's colleague Wallace Beatty, at the Adelaide Hospital. The latter was consulted on 7 October 1891 by a forty-five-year-old married woman who presented with unmistakable myxoedema of five or six years' duration. After consultations with Professor John Mallet Purser and Dr Henry H. Head, it was decided to give her thyroid juice.[28] The first injection was given on 11 December and Beatty noted that the result 'has been really marvellous'.[29]

Little decided on a trial of injections of sheep's thyroid juice but, surprisingly, postponed this until after the holiday season by which time Hector Mackenzie had actually reported from London that excellent results could be obtained by feeding patients with fresh thyroid glands.[30]

On December 4th [Little wrote] I gave the first injection of thyroid

---

[26] J. W. Moore, *ibid.*, p. 540. Little's 'Note on the Power of Saccharine in Preventing Ammonical Change in Urine in Chronic Cystitis' was presented on the same occasion: *ibid.*, p. 493.
[27] G. R. Murray, 'Note on the Treatment of Myxoedema by Hypodermic Injections of an extract of the Thyroid Gland of a Sheep', *Brit. Med. J.* (1891); 2: 796–7.
[28] Not to be confused with his London namesake, Henry Head was physician to the Adelaide Hospital.
[29] Wallace Beatty, 'A Case of Myxoedema Successfully treated by Massage and Hypodermic Injections of the Thyroid Gland of a Sheep', *Brit. Med. J.*, (1892); 2: 544–5.
[30] Hector Mackenzie, 'A Case of Myxoedema Treated With Great Benefit by Feeding with Fresh Thyroid Glands' *Brit. Med. J.*, (1892); 2: 940–1.

juice, and I continued the administration until January 9th. She had altogether twenty-six injections; at first I gave two each week, but afterwards three. The fluid was kindly prepared for me by Dr. J. Alfred Scott with elaborate precaution.[31]

After a few injections were given, Little noticed that he no longer had difficulty in pinching up the skin; other signs of improvement quickly followed. 'She took part in conversation as she had not done for years.' She no longer felt the cold acutely and she could complete her needlework neatly. Within two months of the discontinuation of the injections, however, the family noticed that her face was becoming puffy and her voice was again hoarse. Little then advised that thyroid glands should be taken orally and this was readily arranged.

The butcher who supplies her family has learned how to remove the glands and sends them to her fresh. Each week she uses two glands—half a one, say, on Monday and Tuesday, and again half a one on Thursday and Friday; she chips up the half gland, cleared of fat and capsule, and putting it in a spoon moistens it with a little beaune and swallows it after breakfast.[32]

There was a full symptomatic recovery.

Gastric ulcer

Little opened the section of medicine's discussion on gastric ulcer on 18 January 1907 by referring to his experience of the condition prior to the advent of surgical treatment: he recalled cases who died from perforation[33] but he had never seen a death from haemorrhage. 'I have several time seen a young woman who seemed just about to die from bleeding, but I cannot recall one who did die.'[34]

Gastric ulcer he had found commoner in young chlorotic women who were hospital patients; patients with duodenal ulcers, middle-aged males, were usually seen privately. On the subject of diagnosis he felt the diagnosis of gastric ulcer could not be made until the patient had vom-

---

[31] Little, 'Sequel of a Case of Myxoedema Treated by Thyroid Juice' *Dublin J. Med. Sc.* (1894); 97: 293–6. (John Alfred Scott was professor of physiology in the RCSI and pathologist to the Adelaide Hospital).

[32] *Ibid.*, p. 295.

[33] Dr Alfred Parsons, in his second contribution to the Academy on 6 May 1892, made a passionate plea for surgical intervention in perforated gastric ulcers. He recalled that as he had stood at the bedsides of dying patients only one thought had occupied his mind: 'To save such cases one must open the abdomen and open it EARLY.' A leading surgeon in the audience stresssed the difficulties and said the sutures would not hold. See J. B. Lyons, 'The Section of Medicine and Medical Developments Over the Century' *Irish J. Med. Sc.* (1983); 152: 14–23.

[34] Little, 'The Treatment of Gastric Ulcer', *Dublin J. Med. Sc.* (1907); 123: 161–70.

ited blood, nor could cancer of the stomach be diagnosed unless the tumour could be felt. Patients with gastric ulcers should rest in bed, on a milk diet and take Dr Hudson's white mixture.[35]

He sometimes reinforced the white mixture with ten minims of liquor morphinae hydrochlorhidri, or one-sixth of a grain of cocaine hydrochloride. He also prescribed bismuth, milk of magnesium and a powder favoured by Sir William Whitla[36]—this consisted of hydrochloride of morphine, 1/18 grain; Finkler's papaïn, 3 grains; carbonate of bismuth, 5 grains; bicarbonate of sodium, 15 grains; and heavy carbonate of magnesium, 20 grains. Little's willingness to prescribe morphine and indian hemp for chronic maladies is interesting, but hardly acceptable.

Other measures recommended by Professor Little include rectal feeding, blisters and leeches. Vomiting was sometimes stopped by 'a morsel of stale bread washed down by a wineglassful of champagne'. Never having seen a death from haemorrhage, he thought that surgical help was seldom required to deal with this complication. The desirability of blood transfusion was not mentioned, for in 1907 this valuable amenity was not yet generally available. The discovery of blood groups by Karl Landsteiner in 1900 had made it a practible procedure; the impetus of the First World would demonstrate its benefits.

College of Physicians

Soon after his arrival in Dublin, Little was admitted as licentiate of the College of Physicians and he was elected FKQCPI in 1867. In due course he served the college as censor, registrar, senior censor and vice-president. On St Luke's Day 1886 he was a unanimous choice as president, and during his term of office the viceroy, the Marquis of Londonderry, dined as his guest in the college. Accompanied by John William Moore, the registrar, Little, in June 1897, presented the loyal address of the president and fellows of the college to Queen Victoria, at Windsor Castle, on the occasion of the golden jubilee of her majesty's reign.

James Little was physician-in ordinary in Ireland to three successive monarchs—Queen Victoria, King Edward VII and King George V. He was crown nominee for Ireland on the General Medical Council, and sometime president of the Royal Academy of Medicine in Ireland and of the Association of Physicians of Great Britain and Ireland. He held the MD *honoris causa* of the University of Dublin, and was elected its regius

---

[35] Potassii nitratis, gr. xii; Bismuthi subnitratis, i drachm; Acidi hydrocyanici diluti, min. xxxvi; Acidici nitrici diluti, i drachm; Mucilaginis acaciae recentis, i fl. oz.; Aquae chloroformi, ad vi fl oz. Shake the bottle and give half an ounce thrice daily half an hour before food.
[36] For an account of this popular Belfast physician see J. B. Lyons *Brief Lives of Irish Doctors* (Dublin: Blackwater Press, 1978), pp. 120–21.

professor of physic in 1898, holding the chair for the remainder of his life. The omission of a knighthood surprised many, but it was an open secret that he had politely declined the honour.

Professor Little cannot be credited with any medical discovery; no syndrome is named for him nor had he access to remedies unavailable to his colleagues. His outstanding success depended, presumably, on a remarkably sympathetic personality that brought comfort and assurance to many. 'What is the best qualification of a doctor?' Little asked John William Moore, supplying his own answer: 'Hopefulness'.

Death

His wife predeceased him in 1914. On 1 July 1916 he had the first intimation of the ill-health that continued to weaken him, resulting in his death on 23 December. A bronze plaque to honour the ex-president was unveiled in the RCPI on 17 January 1922.

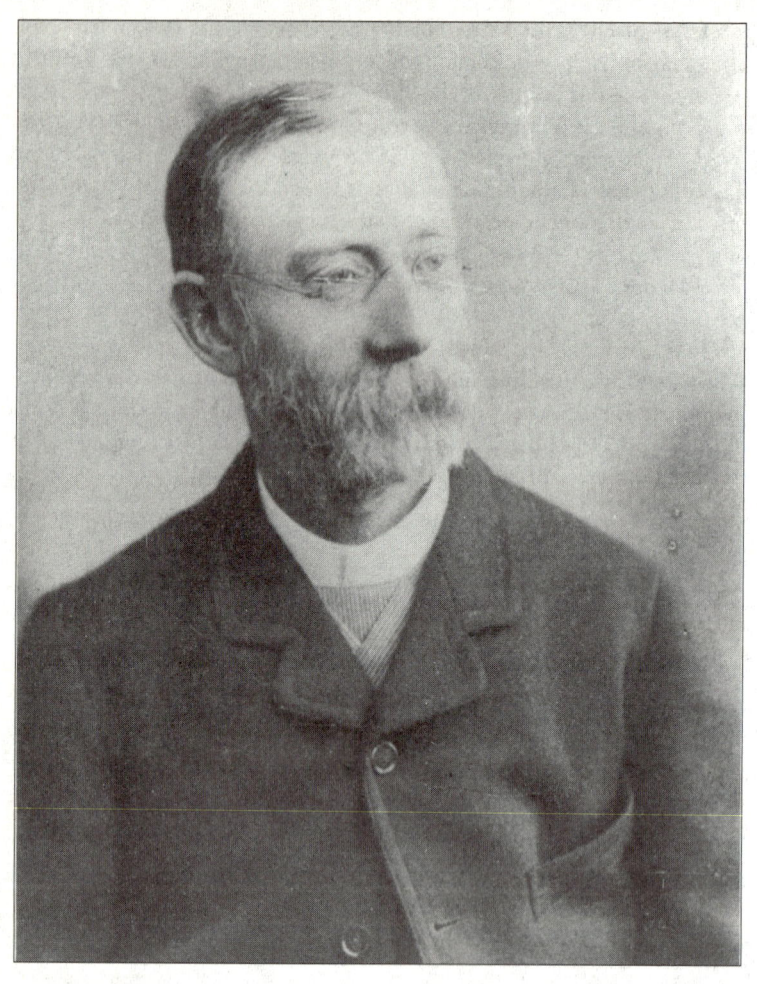

Arthur Wynne Foot, 1838–1900 Professor of Medicine 1883–95 (courtesy Meath Hospital)

Chapter 8: Arthur Wynne Foot, 1838–1900

Sometime in the 1920s, a collection of insects purchased at an auction by a Mrs Jennings was presented to the National Museum. Direct evi-dence of the identity of the original owner, surprisingly, was missing, but looking through an accompanying numbered catalogue, an assistant curator, Arthur Wilson Stelfox (whose grandson in 1993 became the first Irishman to reach the summit of Everest), quickly ascertained that the collector had been a medical man—'witness his capture of a female *Vespa vulgaris* in October, 1870, in the board-room of the Meath Hospital'— with access to the fellows' garden at Trinity College, where on 10 June 1870 he had found eggs of the common Ghost Moth.[1]

Stelfox, an assistant at the museum, noticed that the unknown collector had been in touch with the best entomologists of his period. His favourite collecting-grounds were often mentioned: Portmarnock Sands; Newcastle, County Wicklow; Graiguenamanagh and several places along the River Barrow. Finally on page twenty-six, Stelfox read: 'Blatta . . . 21 Lr. Pembroke St., 8th June, '70.' This was the decisive clue. '"Blatta" is the common Cockroach, and so I argued 21 Lr. Pembroke St. was his residence.'

The Dublin street-directory for 1870 told Stelfox that it was then occupied by Dr A. W. Foot, but left him asking why this forgotten Irish naturalist had risen into prominence as a member of the Dublin Natural History Society in the late 1860s, when he had read many papers to the society, only to disappear sudddenly into oblivion? 'The last entry in the catalogue is of insects caught at Newcastle, Wicklow, in May, 1872.' The conundrum is now easily answered: the young naturalist, who in the immediate postgraduate period published those papers on natural history, had advanced sufficiently in the medical profession to be left without leisure for avocational interests. Nor did the retirement period permit a return to the compelling pursuits of his youth, for he was then enfeebled by illness.

Birth and ancestry

Arthur Wynne Foot, a Dubliner, was born on 22 January 1838, son of a barrister, Lundy Edward Foot and his wife Lelias Caldwell.[2] The family

---

[1] A. W. Stelfox, 'Arthur Wynne Foot, M.D., Irish Naturalist', *The Irish Naturalist's Journal* (1931); 3: 260–1.

[2] His father's first name, a favourite family name for Dublin Foots, derived from a Miss Lundy, an heiress who married Jeffrey Foot, gentleman, c. 1733. See Sir C. Cameron, *History of the Royal College of Surgeons in Ireland*, 2nd ed. (Dublin: Fannin, 1916), p. 95;

had Cornish roots, the Irish branch descending from an ancestor who came to Dublin with William III. Arthur was educated at Portarlington 'under the ferrule of the Rev. J. A. Wall, M.A.'[3] and then apprenticed to Maurice H. Collis, surgeon to the Meath Hospital, where the young man took a number of prizes, including the Pathological Society's silver medal awarded for his dissertation on diseases of the testis. In due course he would be president of the Pathological Society.

He graduated in 1862, taking the diplomas of the Colleges of Physicians and Surgeons, and degrees in arts and medicine at Dublin University, where for eight years he was a demonstrator in anatomy, establishing a reputation for the excellence of his teaching. He proceeded MD in 1865, submitting a thesis on chromidrosis; he was elected FKQCPI in 1866, adding the recently-introduced diploma in state medicine to his qualifications in 1871, one of four enterprising physicians to do so—his fellow-diplomates were John Todhunter, Gerald Yeo and John William Moore.

Ledwich School

Foot was elected physician to the Meath Hospital on 8 April 1871, and towards the end of that year he succeeded James Little as lecturer in medicine at the Ledwich School of Medicine. When it fell to him to deliver the introductory address at the Ledwich School on 1 November 1873 he directed his remarks to the students.[4] He spoke first of his two predecessors, James Little, now professor of medicine at the RCSI, and Henry Eames, the young physician to Mercer's Hospital who had died of fever in March: 'Both have left this place—one with a crown of laurel, the other with a wreath of cypress . . .' Their opposite fates represented the risks and the rewards of the medical profession.

The word *diligence*, he told his audience, included the virtues a student should posssess, while 'Excellence in your Profession' was a high and worthy motive.

> I have not named it Success, because it includes success, and is greater than success, and because success has too much of a commercial smack and of a pecuniary significance wrongly lingering about it, to justify me in putting it before the students of a profession whose generosity is romantic. This profession is not a mercantile one; you do not enter it to amass fortunes, but to do good according to your ability. Fortune may come, and fortune does come to many;

Lambert H. Ormsby, *History of the Meath Hospital* (1888), p. 146–7.

[3] Sir J. W. Moore, 'In Memoriam: Arthur Wynne Foot', *Dublin J. Med. Sc.* (1900); 110: 333–6.

[4] A. W. Foot, 'An Introductory Address, delivered at the Ledwich School of Medicine, November 1st, 1873', *ibid.* (1873); 56: 553–68.

but to few, indeed, unless through their efforts at Excellence.[5]

He reserved his uncompromising hostility for slackers. 'For real idlers I have no sheet lightning of polished and playful sarcasm, but red forked darts of terribly earnest reprobation.' It was they who made a bad name for medical students.

Neurology

Foot published many clinical reports of cases under his care at the Meath Hospital in the *Dublin Journal of Medical Science*. These included examples of Bright's disease, scleroderma, tuberculosis, scarlatina, xanthelesma, hepatic cirrhosis, and a variety of nervous disorders. He gave accounts of two patients with locomotor ataxy (tabes dorsalis), a bachelor doctor and an ex-Liverpool policeman.

The tabetic doctor was unable to manage the considerable practice he had built up on Vancouver Island, being no longer able to ascertain the positions or presentations in his midwifery cases. Returning to Ireland, he consulted Foot and was admitted to the Meath on 16 May 1871. He made no secret of the fact that he had contracted syphilis in 1861, with secondary manifestations in the following year.

> He pleaded guilty [Foot wrote] to sexual excesses, indulged in in Edinburgh, in the year 1865, when under favourable circumstances, he discovered a singular aptitude for repeating the venereal act a great many times within a short period. At this date he used to have connection six or seven times a night three times in the week, and continued to operate at this ratio for nearly a year. Dr. X. often discussed with me the question whether these libidinous excesses were the cause or the result of his disease, and we generally came to the conclusion they were more likely to have been the result.[6]

His gait was described by Foot as 'the embodiment of incapacity and indecision'. He could not stand with his eyes shut, or move in the dark without a light; the knee-jerks were absent. He was unable to differentiate by touch between a shilling, a half-crown and a sovereign, and was unable to fasten buttons without seeing them.

Electrical treatment was started, using Störher's large induction battery, and he was given cod-liver oil and sodium hypophosphite three times daily. He left hospital on 23 August being then well enough to walk slowly to the Phoenix Park, a distance of two miles or so.

Having been deemed unfit for his duties, an ex-policeman came to

---

[5] *Ibid.*, p. 558.
[6] 'Generalised Locomotor Ataxy', *ibid.* (1886); 81: 393–401.

the Meath on 21 March 1872. He was massively built, thirty-four years of age, married with four children. There was no history of syphilis. His legs were numb and unsteady, and he was obliged to use a stick. 'He could not cross a brook using familiar stepping stones without missing the aim of his feet and stepping in . . .' He miscalculated weights, and sometimes picked up light articles with excessive force. His gait was broad-based, and stamping.

Foot cited Romberg's estimation of the average duration of tabes dorsalis as ten years, but the unfortunate policeman developed typhus during his second week in hospital and died on 15 April. An opportunity was taken to examine the spinal cord. 'Throughout the dorsal region the posterior half of the cord felt softened, and appeared shrunken and pale, very pale as compared with the anterior half.'[7]

Dr X was re-admitted to the Meath for further treatment, and by 1873 he was well enough to take a post as ship's surgeon on a steamer sailing to the River Plate. During the voyage he extracted teeth successfully, and was well enough to keep his feet on deck in a gale. Early in 1879 he took over a small practice in Cheshire, but he suffered from bronchitis and died on 28 December 1881.

A case of what would nowadays be called primary generalised epilepsy with tonic-clonic seizures, was classified by Foot as 'gastric epilepsy' on clinical grounds. 'The first nine attacks occurred at or immediately after meals, and appeared to be connected either with the use of unsuitable articles of diet or with an injudicious method of eating ordinary food.' The youth was examined on 5 November 1876 by Dr Charles Edouard Brown-Séquard, during the neurologist's visit to Dublin. An iodine-bromide mixture was prescribed and the severity and frequency of seizures diminished, permitting a return to work but at the cost of severe acne.[8]

For some years, Foot kept buried in his note-books records pertaining to 'a curious case of morbid somnolence' which he was at a loss to categorize, until he encountered the term *narcolepsy*, coined by M. Gélineau in 1880. He presented an account of the little known disorder to the section of medicine of the Academy of Medicine in November 1886, adding two cases collected from the Irish literature.[9]

Graves' disease

Exophthalmic goitre (which in 1868 Trousseau named *la maladie de Graves*) was followed with particular interest at the Meath Hospital. Before coming there with this complaint on 10 April 1890, a twenty-six-

---

[7] 'A Case of Locomotor Ataxy,' *ibid.* (1872); 54: 174.
[8] 'A Case of Gastric Epilepsy', *ibid.* (1888); 85: 384–92.
[9] 'Narcolepsy (Sudden Periodical Sleep-Seizures)', *ibid.* (1886); 82: 465–71.

year-old woman had visited Knock Shrine, in County Mayo, hoping for a miracle cure. Foot prescribed a digitalis and iron mixture; the thyroid gland was painted with linament of belladonna; a light muslin bandage was applied to the eyes at night. The goitre was reduced in size when the patient left hospital on 9 June.

A twenty-two year-old woman from the west of Ireland was admitted under Foot's care on 9 August 1890. She was given digitalis and iron; galvanisation of the cervical sympathetic was carried out daily in addition to electrisation of the eyeballs. Progress appeared favourable, but like the tabetic policeman she had the misfortune to pick up a lethal hospital infection and died on 26 October.[10]

A post-mortem examination was done, and at a meeting of the Pathological Society on 6 November Foot showed the eyeballs, thyroid gland and heart. The eyes were not enlarged, but the retro-orbital adipose tissue was increased. The thyroid gland was 'condensed and firm in structure, as if the congestion to which it was subject had provoked a hyperplasia of the connective tissue of the gland'. Regrettably, a microscopic examination does not seem to have been carried out, though at other meetings in the Pathological Society Foot supported his presentations with histological data.[11]

He examined the cervical sympathetic (then regarded as the cause of the disease) with care, but with negative results. 'It is not at all settled [he concluded] that the seat of the disease is really in the cervical sympathetic.'

A later review[12] shows that Foot saw his first case of exophthalmic goitre in a male patient in 1873, a second in 1890 and a third male case in the following year. He knew that the Mersburg triad of tachycardia, ocular protrusion and goitre, tended to be less marked in men. He was familiar with the way the clinical picture had beeen extended since its recognition. Charcot had added tremor to the principal manifestations making it a *tetrad* of primary phenomena. Russell Reynolds made it a *pentad* by giving an importance to nervous disturbances. The eye signs of Albrecht von Graefe and Stellwag were diagnostically helpful, especially when dealing with *formes frustes*. The presence of skin pigmentation, for instance, when combined with weight loss might suggest Addison's disease.

One of Foot's female exophthalmic goitre patients died suddenly,

---

[10] Foot, 'Two Cases of Graves' Disease', *ibid.* (1880); 70: 452–8.

[11] Foot's accounts in September 1873 of malignant axillary glands, and of a sarcoma, are supported by histological diagnosis. And yet, submitting a myoma of the prostate gland to the Dublin Pathological Society he said that the specimen conformed so closely to the descriptions of Virchow and Billroth that 'he had not thought it necessary to examine it microscopically'. *Ibid.,* (1880); 70: 68

[12] Foot, 'Graves' Disease', *Dublin J. Med. Sc.* (1893); 95: 131–48.

possibly due to digitalis toxicity. When the second autopsy revealed no abnormality of the cervical sympathetic Foot withdrew his support from the theory that attributed the disease to sympathetic nerve dysfunction, accepting now that if galvanisation helped it did so because 'it satisfied the patients that a great deal was being done on their behalf'. He gave adherence, instead, to Sattler, who postulated a lesion of the vaso-motor centres in the brainstem.

He encapsulated the history of the disease for the students: it was described by Graves in a lecture delivered at the Meath Hospital in the session 1834–5, and published in the *London Medical & Surgical Journal* in 1835. Von Basedow described it in 1840 as *Glotzaugenkrankheit* or 'the goggle-eye disease'. Earlier accounts are credited to an Italian, Flajani (1802), and Demours (1818). An English physician, Caleb Hillier Parry of Bath, had observed the disease in a woman aged thirty-seven in 1786 but his publication was posthumous (1825).

The clinical problem remained a mystery in Foot's lifetime. Enlightenment was slow to arrive. The seventh edition of Osler's *Principles and Practice of Medicine* (1909) still entertained the possibility that the disease was 'a pure neurosis', but favoured the view 'urged particularly by Moebius and by Greenfield, that Exophthalmic Goitre is primarily a disease of the thyroid gland'.[13]

Before leaving the subject it may be of interest to allude to certain major events in the history of hyperthyroidism, a term coined by Charles Mayo in 1907. Sir William Withey Gull's seminal paper 'On a Cretinoid State Supervening in Adult Life in Women' was published in 1873; four years later W. M. Ord introduced the term myxoedema. The technique of modern total thyroidectomy evolved in Austria and Switzerland where goitre was endemic in the mountains, but the Reverdins of Geneva, and Kocher of Berne, were appalled to find their patients developing a state which earned the name cachexia strumipriva.

William Smith Greenfield of Edinburgh, who had performed the postmortem examination of one of Ord's cases of myxoedema, was struck by the antithesis it presented to exophthalmic goitre. He advanced this viewpoint in his Bradshaw lecture (1893): 'In thus discussing Graves' disease, even provisionally as a disease of the thyroid gland rather than of the nervous system, I am aware that I am opposed to nearly all English and American physicians of eminence.' But in 1886 Paul Julius Moebius of Leipzig, who noted incomplete convergence of the eyes in exophthalmic goitre, had made a similar suggestion.

Knowledge of a system of endocrine glands was evolving at this time: Claude Bernard introduced the term 'internal secretion' in 1855; Edward

---

[13] William Osler, *The Principles and Practice of Medicine*, 7th ed., (London: Appleton, 1909), p. 765.

Schafer spoke on 'Internal Secretions' at the annual meeting of the British Medical Association in 1895; Ernest H. Starling coined the word 'hormone' for his Croonian lecture of 1905.

At the Mayo Clinic on Christmas Eve 1914, Edward Calvin Kendall crystalized and isolated 'iodine-A', which he later called 'thyroxin'. David Marine proved that iodine is essential for thyroid function, and used it in 1917 to prevent endemic goitre. His observation that cabbage contains goitregens led to a search for other inhibitory substances.

Subtotal thyroidectomy, facilitated by Plummer's introduction of pre-operative iodine, became acceptable treatment for hyperthyroidism in the first half of the present century, until effective medication was introduced. E. B. Astwood reported in 1943 successful treatment of hyperthyroidism at the Peter Bent Brigham Hospital, Boston, using thiourea or thiouracil. Thiourea, incidentally, was synthesised in Dublin in 1879 by James Emerson Reynolds, who was professor of chemistry and physics in the RCSI when he did this work.

As the century progressed, research techniques were refined and they multiplied. The use of paper chromatography enabled the separation of amino acids; investigators could trace the formation of thyroid hormones, and tri-iodothyronine was discovered. Radio-active iodine is a research tool and therapeutic agent.

Some fifty years after Foot's death, a form of hypothyroidism (Hashimoto's disease) was shown to result from an auto-immune process. Current evidence indicates that Graves' disease, too, is a genetically determined auto-immune disorder. An antibody behaving as thyroid-stimulating-hormone stimulates the gland, increasing secretion of thyroid hormones.

Chair of medicine

The amalgamation of the Carmichael College and the Ledwich School with the schools of surgery of the Royal College of Surgeons, led to Foot's election as professor of medicine in the RCSI. He shared his duties with Dr John William Moore. They held the chair jointly until 1895, when increasing ill-health compelled Foot to resign. At the College of Physicians, he held the offices of censor and vice-president.

The Biological Club

On 5 April 1892, Foot, one of the founders of the Dublin Biological Club, presented an account of the history of the club, the concept of which germinated in the minds of a small group of doctors who throughout 1871 met on Thursdays at Foot's house, 21 Lower Pembroke Street.

The Biological Club [he recalled] was formally inaugurated and christened in No. 30 T.C.D., north side of the Belfry-square, on Saturday evening, 6th of January, 1872. On that date a meeting was held there, at 8 p.m., 'to consider the expediency of forming a scientific club.' There were nine present at this meeting . . . Some others who had been invited to attend but were not present at this meeting . . . were co-opted with the nine others to form the original members, making fourteen in all.[14]

Foot spoke of three phases in the club's existence—*infancy* in Trinity College; *youth* in a room in Great Brunswick Street (now Pearse Street); *maturity* reached in the premises of the Royal College of Physicians, Kildare Street—and it may be added that the 'Bi' (sometimes called the 'Senior Bi' to distinguish it from a similarly named undergraduate society) still flourishes, meeting (and dining) in the Kildare Street University Club, St Stephen's Green.

> The club [Foot wrote], now in its twenty-first year, has lived down much vilification, and falsified many predictions. It was prophesied, over and over again, that it would soon fall to pieces, that so many dissentient interests could not cohere long. Instead of that, it seems to have the secret of perpetual youth—not alas individually, for some at least must say of themselves, *non sum qualis eram*. The secret lies in the fact of its being constantly recruited from the ranks of rising merit, and annually renovated with an infusion of the best and freshest blood.[15]

During the first phase, when a barrel of beer and a number of church-warden pipes were kept in a room reserved for the club, the contents of the barrel diminished from week to week with a speed unexpected by the modest drinkers. Nobody was so ungentlemanly as to challenge the 'skip', Tim O'Loughlin, directly, but many speculative explanations were offered. 'It is to be borne in mind [wrote Foot] that the solution of every mystery by a microbe had not been then invented, or perhaps a *Coccus beeriophilus* might have been discovered to be the culprit.'

On 21 November 1876, during the club's second phase, C. E. Brown-Séquard, nowadays recognised as the 'father of endocrinology', attended a meeting, introduced by Mr Robert M'Donnell. 'The illustrious visitor [noted Foot] expressed his approval of what he saw and

---

[14] Foot, 'Reminiscences of the Dublin Biological Club', *Dublin J. Med. Sc.*, (1892); 93: 425–41. The original members were: Edward Hallaran Bennett, James Adams Clarke, Edward Wolfenden Collins, George Frederick Duffey, Charles Edward Fitzgerald, Arthur Wynne Foot, Reuben Joshua Harvey, Thomas Evelyn Little, John William Moore, John Mallet Purser, Richard Rainsford, Henry Rosborough Swanzy, John Todhunter, Gerald Francis Yeo.

[15] *Ibid.*, p. 438.

heard, but made no allusion to the club about his *elixir vitae.*' Here Foot is guilty of a pardonable anachronism. Brown-Séquard's rejuvenation experiments with testicular extracts belong to a period later than the Dublin visit. Foot's throw-away remark, nevertheless, may indicate a lack of appreciation of the potential of the physiologist's research. Foot's own articles on exophthalmic goitre, as we have seen, do not show the least apprehension of that great discovery, the endocrine system, which lay just over the horizon.

Literary stylist

Foot married the eldest daughter of Mr Edward Hunt of Thomastown, County Kilkenny. Sir Lambert Ormsby's *History of the Meath Hospital*, published while the physician was still living observed: 'He is occasionally a little ascetic, is an ardent lover of natural history, fond of taking long country walks, reads and smokes a great deal, and is considered the best read physician in Dublin.'[16] Cameron, with Foot's prolific contributions to medical literature in mind, referred to their erudition and beauty of style;[17] Moore, too, was impressed by their masterly originality, 'written in singularly clear, beautiful, and what may be called *nervous* English'. This is particularly evident in the earnest, if humourless, addresses he delivered in the Meath Hospital at the opening of the academic year in 1885 and 1887.[18] These re-echo the message to the students at the Ledwich School in 1873, promoting diligence, excellence and the necessity to gain clinical knowledge.

> The hospital is your school of experience. It is for each of you a garden of the Hesperides, into which you may at any time enter and pluck the golden apples from the laden boughs. Though the dragon of responsibility is there he will not meddle with you. It is your teachers he keeps his eyes on.[19]

Aware of 'the vocabulary of depreciation' used to ridicule the annual ceremony, Foot selected words that were simple but striking, to impress upon the students the magnitude of their opportunity.

> The object of your study here is Disease in all its relationships, meaning by disease every deviation from the normal condition of the body, either as regards its structure or its function—in other words, the object of your coming here is to learn the Art of how to heal, cure, or minister relief to men, women, or children who may have come to harm from sickness,

---

[16] Ormsby, *History of the Meath*, (note 1), p. 147.
[17] Cameron, *History of the RCSI*, (note 1), p. 595.
[18] He delivered this address in 1871, 1873, 1874, 1877, 1881, 1885, 1887.
[19] Foot, 'Address at the Opening of the Session 1885–6', *Dublin J. Med. Sc.*, (1885); 80: 386–98.

accident, or any other bodily or mental calamity. An endless panorama of disease will pass before your eyes in the wards of this or any other large general hospital, affording realistic presentation of all the ills that flesh is heir to.[20]

Their choice of profession meant that the great problems of existence—birth and death—would be constantly before them, and they must become inured to spectacles that others would view with awe and horror. The learned and the powerful would defer to their opinions, but they would find themselves 'in situations which would draw tears down from the iron cheeks of Pluto'.

He cited Richard Bright and Thomas Addison as examples of men who earned success by attention to minutiae.

> Of Addison we are told that he never reasoned from a half discovered fact, but would remain at the bedside with a dogged determination to track out the disease to its *very* source for a period which constantly wearied his class and attendant friends. So severely did he tax his mind with the minutest details bearing upon the exact exposition of a case, that he has been known to startle the sister of the ward in the middle of the night by his presence. After going to bed with the case present to his mind, some point of what he considered important detail in reference to it occurred to him, and he could not rest until he had cleared it up.[21]

Foot did not pretend that a career in medicine was an easy option.

> I cannot take you up into a high mountain, and show you a promised land of ease and affluence, a land flowing with milk and honey, as a comfort for the evening of your days. To draw such a picture for you would be to cheat your eyes with a mirage, which, when you would seem to be near its confines, would recede still further from your gaze. When Dupuytren was urged to relax his incessant labours, his answer was, *'le repos, c'est la mort!'* Death is the only rest for many medical men; hence, so many of them die in harness—their harness is their uniform, their decoration, their ornament, and they lay it aside only at the bidding of the great Commander. The memorable reply of Dupuytren was not dictated by any necessity to work from pecuniary reasons, for, although at seventeen he was so poor that he had to mend his own clothes, he was afterwards in a position to offer his sovereign, Charles the Tenth, a loan of a million of francs.[22]

Not, indeed, that they could all expect to work in large and pop-

---

[20] *Ibid.*, p. 389.
[21] Foot, 'An Address delivered in the Theatre of the Meath Hospital, 1887–88', *Dublin J. Med. Sc.* (1887); 84: 442–57.
[22] *Ibid.*, p. 454.

ulous centres. Many would join 'the sturdy, warm-hearted, self-sacrificing band of country practitioners' whom Sir Walter Scott had praised for their courage, humanity and professional skill.

Death

Professor Foot was summoned widely in consultation, throughout the country, by former pupils who had worked close to him at the Meath. They idolized him, knowing his worth as a resourceful clinician, his courage in the presence of infection, his instinctive sympathy for the ill. He did not, however, enjoy a large private practice for reasons discernable in the obituary notice written by his friend and colleague Sir John William Moore. Obituarists generally observe the maxim *de mortuis nil nisi bonum* and if constrained, as evidently Moore was, to refer to personality quirks that could not be passsed over, these angularities must have been pronounced.

He was often misunderstood, and the keenness of his intellect coupled with a satiric vein sometimes alienated those whose grasp of medicine was less philosophic, and who approached its practice in a less reverent spirit and a more matter-of-fact fashion. Sham, quackery and cant Foot utterly abhorred, and those who coquetted with such doubtful methods of professional advancement sometimes came under the lash of his epigrammatic sarcasm.[23]

After some years of increasing incapacity,[24] Arthur Wynne Foot sustained a cerebral haemorrhage on 1 September 1900 and died a few hours later. He was then living at 49 Lower Leeson Street where his wife survived him. He left no issue.

---

[23] Moore, 'In Memoriam', (note 3), p. 336.
[24] As Moore states that the malady was 'locomotor ataxy, associated with repeated attacks of haemorrhage due to sclerosis of the arterial system', it is apparent that the obituarist uses the term locomotor ataxy literally rather than with any aetiological connotation, just as Foot himself referred to locomotor ataxy with recovery in diphtheria.

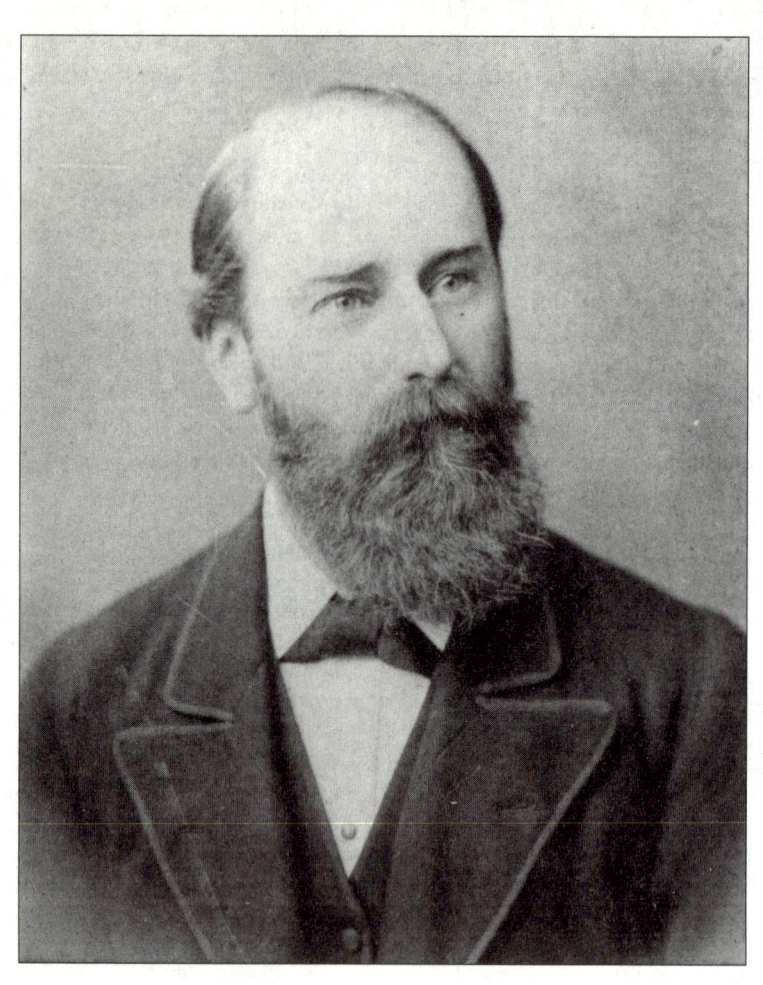

John William Moore in his prime

Chapter 9: Sir John William Moore, 1845–1937

Sir John William Moore, a major contributor to Irish medicine, lacks the full biography he so richly deserves: after his death in 1937 within weeks of his ninety-second birthday, William Doolin[1] who had known him personally presented a vignette of 'that bent figure, with kindly voice and smiling eyes'; more recently, on the occasion of the celebration of the centenary of the Royal Academy of Medicine in Ireland (the resolution that led to its foundation was moved by Moore on a November evening in 1882) C. S. Breathnach's account of Sir John was published in the *Irish Journal of Medical Science* which under an earlier title, the *Dublin Journal of Medical Science*, Moore had edited for forty-seven years.[2] He had been William Stokes's last house-physician, and the great physician's immediate successor on the staff of the Meath Hospital.

Moore was lecturer in medicine at the Carmichael School from 1875. When this school, together with the Ledwich School (the last two surviving private schools), amalgamated with the RCSI in December 1888, rearrangements of staff led to Moore's appointment to the chair of medicine (1889–1916) which for a time he held jointly with A. W. Foot. When well into his eighties he was still physician to the Meath, adding to the general air of antiquity that impressed 'Bob' Collis who joined it in 1930. Entering the mid-morning board room, the paediatrician wondered if he was in an eighteenth-century coffee house. The matron, with a pair of silver sugar-tongs in hand, presided over the cups like a grande dame prior to the French Revolution, while Sir John Moore explained to one of the younger doctors 'something important in the construction of Greek irregular verbs'.[3]

Birth and education

Born on 23 October 1845 at 7 South Anne Street, an area then favoured by tailors, milliners and boot-makers, into a family of Anglo-Irish stock, John William Moore was the eldest child (and elder son) of Dr William Daniel Moore (1813–71),[4] an exceptionally cultured Dublin general

---

[1] William Doolin, 'Sir John William Moore', *Irish J. Med. Sc.* (1937): 654.
[2] C. S. Breathnach, 'John William Moore', *ibid.* (1983); 152: 69–72.
[3] Robert Collis, *To Be a Pilgrim* (London: Secker & Warburg, 1975), p. 72.
[4] William Daniel Moore, LAH, Dublin (1833), LRCS Edin. (1836), MB, TCD (1843), sometime apothecary to the Institute for Diseases of Children in Pitt Street, was born in Dublin in 1813. His flair for languages prompted him to publish many translations, particularly from Scandinavian journals. He also translated Schroeder van der Kolk's essays on the central nervous system for the New Sydenham Society. He was an honorary member

practitioner who was an excellent linguist, and his wife Catherine Mary Montserrat. Christopher Moore, his grandfather, was governor of the Apothecaries Hall; a great-grandfather died in his ninety-seventh year. The earlier ancestors had lived in Ballymahon, County Longford, and in Lancashire.

The boy was educated at the High School, 76 St Stephen's Green South, proceeding to Trinity College. 'A Scholar of the House in Classics in 1865, a Bachelor in Medicine and a Master in Surgery in 1868, a Doctor in Medicine in 1871 of the University of Dublin, he was admitted a Licentiate of the College of Physicians in 1870 and elected a Fellow in 1873.'[5] (The Moores had moved meanwhile to 40 Fitzwilliam Square West, where after his father's death in 1871 from progressive atrophy John William continued to reside and practise.) We have no information about his seven siblings[6] other than the fact that a sister became lady superintendent of the Children's Hospital, Fisherwick Place, Belfast.

At the Meath Hospital in 1865, the young doctor had the good fortune to come under the influence of William Stokes, the celebrated author of *A Treatise on the Diagnosis and Treatment of Diseases of the Chest* (1837) and *The Diseases of the Heart and the Aorta* (1854), and was wise enough to recognise an ideal mentor. 'Those who have seen Dr. Stokes at the bedside of the sick, know how gentle, how refined, how kindly was his bearing towards the patient. Amid all the ardour of clinical observation and research, he never for one moment forgot the sufferer before him—no thoughtless word from his lips, no rough or unkind action ever ruffled the calm confidence reposed in him by those who sought his skill and care.'[7]

Another of his instructors was 'the lynx-eyed' Alfred Hudson. 'He was a master of physical diagnosis; his eye, his touch, and his ear had come to detect signs so slight that they escaped less cultivated senses. Working at the bedsides of the sick from the very beginning of his medical training, and gathering his impressions of disease as much from nature as from books, he displayed in obscure and doubtful cases a singular capacity for diagnosis.'[8]

Moore credited William Stokes with the creation of a diploma of state medicine in TCD (later called the diploma in public health), the

---

of many foreign medical societies.
[5] T. P. C. Kirkpatrick, 'Admission of Sir John William Moore as Honorary Fellow of the Royal Academy of Medicine in Ireland', *Irish J. Med. Sc.* (1935): 133–6.
[6] They were Eleanor Marion, Sydney Jane, Catherine Mary, Charles Johnson (curate of St James' Parish Church, Louth, Lincs), Elizabeth Ruth, Margaret Schröder, Kathleen Marianne.
[7] J. W. Moore, 'In Memoriam: William Stokes', *Dublin J. Med. Sc.*, (1878); LVV: 186–200.
[8] See note 2, Chapter 7.

first of its kind in the United Kingdom: 'He was one of the earliest, ablest, and most disinterested advocates of the doctrines of State Medicine. For many years he used all his powers of mind, and eloquence, and writing, to promulgate and advance these doctrines.'[9] When the examination for the diploma was first held in June 1871 there were, as mentioned in the previous chapter, four successful candidates, Foot, Moore, Todhunter and Yeo.

Hospital appointments

On Stokes' retirement from the Meath Hospital in April 1875, Dr Moore filled the vacancy, but the informal manner in which the appointment was made offended the *Medical Press & Circular*, earning its disapproval.

> Dr. Moore has, though not long entered on his profession distinguished himself already as an ardent worker in science, a physician of great promise and a man of high culture, and it is to be regretted that his appointment to the Meath—which, of itself, would receive unqualified approval should be shadowed by the fact of its being an uncontested 'walk over.' The method of his appointment does credit neither to Dr. Moore nor to the hospital, and must be unqualifiedly condemned as constituting a bad precedent.[10]

It is unlikely that either the Meath Hospital or its new physician paid much attention to the journal's strictures. Dublin's voluntary hospitals generally tended to follow their own counsels when making appointments. By now Moore was also physician to the Molyneux Asylum for Blind Females, and to the Fever Hospital and House of Recovery in Cork Street, a post he was to hold for thirteen years. Later (1875) he became physician to the Coombe Lying-in Hospital.

He was quick to affirm his position at the Meath by publishing 'Cases under the care of J. W. Moore' in the *Dublin Journal of Medical Science*. He described two unusual cases of enteric (typhoid) fever: the first, a twenty-two-year-old maid-servant, developed bullae on the abdomen followed by phlegmasia affecting the right leg; the second, a school-boy, presented the clinical features of macculated typhus while recovering from typhoid. 'On the fourth day a weakening of the heart necessitated the use of wine. I began with marsala, but on the seventh day I changed it for eight ounces of port.'[11] His co-physician at the Meath was Arthur Wynne Foot; the surgeons were Rawdon Macnamara, L. H. Ormsby, R. Persse White, G. H. Porter, P. C. Smyly and J. H. Wharton.

---

[9] Moore 'In Memoriam', (note 7), p. 196.
[10] *Med. Press & Circ.* (1875); 19: 307.
[11] Moore, 'Meath Hospital, Dublin, Cases under the care of J. W. Moore', *Dublin J. Med. Sc.* (1875); 60: 277–82.

Fever

Smallpox accounted for 1,509 of the 2,151 patients admitted to Cork Street Fever Hospital in the year ending 31 March 1879. That dreaded disease, in epidemic form, was responsible for 357 of the 447 deaths. It was apparent that vaccination did not confer complete immunity (and should be repeated after some years), but a discrete form of illness was likely to be seen in vaccinated patients, in whom the mortality rate was significantly lower.[12] Typhus fever (134 cases) and scarlatina (71 cases) caused twenty-five and twenty-two deaths respectively. There were sixty cases of enteric fever, with five deaths; and forty-two cases of measles with nine deaths. Two of the four cases of meningitis died.

Moore's next report for the fever hospital refers to new observation wards. In the year ending 31 March 1881 there had been an epidemic of typhus, 420 cases of which were admitted; the cause of the disease was still unknown.

> It is hard to resist the conclusion that the history of the outbreak might be sketched in this way:—A population impoverished and depressed by a prolonged epidemic of smallpox discovered an unusual receptivity to the poison of typhus, which, if not generated, was at all events spread in the North Dublin Union, where presumably many widows of the victims of smallpox found refuge during a season of unparalleled and general distress. The epidemic was held in check in the summer and autumn of 1880, but rapidly developed in intensity when an early and severe winter favoured the spread of infection, owing to diminished ventilation, and a depression of the vital powers.[13]

In the report for the year ending 31 March 1882, Moore explained that ordinarily the task of compiling the report should have fallen to a colleague, but on the night of 28 December 1881 Dr Reuben Joshua Harvey had died in the prime of life, on the tenth day of petechial typhus acquired while attending a recent case of the disease.

Moore's next report, his patience worn thin, ventilated what was obviously a chronic cause for dissatisfaction: the referral of persons already in extremis. He cited a forty-year-old married woman sent in with typhus on the *fifteenth* day of the illness, to die a few days later. 'At the time, I expressed the opinion that a patient . . . so far advanced in typhus of a severe type could not be safely moved to hospital, and should have been treated and nursed at home.' She was a dispensary patient, and the board of guardians should have arranged to provide a nurse for her. The complaint in due course reached the dispensary doctor who defended himself,

---

[12] Moore, *ibid*, (1879); 68: 24–52.
[13] Moore, 'Medical Report of Cork Street Fever Hospital', *ibid*. (1881); 72: 19.

without explaining the delay in referral. 'I could not at all approve the proposal that fever cases should be retained in their own tenements and nurses obtained for them at the expense of the rates; the other inhabitants of the tenements being turned out, would be most likely to carry infection into other houses.'[14]

Moore saw scarlatina as 'a plague among children of the poorer classes'. He described how when walking from the Meath Hospital to Cork Street he stopped a woman who was carrying a delicate-looking child, and asked her what was wrong with it. Inspecting the mite more closely he saw it was 'peeling'. He told her to go straight to the Fever Hospital. 'Unfortunately, I saw no more of mother or child.'

His propensity to offer advice freely in the public interest is also illustrated by his action on another occasion, when soon after arriving at a hotel in Ryde on the Isle of Wight, Moore heard the unmistakable 'whoop' of pertussis. On enquiry he learned 'that a child suffering from this most catching complaint had been brought for a change of air to the hotel which was crowded, and in which the children of the landlord were living'.

Private hospitals

Speaking in the academy on 19 April 1895 he voiced his disapproval of the 'veritable mushroom growth' of private hospitals in the capital and many provincial towns.

> These institutions [he said] have been started by individual physicians or surgeons, or by a few members of the Medical Profession acting in 'partnership by deed or otherwise,' or by an experienced and fully trained hospital-nurse, or by one or more benevolent ladies without any very special training in sick-nursing. In fact, it seems as though people thought that anyone at all was quite competent 'to run' a private hospital, and that so praiseworthy an ambition should be indulged without let or hindrance.[15]

A house in a noisy, dusty or muddy street, possibly built in the last century as a private residence, was touched up with paper and paint, clean curtains and blinds were fitted 'and—hey presto!—there is our private hospital'. He himself had attended a patient with typhoid in a back drawing-room, while another of his patients with nephritis occupied the front drawing-room, and every sound produced in one room was heard in the other. As a rule there was no management committee; the private hospitals enjoyed 'irresponsible, but reprehensible freedom from governmental, municipal or philantrophic control'.

---

[14] Moore, 'Medical Report of Cork Street Fever Hospital', *ibid.* (1884); 78: 121–130.
[15] Moore, 'Private Hospitals, or Home Hospitals', *ibid.*, (1895); 99: 388–94.

His attack was listened to unsympathetically by Sir William Stokes, FRCSI, who disagreed with him, saying he used at least five private hospitals, and had performed major operations in them quite satisfactorily. Dr Alfred Parsons, too, felt they had to make the best of what they had.

Mens medica

Moore chose 'The Achievement of the Mens Medica' as the subject of an address, on 9 October 1899 at the Meath Hospital where recent improvements included an isolation ward, an extension to the laundry, and a modern operation theatre suited to the triumphs of aseptic surgery. Medical advances included the Widal diagnostic test for enteric fever, and diphtheria anti-toxin.

Speaking directly to the students he said:

> The best physician is the man who, daily witnessing the havoc wrought around him by the hand of Death, from his experience forms the habit of acting with a constant view to death, and develops the earnest desire to shield from its stroke the sick entrusted to his care. 'Perception of distress in others', writes Bishop Butler in *The Analogy of Religion*, 'is a natural excitement passively to pity, and actively to relieve it; but let a man set himself to attend, inquire out, and relieve distressed persons, and he cannot but grow less and less sensibly affected with the various miseries of life, with which he must become acquainted; when yet, at the same time, benevolence, considered not as a passion but as a practical principle of action, will strengthen, and whilst he passively compassionates the distressed less, he will acquire a greater aptitude actively to assist and befriend them.'
>
> This is the 'Mens Medica', which endows the true physician with the God-like power of healing. His compassion, observation, experience, reason, and learning are all enlisted in a self-denying and supreme effort to combat disease and to ward off death.[16]

The 'Mens Medica', he told them, was not to be easily won. It was the Golden Fleece which they, the Argonauts, must win after many trials and perils.

He commended to them, on another occasion, the writings of his contemporary William Osler (whom Moore nominated as honorary FRCPI), which stressed the vital part played by the patient in medical education: 'In what may be called the natural method of teaching the student begins with the patient, continues with the patient and ends his studies with the patient, using books and lectures as tools, as means to an end.'[17] Moore also mentioned Clifford Albutt's *Notes on the Composition*

---

[16] Moore, 'The Achievement of the Mens Medica', *Dublin J. Med. Sc.*, 1899; 108: 372–83.
[17] William Osler, 'The Hospital as a College', address to the Academy of Medicine, New York, 1903.

of Scientific Papers, and warned students against the use of false Latin plurals. 'Such words as "sera", "sanatoria", "curricula", and so on, simply show an ignorance of the Latin language, and should be shunned.'[18]

Being receptive to developments in all branches of medicine, he was impressed by Professor John Joly's lecture on radium on 2 October 1914, and in consultation with Dr Walter Stevenson arranged for a patient under his care at the Meath, with an inoperable cancer of the womb, to be treated with radium. There was a decided improvement, and Moore reported that his patient returned to her home in County Kildare— 'driving off in state' in a taxi which her sons provided.

A younger colleague, T. G. Moorhead, has referred to Moore's value as a member of the many committees to which he was eventually elected. 'He always attended regularly, and took care to be acquainted with whatever business was on hand. He was much learned in precedents, and was a great stickler for procedure, always insisting that everything should be done decently and in order.' As a classical scholar he was painstaking, not to say pedantic, concerning pronunciation of words derived from Greek and Latin. A polyglot, he learned the Scandinavian languages mastered by his father, and believing that as editor of the *Dublin Journal of Medical Science* he should be able to read all the journals which reached him, he equipped himself to do so.

Publications

Richard Hayes[19] credits Moore with 169 articles in Irish periodicals to which must be added his books, *Textbook of the Eruptive and Continued Fevers* (1892), *Meteorology, Practical and Applied* (1894), and scattered publications in English journals. Such an immense body of work cannot be reviewed here comprehensively but it is clear that his principal interests were infectious diseases, state medicine (community health) and meteorology. His first contribution to the *Dublin Quarterly Journal of Medical Science*—'Note on "Mean temperature in its relation to disease and mortality"'—was published in August 1869; sixty-three years later his 'Introductory address delivered at the opening of the session, Meath Hospital, Dublin', appeared in the *Irish Journal of Medical Science*, in October 1932. His longevity placed him in a position to provide 'In Memoriams' for a long line of colleagues, including his mentor, Dr William Stokes; Robert M'Donnell; Aquilla Smith; Sir William Stokes who died from typhoid fever in the Boer War; John Todhunter who forsook medicine for poetry, prompting John Butler Yeats to say that if he were a true poet he would have remained a doctor; Richard Lane Joynt, a pio-

---

[18] Moore, 'Clinical Case-Taking', *Med. Press & Circ.* (1905); 80: 398–401.

[19] Richard J. Hayes, (ed.), *Sources for the History of Irish Civilisation*, vol. 3 (Boston, Mass., 1970).

neer in radiology; and many others.[20]

His obituaries of Queen Victoria (1901) and King Edward VII (1910) should also be mentioned, if only as confirmation of his unquestioning support of the establishment. An exemplary Victorian, he mourned the passing of 'the womanly Queen and queenly Woman who was privileged in God's good providence to rule the destinies of the British Empire for more than three-and-sixty years'. He mentioned medical advances that had appeared in her reign: anaesthesia ('the Queen herself took chloroform at her last confinement'), antiseptic surgery, bacteriology, preventive medicine, the reform of nursing and other benefits.

Edward VII, according to Moore, 'had suffered for years from pulmonary emphysema', aggravated by 'smoker's throat' and causing heart-failure. Earlier illnesses included enteric fever in 1871, and 'perityphilitis' [appendicitis] in 1902 on the eve of his coronation. A fractured patella in 1898 was diagnosed as the result of 'a Rontgen-ray photograph'. In the course of his presidential address to the seventh international congress of hygiene and demography in London in 1891, Edward, then Prince of Wales, asked 'the now famous epigrammatic question—"If preventable, why not prevented?"'

Book reviews were usually unsigned in the *Dublin Journal of Medical Science* and it was a measure of Moore's enthusiasm that he added his name to his notice of T. H. Parke's *My Personal Experiences in Equatorial Africa* (1891). 'We have read this book from cover to cover', he began, whetting readers' appetites with an outline of an incredible journey undertaken for the relief of the enigmatic Emin Pasha. And in conclusion: 'we have a warrantable pride in reflecting that it was an Irishman—an Irish physician and surgeon—who played a hero's part . . . and shed a fresh lustre upon the medical profession.'[21]

Tragedy

The fairy-godmother who appears to have presided over John William Moore's birth, seemed still to have been in attendance on 4 January 1876 when the thirty-one-year-old doctor married Ellie Ridley in St Stephen's Church. It was a stylish wedding and the twenty-one-year-old bride, a doctor's daughter from Tullamore, must have quite happily taken over

---

[20] Moore also wrote obituaries for Sir George Porter, Thomas W. Grimshaw, William Moore, Henry G. Croly, Sir George F. Duffey, Sir Philip Smyly, Austin Meldon, Sir John Banks, Sir Arthur V. Macan, Gerald Yeo, Sir Francis Cruise, Arthur H. Benson, Sir Henry Swanzy, Sir Christopher Nixon, Sir Charles Bent Ball, Charles Edward FitzGerald, Frederic Kidd, Sir James Acheson MacCullagh, Charles Molyneux Benson, Richard Dancer Purefoy, Sir Arthur Chance, Sir John Hawtrey Benson.

[21] Moore, review of T. H. Parke's *My Personal Experiences in Equatorial Africa*, *Dublin J. Med. Science* (1892); 93: 386–94. See also J. B. Lyons, *Surgeon Major Parke's African Journey 1887–89* (Dublin: Lilliput Press, 1994).

the running of her husband's large house in Fitzwilliam Square, where lawyers were then more numerous than doctors. It was there that her baby daughter was born on 9 April 1878, but tragedy struck and Ellie Moore paid the price not uncommonly demanded of nineteenth-century mothers, but exceptionally ironic when involving the family of a specialist in fevers. The widower re-married on 15 March 1881; his second wife, Louisa Emma Armstrong was to survive him with their family—a son, Surgeon-Commander Maurice Sydney Moore, RN, and three daughters. Two sons predeceased him: William Edmund Armstrong (1882–*c.* 1922); Arthur Robert, MC (1883–1917) died of wounds.[22]

Editor

Moore assisted Dr James Little in 1873 as editor of the *Dublin Journal of Medical Science*, and in the following year he took over the editorial chair which he held until replaced by Arnold K. Henry in 1920. He was consulting physician to Drumcondra Hospital from 1889. Having served as vice-president (1881–2), and registrar (1882–91), he was president of the Royal College of Physicians of Ireland from 1898 to 1900, in which year he was knighted. Sir John represented the RCPI on the General Medical Council from 1903 to 1933, and he was a founder member of the Association of Physicians of Great Britain and Ireland in 1907. The honours bestowed on him included the honorary D.Sc of Oxford University (1904), the honorary LL.D. NUI (1933), and the honorary fellowship of the Royal Academy of Medicine in Ireland (1935). He had been president of the academy since 1918 after many years as a vice-president and secretary for foreign correspondence.

Infectious diseases

The chasm separating the 'miasmaists' from the 'contagionists' has been referred to earlier. Moore was fortunate to commence his studies at a time when the problem of infection was being put on a scientific basis. Editing William Stokes's *Lectures on Fever* (1874), he felt obliged to concede this was 'the least happy' of the great physician's publications, being largely devoted to the advocacy of the no longer tenable belief of a common identity for typhus and typhoid fevers. 'At first it is not easy to understand how so accurate and admirable an observer as Dr. Stokes failed at once and completely to isolate these two forms of continued fever. But it is probable that the admixture of cases of both fevers in the

---

[22] The medical line continues through Maurice Moore, MD (1886–1972), whose sons, John and Richard are doctors. When Richard Moore (b. 1930), MB, FRCCGP, visited the Mercer Library in 1998 he was delighted to find his beloved grandfather, whom he used to visit in childhood, so well remembered. Richard has a son, James (MB FRCGP) and a daughter, Jane (MB MRCOG) in the profession.

same wards, without any attempt at isolation of those suffering from typhus, led to the frequent occurrence of typhus in typhoid patients, and to the all but necessary confusing of the two diseases.[23]

Seeking a subject for the opening address at the Meath Hospital in the autumn of 1879, Moore decided it would be 'neither uninteresting nor uninstructive' were he to speak on 'The Microcosm of Disease' and discuss what were variously called 'Zymotic disease', 'blood-poisoning', 'germ theory of disease' etc.[24] At the appointed hour he conducted his audience to the most active frontier of medicine, illuminating a sombre area with lamps lighted by Pasteur, Koch, Klebs and others.

> It is now many years since the terms 'Zymosis' and 'Zymotic Diseases' were reintroduced into medical nomenclature. In the first instance, these words which were derived from the Greek, 'leaven', were employed to denote a class of diseases, the process of development of which was regarded as analogus to the vinous fermentation. In this form of fermentation, as is well known, the introduction of the yeast plant—a microscopic fungus called *torula cerevisiae*—into a saccharine fluid causes the conversion of the sugar contained in such a fluid into alcohol and carbonic dioxide or carbonic acid. The yeast plant itself flourishes and multiplies provided it meets with a suitable soil, containing nitrogenous elements to supply it with nutriment. Now, in certain diseases there is good reason to believe that minute living bodies or organisms—called 'microzymes' by Dr. Burdon Sanderson, 'microdemes' by Dr. Billings, and less accurately 'bacteria' by many writers—if introduced into the blood are capable, *under certain circumstances*, of inducing a process of fermentation accompanied by the formation of a poison or virus, which in turn produces in each disease a special train of symptoms.[25]

The 'Malignant Pustule' was now known to be caused by the *Bacillus anthracis* and in 1876 Koch had shown the existence of spores which having resisted extinction for years gave rise to a new generation of organisms. Almost unbelievable, perhaps, and yet not any more wonderful than changes accepted to take place in seeds, in animal ova and in roots, changes referred to by Robert Graves.

> 'Thus,' says Dr. Graves, 'the curious fact has been observed of a bulbous root, taken from the hand of an Egyptian mummy, having germinated when placed in the soil. How happened it that this bulb remained for several thousand years in contact with the fingers of death, without its own vital principle being either extinguished or called into active operation? What power at once preserved that principle and held it in abeyance? And yet so it was. And age after age passed away without summoning into action that wondrous

---

[23] Moore, 'In Memoriam', (note 7).
[24] Moore, 'The Microcosm of Disease', *Dublin J. Med. Sc.* (1879); 68: 370–86.
[25] *Ibid.*, p. 372.

spell which could thus convert this long-enduring tenant of the tomb into the lily of the field, the Scriptural emblem of beauty, and the honoured type of the glories of vegetable life, beside the purity and brightness of whose hues even the raiment of Solomon appeared dull and faded.'[26]

Relapsing fever is caused by a spirillum, smallpox by infective particles so minute 'that they can be readily diffused through a fluid or remain suspended in the air for a considerable time, like the tiny motes seen floating in a sunbeam'.[27] The contagia responsible for measles and scarlatina had not yet been isolated. Septicaemia ('Blood-poisoning') though 'an ever-present danger especially in surgical and puerperal cases', could be prevented in most instances.

The practical importance of these researches, Moore emphasized, was that they made prophylaxis possible, but in saying so he evidently felt it necessary to placate a minority group.

> It is true [he said] there are some men even at the present day—conscientious, intelligent, and otherwise well-informed men—who object to the use of such a phrase as 'Preventable Disease' on the ground that it is—to say the least—irreverent. They point to that close analogy which exists between the moral nature and the physical nature of man, both subject to laws which cannot be broken or violated with impunity. Any infringement of the Divine Moral Law is followed by spiritual disease and death. No less certainly will the violation of the equally Divine Physical Law, subject to which we live and move and have our being, be followed by bodily diesase and death. 'The soul that sinneth, it shall die!' Ah, yes, but do those who use this argument, so solemnly, so fatally true, forget the glorious antithesis—God is *not willing* that *any* should perish'? And so I believe that every earnest effort made to prevent disease, and the misery it brings in its train, has the Divine sanction and approval.[28]

Aware of the undesirability of prolonged detention of patients in hospital, Moore emphasised the necessity of adequate isolation of convalescents to prevent the spread of disease. 'The convalescent . . . must be kept separate until the days of his purification are accomplished—in the words of the Mosaic law, "He shall dwell alone; without the camp shall his habitation be."' [190] The only answer to the problem, Moore believed, was the provision of properly designed, rate-supported convalescent homes for patients recovering from smallpox, scarlatina, typhus and measles. Unapologetically, he advocated the costly measure of building

---

[26] R. J. Graves, *Studies in Physiology and Medicine*, ed. William Stokes (London: Churchill, 1863), p. 211.
[27] Moore, review of Parks, *Dublin J. Med. Science* (1892); 93: p. 382.
[28] Moore, *ibid*, p. 384.

convalescent homes on airy sites outside towns: 'In one scale of the balance lies the gold and the silver—in the other are precious lives of fathers, mothers, children rescued from disease, or, it may be death. Can we doubt for a moment to which side of the beam the balance will incline?'

Tuberculin

Koch, the German scientist who in 1882 isolated the tubercle bacillus, the cause of tuberculosis, announced a cure for the disease at the Tenth International Congress of Medicine in Berlin in 1890. This was sensational, and soon patients and doctors were flocking to Germany, the former seeking the miraculous remedy the latter hoping to study Koch's newly-developed therapy. But sadly it emerged that the bacteriologist had been pressurised into making a premature claim before his 'lymph' (later called Tuberculin) was adequately tested. Virchow revealed damning evidence of pneumonic extension, and in cases who had died miliary spread was demonstrated.

Moore was one of many Dublin doctors who started therapeutic trials, urged to do so by Sir William Stokes who after visiting Berlin lectured on Koch's method at the Meath on 5 December 1890. Reporting the condition of six treated cases to the Academy of Medicine on 30 January 1891, Moore said that even in small doses Koch's fluid produced severe constitutional and local symptoms; it did have diagnostic value; its use in advanced phthisis was inadmissable; in early pulmonary tuberculosis 'there is reason to believe that its use is beneficial'.[29]

This preliminary report was made 'without prejudice, and in a calm, philosophic spirit'; but speaking on 'Tuberculosis: its Prevention and Cure' at the British Medical Association's annual meeting in Carlisle on 31 July 1896, Moore said that Koch's premature announcement had aroused 'a wave of enthusiasm which was doomed swiftly to spend itself in a reaction almost of despair'.[30]

In the decennial period 1871–80 phthisis was a major cause of mortality in Ireland, causing 103,528 deaths; it was far commoner in Belfast and the North Dublin Union than in 'the storm-swept wilds of Belmullet Union, Co. Mayo'. Preventive measures included bright, airy houses protected against damp—sunlight sustains the man and kills the microbe—exercise to ventilate the lungs, hygienic disposal of sputum. 'By any, or by all means—*Delenda sunt Sputa!*'

Prior to the availability of x-rays, the early diagnosis of consumption was an onerous responsibility. Moore lists signs that no longer remain in medical textbooks: the 'tuberculous red line along the gums'; myotatic

---

[29] Moore, 'A Series of Six Cases of Pulmonary Disease Treated by Koch's Method', *Dublin J. Med. Sc.* (1891); 91: 205–12.
[30] Moore, 'Tuberculosis: its Prevention and Cure', *ibid.* (1896); 102: 290–320.

irritability of the pectoral muscles; 'cogwheel inspiration'; apical tenderness. Milk, eggs, butchers' meat and fish should form the staple diet of the consumptive, and cod-liver oil was a useful additive. Asses' milk and goats' milk were favoured by some. The climatic treatment of tuberculosis was expensive, and limited to those who could pay for it; one of Moore's patients, a Dublin barrister, spent two winters at Davos, and was cured.

At that period, Moore seemed relatively indifferent to the notification of tuberculosis: it appeared in so many forms; it was generally chronic and disinfection would be purposeless while the invalid continued to occupy the same room or dwelling. He was increasingly unhappy, however, with the practice of treating active tuberculosis in the wards of the Meath Hospital: 'Year by year the conviction grows stronger that in treating this fell disease in the wards of a general hospital we are committing a grave hygienic error.' The consumptive may infect others; he occupies a bed month after month that could have been used for a succession of other patients; the air and the diet may not suit him. The solution lay in the provision of special wards for tuberculosis; sanatoriums and refuges for those dying from the disease.[31]

Between 1874 and 1883 inclusive, 738 patients with scarlatina were admitted to Cork Street Hospital and the epidemics obeyed 'the law of seasonal prevalence', increasing in the second half of the year, attaining a maximum in the December quarter, then decreasing. Mortality was higher in epidemics and in young children. 'In some cases life was extinguished almost in a few hours by the malignancy of the fever poison.' Nephritis was a common complication.[32]

Text-book

In the spring of 1891, Moore lectured on fevers to the 'Jubilee Nurses'. Having compiled a set of notes for the purpose, it seemed natural to a man of his literary gifts to extend his 'important and fascinating theme' in a *Text-Book of Eruptive and Continued Fevers* (1892).[33] This is an unrecognised classic, presenting vivid depictions of diseases no longer known to most doctors, rich in aphorisms and recollections of the teachings of Corrigan, Graves and Stokes. It is also an etymological gem; reviewing it in the *Medical Press & Circular*, Dr John Knott suggested that the polyglot author 'was probably inspired by the Muse of Fever on the day of Pentecost'.[34]

The constantly-menacing diseases were palpable occasions of shock

---

[31] Moore, *Dublin J. Med. Sc.* (1899); 108: 381.
[32] Moore, 'The Present Epidemic of Scarlet Fever', *ibid.* (1884); 77: 364.
[33] Moore, *Text-Book of Eruptive and Continued Fevers* (Dublin: Fannin, 1892).
[34] [John Knott] *Medical Press & Circ.* (1892); 105: 226–7.

and mystery to all concerned. Typhus—'the Irish Ague'—had its peculiar odour, likened to 'the smell of rotten straw'.[35] The typhoid patient 'wears an expression of languor, ennui, and even sadness'.[36] Smallpox, if it spared its victims' lives, not infrequently left them blind or so hideously scarred that, in Lord Macauley's words, 'it turned the babe into a changeling at which the mother shuddered, and making the eyes and cheeks of the betrothed maiden objects of horror to the lover'. With the intention of reducing scarring, William Stokes used to apply light poultices to the entire face, or a lint mask steeped in glycerine and water and covered with oiled silk.

The appalling suffering of confluent smallpox, as experienced by a robust medical student at the Meath in the 1860s, was vividly described by Stokes, as Moore recalled:

> Delirium set in, and the patient tore off the dressings from his face so often that we desisted from their further application, After the tenth day the condition of the patient was most appalling. The delirium continued, the circulation became every day weaker and more rapid, notwithstanding the free use of stimulants; the crusts were not only black, but on the legs where here and there there was less confluence, the blackness of the worst purpura appeared—a condition held by Hebra to be always fatal. The body was one universal ulcerous sore, and the agonies of the patient from the adhesion of the surface to the bed-clothes were not to be described. In addition to the usual foetor of smallpox in the stage of decrustation, which was present in the highest degree, there was an odour of a still more intensely pungent and offensive character, which seemed to pass through the bystander like a sword. I never before or since experienced anything similar. Stimulants alone, freely and constantly applied, seemed to preserve the patient alive; the pulse was rapid, weak and intermittent, and for several days we despaired of his life.[37]

Stokes happened to mention the case to a surgical colleague, Mr Philip Smyly, who suggested putting the afflicted student into a warm bath. There was instant relief. The delusions ceased, the foetor disappeared. '"Thank God! thank God!" the patient exclaimed. "I'm in heaven, I'm in heaven! Why didn't you do this before?"' He made a full recovery.

Moore acquired a vast clinical experience of smallpox during his years at Cork Street Fever Hospital, and contributed a chapter on the disease to Volume XIII of *Twentieth Century Practice* (1898), an international encyclopaedia edited by Thomas L. Stedman. He attributed the decline in the prevalence and mortality of smallpox, that had come about in his

---

[35] Moore (1892), *op, cit.* (note 33), p. 272.
[36] Moore, *ibid.*, p 369.
[37] William Stokes, cited by Moore, *ibid.*, p. 119.

own time, to vaccination, and 'grave indeed is the responsibility incurred by those who do not accept it' or seek to discredit it.[38]

It has been said that to Sir William Gowers, a leading London neurologist, 'the neurological sick were like the flora of a tropical jungle and his keen eye and collector's flair enabled him to identify, arrange and classify'.[39] Moore, likewise, knew the full clinical repertoire of infectious diseases, the weather that bred them and the polluted streets favouring their spread. Bride Street and Francis Street, with the neighbouring lanes and alleys, provided an endless series of cases for Cork Street Fever Hospital. And there were other incriminated areas.

> Mapas-street is very unhealthy—the houses are old and dirty, ill-stained and dilapidated. The street runs down to the bottom of a valley, through which a small tributary of the Poddle river flows sluggishly. The district is a prolific hotbed of disease.[40]

On 6 December 1907, Sir John Moore spoke in the Academy of Medicine on what he called 'Diphtheritic Fever' to distinguish it from classical diphtheria. He reported eighteen cases of sore throat in a Dublin girls' school, a private concern in a sound sanitary condition. The Klebs-Lôffler bacillus was isolated in the cases examined, but no girl developed the characteristic false membrane. It appears that he was dealing with an epidemic due to what was called a *mitis* strain when it became customary to grade the *Bacillus diphteriae* into *gravis*, *inter-medius* and *mitis* types.[41]

Prompted by references in the recent literature 'to an apparent close connection between chickenpox and shingles', Moore published 'An Old-Time Note on Varicella and Herpes' in the *Irish Journal of Medical Science* in September 1930. He cited brief records written in his father's 'Case-Book' in October and November 1852, which 'may be quoted in corroboration of the view that herpes zoster and varicella are clinical manifestations of one and the same acute infection'.[42] This was his last publication on infectious diseases.

Meteorology

Every morning and evening for seventy years, Moore read his barometer and thermometer and recorded the rainfall, sometimes stealing away from

---

[38] Moore, 'Why has Small-pox declined in Prevalence and Fatality?', *Dublin J. Med. Sc.* (1910); 130: 106–28.
[39] Macdonald Critchley, *Sir William Gowers 1845–1915* (London: Heinemann, 1949), p. 30.
[40] Moore (1892), *op. cit.* (note 33), p. 361.
[41] Moore, 'Diphtheritic Fever', *Dublin J. Med. Sc.* (1908); 125: 10–20.
[42] Moore, 'An Old-Time Note on Varicella and Herpes Zoster', *Irish J. Med. Sc.*, (1930): 518–9.

an academy meeting to do so. He was chairman of the GMC's public health committee for twenty-three years. A second edition of *Meteorology, Practical and Applied* appeared in 1910 and he wrote a daily weather report for a Dublin newspaper.

His earliest public exposition of this interest may have been a lecture, 'Meteorology in its bearing on Health and Disease', given in the lecture hall of the Royal Dublin Society in April 1873.[43] Being aware that weather is a 'break-ice topic of everyday conversation', the young doctor was at pains to explain briefly to his audience the *scientific* aspects of meteorology; providing reasons for the climate of the British Isles in summer and winter—so different from conditions in countries with continental climates, where the inhabitants are destined to suffer the torments of Dante's 'Purgatory' in summer and, in Milton's words, 'From beds of raging fire to starve in ice'.[44]

The works of Hippocrates contain passages relevant to the influence of meteorology on health and disease, and Moore cites some of these—'Different diseases prevail at different seasons, or again subside'; 'Some constitutions fare well or ill in summer, others in winter'. These observations, Moore believed, had been largely forgotten or replaced by others ('A green Christmas makes a fat churchyard') with which he disagreed. A paper by Dr William Heberden junior, FRS—the first modern paper on the subject—had shown that the number of deaths increased in a cold winter.[45]

The tendency to sickness and death from respiratory diseases is greater in winter months; morbidity and mortality from diarrhoea and dysentery are greater in the summer. The low summits of repiratory death-curves corresponded with the mild winters of 1867–8, 1868–9, and 1871–2. 'Children under five years and the aged go down like grass before the scythe, when the keen frost-wind or the fiery heat of summer sweeps across the land.'

Apart from the cholera year 1866, the abdominal [diseases] death-curve

---

[43] *Lectures on Public Health delivered in the Lecture Hall of the Royal Dublin Society* (Dublin: Hodges, Foster & Co., 1874). The committee of science of the RDS selected 'Public Health' as a theme for the fourth annual series of afternoon scientific lectures in April and May 1873 with William Stokes as opening speaker ('Introductory Discourse on Sanitary Science in Ireland'). The other lecturers were J. Emerson Reynolds, 'On the Discrimination of Unadulterated Food'; James Little, 'On the Geographical Distribution of Disease'; Thomas W. Grimshaw, 'On Zymotic and Preventable Diseases'; Alfred Hudson, 'On Liability to Disease'; Robert McDonnell, 'On Antiseptics and Disinfection'; Edward Dillon Mapother, 'The Prevention of Artisans' Diseases'; George Carlisle Henderson, 'On the Construction of Dwelling Houses with Reference to their Sanitary Arrangement'; Robert O'Brien Furlong, 'On Sanitary Legislation'.

[44] Moore, *ibid*, p. 36.

[45] Moore, *ibid*, p. 39.

shows high summits in 1865, 1868, and 1870. The majority of my audience will not have forgotten the wondrous September of 1865, with its July temperature and absolute drought; the burning sun of the summer of 1868; and the glorious weather of July, August, and September, 1870.

The mortality from diarrhoea in the summer of 1868 assumed alarming proportions, but in the middle of August, providentally, there was torrential rain—'amounting in one week to 302 tons of water on every acre'—and within a few weeks the epidemic was over.

Measles is a disease of the spring and summer quarters, mean air temperatures above 60° and below 42° tending to arrest its spread. Whooping-cough is a disease of winter, 'the greatest mortality generally occurring in the first quarter of the year'. From his analysis of the weekly death-rate for scarlatina over a period of nine years, Moore found the disease to be most fatal (8.2 deaths) in the forty-sixth week, least fatal (1.9 deaths) in the twenty-fourth week.

Among the causes of scarlatina's increased frequency in colder months diminished ventilation is important. 'Every chink and crevice through which the outer air might gain access to the overcrowded tenements is eagerly sought out and effectually closed.'[46] The disease spreads like wildfire in the poorer parts, and because of its contagious nature the richer and more affluent areas also suffer.

But overcrowding, Moore emphasized, moving to his peroration, is just another name for poverty entailing lack of fuel, food and clothing—the neccessities of life.

> And so it is. Our poorer fellow-citizens have to do battle with snow and ice, hail and tempest. Their weapons of defence in this otherwise unequal warfare must be raiment, food and warmth. Lo! there on the journey of life lies the wounded, the helpless wayfarer, cold, and naked, and hungry—be you the good Samaritans.[47]

When the congress of the Royal Institute of Public Health was held in Dublin in August 1898, Moore took the chair at the inaugural meeting of the section of chemistry and meteorology. He spoke on 'Ireland: Its Capital and Scenery', opening with a brief historical introduction, and described Dublin as 'a handsome, and in parts a picturesque city', well supplied with open spaces, but with the grave defect of insanitary housing for the poorer classes, a large proportion of whom lived in unwholesome tenements. A detailed account followed, of the meteorological factors which determined the city's climate. He closed by recalling a re-

---

[46] Moore, *ibid*, p. 56.
[47] Moore, *ibid*, p. 61.

cent tour of Ireland.

> In the spring of the present year it was my happiness, accompanied by my wife, to travel through the south and south-west of Ireland, from Waterford to Lahinch and Lisdoonvarna, in Co. Clare. The most ample facilities for transit by rail, and road, and water now exist, and the serious hindrance to travel which inadequate and uncomfortable hotel accommodation presented in bygone days is fast being removed. The Southern Hotels in Kerry and the Golf-Links Hotel at Lahinch, on Liscannor Bay in Clare, leave nothing to be desired in respect to site, accommodation, and moderation in charges.[48]

Whether this was quite the thing for a scientific occasion seems a valid question, but no doubt Dr Moore's personality added grace to his travelogue, and in the pre-motoring age his itinerary was novel and enterprising.

Climatic change

The possibility of climatic change affecting the British Isles, a topic frequently considered in the present decade, was discussed by Moore before the British Association for the Advancement of Science on 7 September 1908. He had studied the matter fully, using his own data and the records of Merle, Boate, Rutty and others. The oldest evidence available was a small vellum folio containing observations made by Rev. William Merle, fellow of Merton College, Oxford, between 1337 and 1344.

> A.D. 1342. Merle writes:—'It is to be noted that there was dryness about April this year, as there was in the year of Christ, 1333 and 1340. It is also to be noted that there was spring-like weather the whole time between September and the end of December, except on these days to which frost is ascribed, so much so that in certain places the leeks burst forth into seed, and in certain places the cabbages blossomed.[49]

With the assistance of his brother Arnold, a Dublin medical practitioner, Dr Gerard Boate, state physician to Cromwell's army in Ireland, made observations on climate and diseases. Dr Thomas Rutty's *A Chronological History of the Weather and Seasons* published in 1770 was also cited by Moore, as providing evidence that the weather in the early years of the eighteenth century closely resembled the weather of the twentieth century.

> 1731. 'April. An unusually dry and cold month for the most part: a little

---

[48] Moore, 'Ireland: Its Capital and Scenery', *Dublin J. Med. Sc.* (1898); 106: 299–314.
[49] Moore, 'Is Our Climate Changing?', *Dublin J. Med. Sc.* (1908); 136: 254–77.

snow. The 15th, 16th, and 25th, rainy... May. The cold weather continued to the thirteenth day...'
1735. 'On Christmas Day some pear trees were in blossom.'
1735-1736. 'Summary. Of the spring the two first months were pretty open; but succeeded by a cold and dry May. The summer cold and wet like winter. Autumn wet. Winter open.'
1736. 'June. Mostly fair and very hot, the hottest June that is remembered since the year 1723. The principal winds E., S.E., N.E., W. and N.W. ... This summer was as remarkable for heat as the preceding one had been for coldness and moisture.'[50]

A description of 20–21 January 1802, a night to rival 'The Night of the Big Wind' (6–7 January 1839) is taken from John Underwood's *Diary of the Weather ... at the Botanic Garden of the Dublin Society*: '"Last night the wind was very high; about eleven at night, it encreased to a terrible tempest; from one o'clock this morning, to six, was supposed to be the most dreadful hurricane ever remembered by any of the present age."'[51]

The detailed evidence presented by Sir John Moore supported his conclusion that 'within the past six centuries at all events, no appreciable change has taken place in the climate of the British Isles.'

State medicine

The term 'state medicine' and its earlier synonym, 'political medicine', have been replaced by more explicit terms: 'public health', or 'community medicine'. Henry Maunsell, as we have seen, was appointed professor of political medicine at the RCSI in 1841; Moore and his fellow diplomates at TCD were relative latecomers in a field of endeavour that despite its enormous scope and importance has never had the same attraction for practitioners as the immediate care of sick persons. Maunsell, in 1839, called the leading doctors of his day 'professional traders'; he rebuked them for having 'abandoned the higher and more honourable walks of their profession', i.e. preventive medicine, to become 'the servants of individuals'.

Moore succeeded Dr Thomas Grimshaw, the registrar general for Ireland, and Dr (later Sir) Charles Cameron, MOH for Dublin, as president of the sub-section of state medicine in the Academy of Medicine for the session 1884–5; re-elected two years later he held office for a third time in 1903–4. His inaugural addresses (1885, 1887, 1904) dealt with outstanding public health problems at the turn of the century. These included the notification of infectious diseases, tuberculosis, housing for

---

[50] Moore, *ibid*, p. 264.
[51] Moore, *ibid*, p. 265.

the poor, workhouse reform, the poor-law medical service.

On 8 August 1878 the Public Health (Ireland) Act received the Royal Assent. It was intended to consolidate into one Act the several relevant Acts, twenty in number, previously in force in Ireland, with suitable amendments. But despite its splendid Sanitary Code, Moore's judgement in 1885 was that it had failed to bring about the expected benefits. 'So far as its medical aspect is concerned, it has signally failed, mainly from two causes—first, want of independent supervision; and, secondly, inadequate remuneration.' The dispensary medical officer, the MOH for his district, could not act independently of the board of guardians that employs him, and pays him a shameful wage.

> What political economy is here! The bread-winner of a family perishes of enteric fever or of typhus—preventable diseases. His widow and orphans are thrown upon the rates at a cost to the ratepayers of, perhaps, ten times the yearly salary offered to the medical officer of health—looked upon as 'passing rich' not 'on forty', but on five 'pounds a year', or threepence farthing a day.
>
> But how came it that the local authorities were permitted to fix such inadequate salaries? Let the eleventh section of the Act supply the answer:— 'Every medical officer of a dispensary district shall be'—note the *compulsory* phrase—'a sanitary officer for such district, or for such part thereof as he shall personally be in charge of, under the title of medical officer of health, *with such additional salary as the sanitary authority thereof may determine, with the approval of the Local Government Board.*' Surely it was the bounden duty of the controlling authority to refuse to sanction nominal salaries to medical officers of health, whose duties would be the reverse of nominal unless the Public Health Act was to be rendered null and void. The blame rests with the Local Government Board.[52]

Nineteen years later, Moore was still concerned with the unenviable lot of the overworked and underpaid Irish dispensary medical officer. In respect of his public health committment the DMO was little better than a sanitary sub-officer, though deserving to be better appreciated and properly remunerated.

Moore was a fervent advocate of the compulsory notification and registration of infectious diseases, long accepted in the Scandinavian nations and more recently enforced by certain English towns. Convinced of their potential, he stressed the urgency of the *notification* of infections whereas their *registration*, facilitating the compilation of vital statistics, could be effected at leisure. Isolation and disinfection were much talked of in Ireland, but he ventured to recall an eighteenth century-cookery

---

[52] Moore, 'Sanitary Organisation in Ireland in its Medical Aspect', *Dublin J. Med. Sc.* (1885); 79: 211–12.

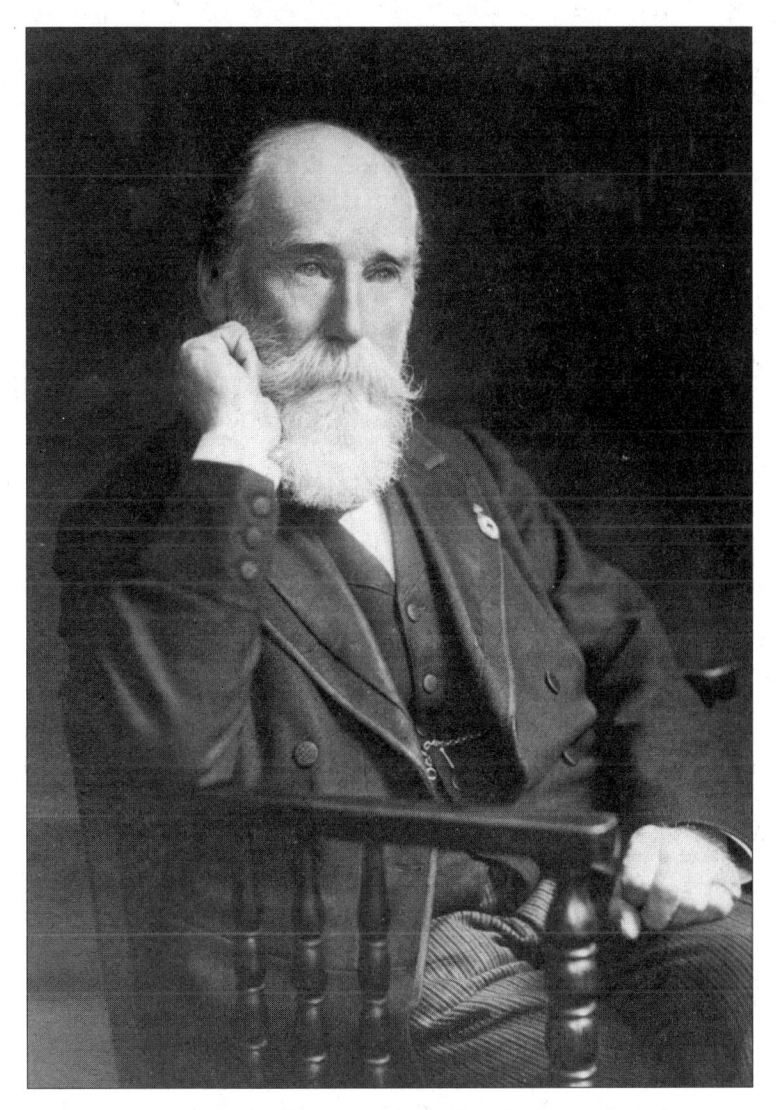

Sir John William Moore, 1845–1937 Professor of Medicine 1889–1916

recipe for hare soup: 'first catch *your hare*, and then skin it!' Prompt notification was life-saving. This had been proven in Leicester, after the Leicester Corporation Act came into force.

He favoured direct notification by the doctor, but would accept a modification in which the medical attendant signed the certificate, and handed it to the person in charge of the patient to forward to the sanitary authority. The doctor, he insisted, should be adequately remunerated. 'To offer a member of a learned profession one shilling in return for an important public service is an injustice and an insult.' Smallpox, scarlatina, measles, typhus, typhoid, relapsing fever, erysipelas, diphtheria, whooping-cough and cholera should be notifiable.

Moore complained repeatedly of the way the medical profession was exploited in regard to medical certification, being usually offered paltry fees or none at all.

> My object is to draw attention to what I regard as a serious professional grievance—namely the demand made upon the time, patience, and responsibility of registered medical practitioners in respect of medical certification for State purposes at a nominal fee, or, as in the case of Medical Certificates of the Cause of Death, for no fee at all.[53]

Having deplored the medical profession's uncompromising opposition to compulsory notification in 1887—'Rightly or wrongly, a grievous stumbling-block has been placed in the way of general legislation on the subject, and year by year an incalculable amount of injury to life and property is being done by systematic concealment of the presence of preventable disease among the population'—it gratified him to say in 1904 that the 'Infectious Disease (Notification) Act 1889' had been enthusiastically adopted, with untold benefit to the public health. The 'Infectious Diseases (Prevention) Act, 1890' enabled the application of preventive measures, and Moore saw these Acts as 'the Magna Charta of Public Health.' They had been eagerly received and worked by the medical profession, 'who with a noble self-denial have once more admitted the truth of the adage—*Salus Populi, Suprema Lex.*'[54]

The discovery by Koch in 1882 of the *Bacillus tuberculosis* had been a major achievement. 'Stated briefly [Moore said] tuberculosis is a parasitic disease—the parasite is a bacillus, which may be distinguished from all other bacilli by its remarkable behaviour towards the colouring reagent "vesuvin".'

Figures for 1902 showed an annual death-rate from tuberculosis in

---

[53] Moore, 'The Exploitation of the Medical Profession in regard to Medical Certificates', *ibid*, (1915); 139: 338–46.
[54] Moore, 'Some Public Health Problems', *ibid.* (1904); 117: 178–88.

Ireland of 2.7 per 1,000 of the population, the lowest death-rate recorded in Ireland since 1896. Phthisis was responsible for 9,400 deaths in 1902 and Moore, speaking in 1904, outlined a scheme to check the ravages of consumption based on compulsory notification, accurate bacteriological disgnosis, hospitalization, inspection and disinfection of the houses of the tuberculous, and public education.

The Tuberculosis Prevention (Ireland) Act, 1908, generally called 'Birrell's Tuberculosis Act', introduced to Ireland on 1 July 1909, the principle of notification of tuberculosis, leaving it up to each sanitary district to apply compulsion or not. By 1914 only fifty-five out of 311 districts had opted for compulsory notification. And in Dublin, where compulsory notification was in force, the death-rate when compared to the notifications left little doubt that notification was incomplete.[55]

Sir John Moore circularized Dublin newspapers on 18 October 1916 with a letter of complaint, when, as a wartime economy, the Local Government Board took the unilateral decision 'to whittle down' the customary fee of two shillings and sixpence to a shilling, 'which practically amounts to a war tax on notifications fees of 60 per cent'. 'Is it not a fact', he asked, 'that the members of the House of Commons are still drawing their salary of £400 a year without any deduction whatever?'

The octogenarian physician addressed the Royal Institute of Health's section of epidemiology at its Dublin meeting on 16 August 1928, his subject 'Epidemiology in Ireland: Past and Present'. His information for past epidemics—including the first recorded pestilence which killed nine thousand in a week at Tallaght—was taken from the *Annals of the Four Masters*, Sir William Petty's *Bills of Mortality*, Joseph Rogers' *Essay on Epidemic Diseases* (Dublin, 1734), Rutty's *Chronological History of the Weather . . . and of the Prevailing Diseases in Dublin* (1770), Sir William Wilde's *Census Report for the Year 1851*, etc., but his personal experience of epidemics extended back to the third cholera epidemic. Referring to it he said: 'Of the third—and may God grant that it should prove the last epidemic of cholera in Ireland, I was myself an eye-witness as a medical student in the winter of 1866–1867.'[56]

That epidemic, as we have seen, began with the death on 22 July 1866, in a house at City Quay, of a fifteen-year-old girl, a recent passenger in a Liverpool steamer. Four days later another child died in the same house, and within twenty-two weeks cholera carried off 1,459 victims in Dublin. When the wards at the Meath Hospital proved unsuitable, wooden sheds were erected, but they were not ready for the reception of patients until December. The mortality rate in the airy fever sheds was

---

[55] Moore, 'Notification of Tuberculosis in Ireland: its Failure and the reasons therefor', *ibid.* (1914); 137: 331–40.
[56] Moore, 'Epidemiology in Ireland: Past and Present', *Irish J. Med. Sc.* (1928): 629.

lower than in the small, ill-ventilated wards, but for those who attended the cholera cases the experience was unforgettable, as Moore testified some sixty years later.

> The clinical picture presented by the ill-fated victims of that dread disease left an ineffacable, a life-long, impression on my memory. To this day I see in my mind's eye the wasted, icy cold, blue-tinted, yet withal conscious, pain-stricken, hapless sufferers for whom medical skill could do so little in their sore extremity. The use of the clinical thermometer was then in its infancy, but collapse temperatures of $95°$ or lower were often recorded, and a rise of body temperature to fever heights was one of the earliest signs which gave a dawn of hope that the patients might perchance recover.[57]

In the mild smallpox epidemic of 1865–6, which caused 103 deaths in Dublin, Moore had an attack of 'varioloid' to which he attributed his subsequent life-long immunity to smallpox, for he was never re-vaccinated although called upon to deal with patients at Cork Street Hospital during the epidemics of 1871–2, and the 'really terrible epidemic' in 1878 and 1879. 'The deaths from the disease registered in Dublin city and county were 10 in 1876, 42 in 1877, 568 in 1878, 555 in 1879, 282 in 1880, 14 in 1881, and 1 in 1882—1,490 deaths in all.'[58]

The last great typhus epidemic occurred during the famine. Moore's personal acquaintance with the disease began in 1865 at the Meath Hospital, when nothing was known of the part played by lice in its transmission. The last case he saw was sent to the Meath in 1922 misdiagnosed 'enteric fever'. Moore's diagnosis of typhus was verified when a probationer-nurse who attended the patient developed typical typhus. Both patients recovered.

Enteric fever was endemic rather than epidemic. Moore recalled that after his family moved to 40 Fitzwilliam Square in 1867, an aunt who lived with them sickened and died from typhoid fever. A domestic servant was infected but survived. At the time the city's water was taken from the Grand and Royal Canals, but the Vartry waterworks was nearing completion, and from 1868 supplied potable water to the city and suburbs.

Moore's article, 'The Water Supply of Dublin', recounts how the River Vartry, which rises at Calary Moor at the foot of Djouce and the Sugar Loaf Mountains, was turned from its course through a tunnel under the main embankment of a vast storage reservoir near Roundwood, County Wicklow. Sir John Gray, MD (whose statue stands in O'Connell Street), chairman of Dublin Corporation's waterworks committee, was

---

[57] Moore, *ibid.*, p. 630.
[58] Moore, *ibid.*, p. 631.

knighted by the lord lieutenant on 30 June 1863. By 1893 the average daily consumption was around 14 million gallons, and critics who impugned the purity of the water were answered by an English expert: he reported to Sir Charles Cameron that 'the Vartry water complies with the most stringent demands of modern sanitary science'.[59]

Moore remained alert to the importance of water in the transmission of disease, having described an outbreak of illness in a Dublin school resulting from secondary contamination of Vartry water.[60] His epidemiological survey included encouraging figures for the half century between 1872 and 1921 inclusive. Deaths in Dublin city and county from typhus and typhoid respectively, were 1,727 and 4,419 in the first twenty-five years of that half century; in the following twenty-five years there were 102 deaths from typhus, 1,937 from typhoid. Between 1921 and 1926 inclusive there was only one death from typhus, fifty-six from typhoid.

Preventive medicine had reaped its rewards. 'But [said Moore] "there remaineth yet very much land to be possessed."' Measles, scarlatina, diphtheria and pneumonia were rife; no summer passed without an epidemic of diarrhoea; anterior poliomyelitis (infantile paralysis) had not yet invaded the capital in epidemic form, as it had done in Counties Armagh, Cavan, Down, Monaghan and Tyrone in the autumn of 1916. And a recent housing report showed that 22.9 per cent of Dublin's population lived in one-room tenements.[61]

Insulin

When the first number of a new series of the *Dublin Journal of Medical Science* came out in February 1920 it carried a farewell message from the retiring editor. Moore had held office for forty-seven years, far longer than any of his predecessors, editing ninety-four volumes.

> The Editor cannot relinquish his office, which he ever regarded as one of great honour, as it surely was one of grave responsibility, without recording his grateful sense of the generous help at all times afforded him by his colleagues on the staff of the Journal.
> He would also thankfully acknowledge the loyalty and patriotism which his professional brethren ever placed at his service. With their valued aid, he has tried—not altogether unsuccessfully he is bold enough to think—to render a Medical Journal, which dates from the year 1832 and includes in its Roll of Editors the names of Graves, Stokes, Wilde, Kidd, and James Little—worthy of Ireland and of its capital.[62]

---

[59] Moore, 'The Water Supply of Dublin', *Dublin J. Med. Sc.* (1899); 108: 176–87.
[60] Moore, 'An Outbreak of Disease Traceable to the drinking of Impure Water, *ibid.* (1882); 73: 131–37.
[61] Moore, 'Epidemiology in Ireland: Past and Present', *Irish J. Med. Sc.*, (1928): 626–39.
[62] Moore, 'A Message of Farewell', *Dublin J. Med. Sc.*, 4th series (1920); 149: 1.

He offered his best wishes to his successor, Arnold K. Henry, who within an unexpectedly short time resigned, in order to take up the post of professor of surgery in Cairo, handing over his editorial duties to William Doolin, then assistant surgeon to St Vincent's Hospital. The latter, in due course, acknowledged his indebtedness to Moore, his neighbour across Fitzwilliam Square, for many acts of courtesy and words of encouragement.

> He cannot lightly forget an informal visit paid to him by Sir John within the first few weeks of his appointment, to bring a message of congratulation on the appearance of his first editorial review—a venturesome innovation in the Journal's production at the time. Such a gesture from the *doyen* of the profession—typical of the chivalrous gentleman—meant much to the novice, secretly apprehensive of the wisdom of the step which he had undertaken. It was the first of many visits, many talks, either in the study or in the Square, where he so greatly loved to walk. There on those quiet paths that bent figure, with kindly voice and smiling eyes, was known and daily greeted as a friend by all the children of his colleagues, many of whom he had known playing there as children too.[63]

Doolin, we may presume, spoke for many, when he described Moore as 'the embodiment of kindliness', the possessor of 'an old-world, unhurried courtesy of manner which endeared him to all'.

At the Academy of Medicine on 24 November 1922, Moore presented the case-history of a patient with diabetes complicated by xanthoma diabeticorum, a child who had recently been under his care in 1922 at the Meath Hospital, dying there on 8 October. Concluding the presentation he regretted that while she was attending him he was unaware that 'insulin' an antidiabetic hormone had been isolated in Toronto. The Medical Research Council had taken the matter up and a supply of insulin should be available shortly.[64] In the event, Henry Moore (physician to the Mater Hospital and unrelated to Sir John) was the first Dublin doctor to use insulin: 'My personal experience with Insulin [he wrote in the *Lancet* in April 1923] is brief and confined only to two cases, owing to the difficulty in obtaining the substance.'

Treatment of children

When the practice of delivering an introductory address at the opening of the teaching session was revived at the Meath Hospital in 1926, Sir John

---

[63] Doolin, 'Sir John William Moore', (note 1), p. 654.
[64] Moore, 'Some Recent Clinical Records', *Irish Journal of Medical Science* (1922–3): 507–14.

Moore was invited to speak on 'The treatment of Children'.[65] He discussed 'Childhood in the Home and in the Hospital', under which heading he referred to ante-natal care, early feeding—breast-feeding preferably—and personal cleanliness; 'the successful crusade against body-vermin has been one of the chief elements in the total disappearance from our Bills of Mortality of typhus fever'. Dublin's open spaces were 'a powerful asset to health', and he regretted that Leinster Lawn was no longer open as a children's playground. He inveighed against 'that abomination the "infant comforter"', and against flies, 'subjects of Beelzebub'. He said that a high infant mortality deadened the natural affections and blunted the sense of bereavement.

Moore recalled that in 1873, making a tour of inspection on behalf of the Freeman's Journal Sanitary Commission, he asked in a tenement was there much sickness about to be told, 'Oh, no, there's only a child with the chincough,' 'Only a child!' Moore exclaimed. 'Those words grated harshly on my ears, and yet they were uttered in good faith by the speaker.'[66] One out of every six patients at the Meath was a child, and the greatest scourge was tuberculosis. 'Even forty-four years since its exciting cause became known through Robert Koch's research!' Comparatively rare as 'consumption', tuberculosis slew children in Dublin by causing peritonitis or meningitis, and disabled them by crippling limbs and joints. These conditions were not notifiable.

Moore did not fail to discuss how the doctor, if he is to succeed in the treatment of children, must be able to capture the fortress of the sick child's heart. He should have a smile on his lips—or better still, in his eyes—and there were obvious stratagems, an orange or a banana or 'the offer of a gift of "siggers" [cigarette pictures]', a word he had recently acquired. 'Let the child's physician take as his watch-word: "Faith, Hope and Love, but the greatest of these is Love."'

A keen swimmer and oarsman in his youth, Sir John William Moore enjoyed walking in his later years and having got rid of his victoria, he rarely used a tram. C. S. Breathnach has mentioned his daily walk from Fitzwilliam Square to the Meath Hospital. 'To all whom he met he gave a cheery greeting and salutation. His brisk step belied the bent figure and full white beard of his years, his pleasant smile and friendly greeting were not restricted to ward-rounds. On Sundays a minor detour past Marsh's Library, where his son William Edmund was assistant librarian, brought him to St. Patrick's Cathedral.'[67]

He was still a consultant to the Coombe Lying-in Hospital when well into his eighties, and Bertie Corbet who was assistant master in 1929

---

[65] Moore, 'The Treatment of Children', *ibid.*, (1926): 671–82.
[66] Moore, *ibid.*, 674.
[67] Breathnach, 'John William Moore', (note 2), p. 70.

remembered him as a 'little bent figure in a black frock coat, a long white beard, a ruddy healthy complexion and very bright eyes. He was courtesy itself in consultation.'[68]

Last years

As his eighty-seventh birthday approached, Sir John William Moore was again invited by his colleagues at the Meath to deliver the introductory address. It was a duty he had eagerly performed for the first time on 2 November 1875, speaking of the history of the hospital, and it is probable that his mood when he faced his audience on 14 October 1932 was a mixture of nostalgia and optimism. He spoke now, as William Stokes had done, of the doctor's responsibility to his patient—'That patient must be spared all bodily fatigue or pain while he is being examined'— and of the development of modern scientific medicine as he himself had witnessed it; the emergence of vitamins and hormones; the expansion of preventive medicine; the discoveries of Pasteur and Lister which had ushered in a new era.

He spoke, too, of the individual doctor's duty to his colleagues and of the medical vocation:

> No other calling—the Church not excepted—demands so much self-denial, patience, and—with reverence I say it, prayer. Armed with such a panoply, the physician is fully equipped for the battle with disease and death. Should he suffer defeat in what may prove to be an unequal conflict, vanquished indeed he may be, but with untarnished honour and without disgrace. He has fought the good fight.
>
> Considerations such as these should weigh with every member of the great, the noble and ennobling profession to which may of us have already the honour to belong, or—as is the case of many whom I am now addressing—to which, as medical students, they aspire.
>
> And yet are not all of us in a very special sense still medical students? Not a day passes in our professional life that an opportunity does not offer of learning something new, of testing that 'something' and of making use thereof.[69]

Leaving the podium his race was not yet quite run. He resigned from the Meath in 1933, but continued to visit the hospital daily until close to his death. On 21 February 1935 Mr Richard Atkinson Stoney admitted him to the honorary fellowship of the Royal Academy of Medicine in Ireland, and presented him with his portrait drawn in coloured crayons by Seán O'Sullivan, RHA. He marked the seventieth anniversary of his

---

[68] R. M. Corbet, 'Reminiscences of the Coombe Hospital, *J. Irish Med. Assn.* (1967); 60: 291–96.
[69] Moore, 'Chronicle', *Irish J. Med. Sc.* (1932): 616–18.

election as a scholar in the University of Dublin with an after-dinner speech on Trinity Monday.

Sir John William Moore died at his home in Fitzwilliam Square on 12 October 1937, from pneumonia which followed the cerebral thrombosis that had confined him unwillingly to bed a few weeks earlier. 'One finds it difficult to think of him as gone', wrote William Doolin,[70] who saw him as the personification of Chaucer's pilgrim:

And though that he were worthy, he was wys,
And of his port as meek as is a mayde.
He never yet no vileinye ne sayde
In al his lyf, unto no maner wight.
He was a verray parfit gentil knight.

---

[70] Doolin, 'Sir John William Moore', (note 1), p. 654.

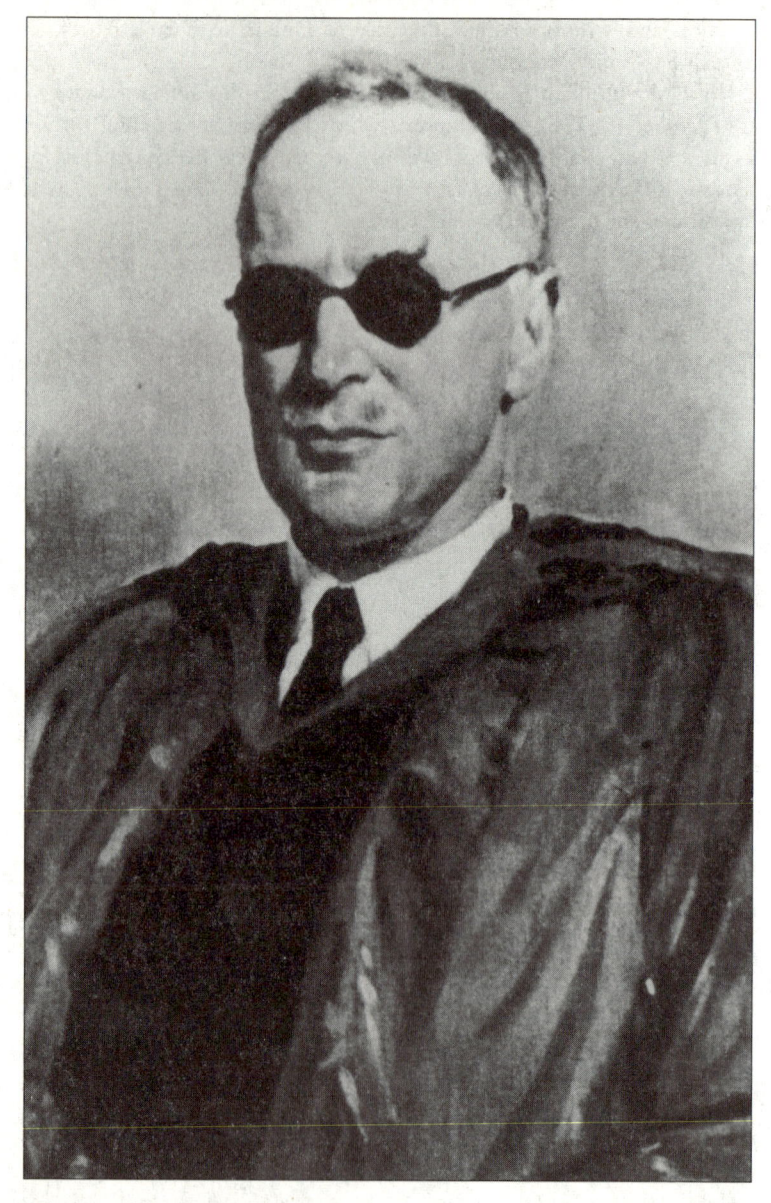

Thomas Gillman Moorhead, 1878–1960 Professor of Medicine 1916–17 (portrait by Leo Whelan, courtesy RCPI)

Chapter 10: T. G. Moorhead, 1878–1960

Thomas Gillman Moorhead's career falls neatly, and tragically, into two phases: in the first he had effortlessly attained an enviable position as one of Dublin's leading physicians; the second phase, ushered in suddenly as the result of an appalling accident in 1926, found the middle-aged doctor cast into the sightless world of the blind, where he quickly learned to move with remarkable equanimity and assurance.

The son of Dr William Robert Moorhead and his wife Amelia Davis Gillman of Oakmount, County Cork, he was born in Benburb, County Tyrone, on 15 October 1878 and grew up in Bray, County Wicklow, where his father established a practice. From Aravon School he entered TCD, and after winning many prizes took a medical degree in 1901. He proceeded MD in the following year, became MRCPI in 1905, and was elected FRCPI in 1906. Meanwhile he had visited Vienna as a graduate student.

His eldest brother James Herbert, and a younger brother William St Leger Moorhead, also entered the medical profession and practised in Birmingham and London respectively.

Early success

T. G. Moorhead married Mai Beatrice Quinn, a daughter of Robert Erskine Quinn, in 1907 and they lived in 23 Upper Fitzwilliam Street. A younger colleague recalled 'the stacks of bicycles ranged against the railings of his house, set there by Trinity students who flocked to his tutorial classes in every subject from biology and physiology to materia medica and internal medicine'. His clinics at the Royal City of Dublin Hospital and Sir Patrick Dun's Hospital, where he was visiting physician, were well attended. His popularity was summed up by a student who said: 'the great thing about Moorhead is that you'll never find him throwing his weight about.'[1]

He was co-editor of the *Dublin Journal of Medical Science* from July 1907. He published several articles from his own pen; these dealt with a variety of subjects, which included the teaching of anatomy and accounts of recent advances in medicine. A report to the Academy's section of pathology of a case of bacterial endocarditis was made on Moorhead's behalf in 1913 by Adrian Stokes, then a trainee pathologist. The autopsy showed ulcerative endocarditis of the heart valves, from which Stokes

---

[1] William Doolin, 'In Memoriam', *Irish J. Med. Sc.* (1960): 438; see also J. B. Lyons, *Brief Lives of Irish Doctors* (Dublin: Blackwater Press, 1978), pp. 140–1.

obtained what he called a pure culture of 'a cross between streptococcus and pneumococcus'.[2]

Moorhead's avocations included bridge, fishing and mountain climbing of which he gained some experience in Switzerland and France. He was interested, too, in the history of medicine and published 'A Sketch of the History of Medicine in Ireland'[3] and *A Short History of Sir Patrick Dun's Hospital* (1942).

War service

Sir Patrick Dun's Hospital, in common with other Dublin voluntary hospitals, opened its wards to war casualties in 1914. This opportunity to be of service satisfied Moorhead, until in the summer of 1915 it was clear that the armies in Gallipoli were beset by diseases. He joined the RAMC with the rank of temporary captain, and reached Alexandria, the primary medical base for Gallipoli, on 31 December. The evacuation of troops from the Gallipoli peninsula had by then been almost completed.

At Alexandria there were four large hospitals for European and Anzac troops; two for Indian troops, and a local Egyptian government hospital. Moorhead was posted to the largest general hospital, which accommodated 2,500 patients, and had a staff of forty medical officers who lived in tents. The officer in command, Colonel Healy, was a Dubliner; the matron, an Irish nurse, had trained at St Vincent's Hospital.

Unaccustomed to military rules, Captain Moorhead found the organization of the RAMC bewildering, but he rapidly accustomed himself to think in military shorthand, accepting 'that names and forms at first perplexing were useful and part of a dovetailed system'. He noticed how much time was gained in the military hospital because the long explanations expected in civil practice were unnecessary. 'The soldier, with few exceptions, receives his treatment without question, content that the best is being done for him, and, indeed, sometimes appears too machine-like.'[4]

The great summer heat at Gallipoli, and the abundance of flies, had made conditions especially trying for sick men who had been obliged to remain for days in trenches, before they could be evacuated by sea to the base hospitals. Sanitary conditions were bad, and for this Moorhead blamed the War Office, as newly-qualified doctors had been sent out without instructions on camp sanitation. Anti-typhoid innoculation was successful; few genuine typhoid cases were admitted under Moorhead's care in Alexandria. Neurasthenic patients were numerous; most were

---

[2] A. Stokes, 'Malignant Endocarditis', *Dublin J. Med. Sc.* (1913); 136: 216.
[3] T. G. Moorhead, 'A Sketch of the History of Medicine in Ireland', *ibid.*, (1908); 126: 417–40.
[4] Moorhead, 'Some experiences in a Base Hospital in Egypt', *ibid.* (1916); 142: 412–14.

invalided home, and as these men had had an adequate cause for the breakdown he hoped they would make full recoveries.

Moorhead was faced with an epidemic of 'camp jaundice'. This ill-understood condition resembled what was called catarrhal jaundice at home, but others regarded it as mild Weil's disease. During a three-month period, sixty cases of jaundice were admitted under his care, most coming from local camps, a minority from distant stations. The illness was characterized by anorexia, malaise, vomiting, headache and gradually increasing jaundice; stools were clay-coloured, the urine dark with bile. Pyrexia was moderate, and when the pain of an enlarged liver abated the pulse was slow. Jaundice diminished after a week, and most patients left hospital within a month of admission.[5]

The clinical picture was, indeed, identical with that of so-called catarrhal jaundice (later recognised as a viral infection, Hepatitis A), but instinctively Moorhead and his colleagues looked for 'some bacterial source'. Yet, having correctly accepted infection as the cause, they hankered after the older model of pathology, so tenacious are accepted teachings:

> Although, doubtless, there is a definite bacterial cause for the disease, predisposing factors should not be lost sight of, and in this connection the importance of diet and of exposure to cold must be remembered. The initial symptoms point strongly to an acute gastro-duodenitis as the primary pathological lesion. This is almost certainly followed by a catarrh of the common bile duct, which probably extends upwards and involves many of the smaller bile channels within the liver. Whether the condition should be regarded as identical with Weil's disease or not is more a question of terminology than anything else, as nothing definite is known concerning the bacteriology of Weil's disease.[6]

From the speakers' platform at the annual meeting of the RCSI's Biological Society, Captain Moorhead said the duty of students who graduated while the war continued was to join the RAMC immediately. Every Irishman should do his part in the defence of the empire.

Later he served at a base hospital in France, with the rank of temporary lieutenant-colonel. He described the results of poisoning by mustard gas. 'Out of 189 cases during my stay at the hospital there were only five fatalities showing that however disabling the gas may be, it is less fatal than many of the other poisons employed by the Boche.'[7]

---

[5] T. G. Moorhead and G. D. Harding, 'Notes on Camp Jaundice', *ibid.* (1916); 142: 1–8.
[6] *Ibid.*, p. 8.
[7] Moorhead and Harding, 'The Clinical Results of Poisoning by Mustard Gas', *Dublin J. Med. Sc.* (1919); 147: 1–7.

Chair of medicine

While on leave from Egypt in July 1916, he was elected to the chair of medicine in the RCSI. William Doolin, a former pupil, felt that Moorhead's 'destiny was marked out as an academic teacher', and recalled him in that capacity at the bedside—'intent and earnest, never over-critical or sarcastic, but always insistent on two things in handling a patient, *viz.*, accuracy in case-taking and consideration of the patient's comfort and understanding during the course of the examination'.[8]

He held the post for one year only, and submitted his resignation in a letter to the registrar on 6 June 1917:

> Owing to the severe pressure of work I am regretfully forced to the conclusion that it would be quite imposible for me to continue to hold the post. At the time when I applied for it I was under the impression that I would be able to carry on the duties for some years, but the adddition now of military to my ordinary civil work, renders it quite impossible for me to do so.[9]

An adequate explanation, perhaps, for his intended resignation? But somehow one is reminded of Henry Maunsell's complaint, in a slightly different context, that the leaders of the profession (attentive to their private practices) had 'abandoned the higher and more honorable walks of their profession . . . to pursue exclusively, the less exalted, though more profitable trade of the empirical curing of disease'.[10] But, in any case, Moorhead's real interest lay in his alma mater where he was appointed regius professor of physic in 1925.

Academy of Medicine

During Moorhead's term of office (1922–4) as president of the section of medicine of the Royal Academy of Medicine in Ireland, there were a number of important and historically interesting meetings, including those to discuss hyperthyroidism and diabetes. His inaugural address on therapeutics[11] was delivered in 1922, against a background of momentous happenings.

> We stand now [he said] at the beginning of our 41st Session, at the beginning also of a most important epoch in our national affairs. A new era is opening out, and with animosities both old and new, laid aside, men of good-will look forward to years which they trust will be marked by a general renaissance. If their hopes are fulfilled, and I personally have every confi-

---

[8] Doolin, *op. cit.* (note 1).
[9] College minutes, 1917.
[10] H. Maunsell, *Political Medicine* (Dublin: Fannin, 1839), p. 2.
[11] Moorhead, 'Remarks on the Principles of Therapeutics', *Irish J. Med. Sc.* (1923): 479–94.

dence that they will be fulfilled, and that through much travail our country will before long emerge, honouring its pledges into a new life; in which, while not forgetting old friends it will by its own powers make many new friends throughout the world, and achieve a name honourably standing for progress and high endeavour. In such progress, medicine and the allied sciences must take a part.[12]

The paper on the principles of therapeutics broke no new ground, but provides an interesting retrospect of what were then recent achievements: the introduction of emetine in amoebic dysentry; '606' for syphilis; diphtheria and tetanus antitoxins. 'The advances of medicine are not so dramatic as those of surgery', the physician conceded. 'The reason is that they save by the thousand, while surgery saves only individuals.'[13] The availibility of emetine, for instance, outweighed in life-saving powers all the recent advances of surgery.

The work of Ehrlich and his co-workers promised to offer a group of anti-parasitic drugs, and 'enables us to foresee a time when by means of some specific chemical remedy, we will be able to destroy every pathogenic organism without injury to its temporary host, the patient'.[14] Sound therapeutics, he pointed out, are based on exact diagnosis. They demand a knowledge of the natural history of the ailment treated, and the effects of the drugs must be fully known. One must not argue from the particular to the general, and *primum non nocere* is a maxim to be kept ever in mind. Departures from it, such as the great wave of unnecessary colectomies, and the teeth extracting campaign should not be forgotten.

Organo-therapy, a comparatively recent development, was at once, in Osler's words, a major scientific triumph 'and the very apotheosis of charlatanry'. The effects of every conceivable organic product, Moorhead continued, are lauded as cures for every imaginable illness, until one feels back at a time 'when lions's heart was prescribed for cowardice, and fox's lung for dyspnoea'.[15]

Hyperthyroidism

Moorhead opened a discussion on Graves' disease, commonly called hyperthroidism now that it was known to be the result of 'an excessive and possibly morbid secretion from the thyroid gland'. The actual cause of the excessive secretion was unknown; the relationship to the commonly associated enlarged thymus gland was also a mystery. He had carried out

---

[12] *Ibid.*, p. 480.
[13] *Ibid.*, p. 494.
[14] *Ibid.*, p. 493.
[15] *Ibid.*, p. 493.

experiments in an attempt to develop an anti-thymic serum but details are not given.[16]

He referred to the frequency with which sudden physical or mental shock precipitated the disorder. He was obviously familiar with the broad range of manifestations (warning that hyperthyroidism may masquerade as intestinal disease), but did not mention its presentation as myasthenia. If diagnosis is uncertain, 'a determination of basal metabolism will decide'.[17] He admitted that he had no actual experience of this test, which Professor Fearon promised to make available. Exophthalmos was the important eye sign; the galaxy of minor eye signs so frequently discussed at the final medical examination were really unimportant. He was particularly interested in those rare cases that exhibited phenomena of both myxoedema and Graves' disease.

Graves' disease was often referred to as a condition 'from which no one can recover and of which no one ever dies', a useful aphorism but one that overstated the facts.[18] Acute toxic varieties of hyperthyroidism, which may be fatal, are occasionally seen. A considerable percentage recovered spontaneously in the fullness of time. Gain of weight and slowing of the heart were favourable signs.

Moorhead was decided in his preference for 'medical' rather than surgical treatment, remarking: 'I can conscientiously say that if dealing with a relative of my own, I would unhesitatingly select medical treatment, unless the case was one of the most severe varieties—in such a case I might hesitate.'[19] He could guarantee cure within six months in eight out of ten cases.

His patients had never responded to the milk of thyroidectomised goats, the dried blood of goats injected with thyroid extracts, or cures of that kind. He insisted on admission to a nursing home where during the first week complete rest was enforced, and few visitors permitted. An ice bag was applied to the goitre; focal infection eliminated; bromides were given and a vegetable diet imposed. During the next three weeks, the patient received a daily exposure of thyroid and thymic regions to x-rays, under the direction of 'an expert x-rayist'. At the end of the first month's treatment the patient was allowed home, but recalled after four weeks for a further course of x-ray treatment.

Diabetes mellitus

Banting's and Best's 'epoch-making' discovery—not by any means a lucky fluke but 'the happy result of a well-planned and splendidly exe-

---

[16] Moorhead, 'Remarks on Hyperthyroidism', *Irish J. Med. Sc.* (1923): 107–17.
[17] *Ibid.*, p. 111.
[18] *Ibid.*, p. 112.
[19] *Ibid.*, p. 117.

cuted scheme of investigations'—was discussed at the Academy on 9 November 1923. (Dr Henry Moore, visiting physician to the Mater Hospital, had already spoken on insulin in the previous session.) Moorhead admitted that he had 'neither the time nor skill' to carry out the necessary laboratory tests, which would be discussed by Dr R. H. Micks.[20]

Insulin was in short supply, and it was expensive. Hospitals throughout the country were 'beseiged by glycosurics of every type' clamouring for admission. 'Personally [Moorhead said], if I acceded to all the requests made to me, I could keep filled all my available beds, and still have an extensive out-patient clinic for those whom I could not admit.'[21] He discriminated carefully, giving preference to acute cases and those presenting urgent symptoms. He refused admission to 'the more abundant chronic cases', to whom he would only give insulin if control was not achieved by dieting.

The question of cost had to be faced—and there were other fundamental issues:

> The community must first, indeed, decide whether from the eugenic outlook it is desirable to maintain the life of diabetics. Diabetes is a disease which is often transmitted in families, so that it is possible that our present methods of treatment may lead to an increase in the incidence of the disease in future generations. Further, the community must decide whether from the purely economic point of view it is willing to provide the funds necessary to keep alive individuals who are likely to be uneconomic units.[22]

One is relieved to find that having delivered himself unevenly of this stark prediction of the possible outcome (quite reminiscent of H. G. Wells or George Bernard Shaw), Moorhead was, after all, on the side of the angels, believing that most people would decide the question 'not from a eugenic or economic but from a humanitarian standpoint'. Still, the money had to be found, and the provision of an 'Insulin Fund' would be worthy of support. And if the State is willing to pay for the cure of venereal disease should it not provide insulin for a disease 'which is a misfortune and not a fault'?

He referred to the thirty-one cases of diabetes he had seen in the past seven months. The actual number that received insulin is unclear but Dr Micks, who carried out the blood-sugar estimations, said he had records of twelve of Moorhead's cases. The latter found the response to insulin in acute cases 'miraculous'; in other cases he was impressed by 'the increased

---

[20] Moorhead, 'Introductory Remarks on the "Modern Treatment of Diabetes"', *Irish J. Med. Sc.* (1923): 396–405.
[21] *Ibid.*, p. 398.
[22] *Ibid.*, pp. 398–9.

sense of well being and increased capacity for work', and by the rapid clearance of thirst and glycosuria. Inevitably some patients were disappointed that insulin is not 'a permanent and magical cure'. Moorhead's doses were economical; he gave courses of, say, three weeks duration rather than continuous administration.

R. H. Micks outlined techniques for blood-sugar estimation; he described the glucose tolerance test, gave details of blood-sugar levels in twelve of Moorhead's cases, and concluded by observing that the doctors' duty was to determine the need for insulin in particular cases, and 'to lead the nation in its duty of providing it for our poor'.[23]

Sued for assault

An assault suit was taken against Moorhead by Miss Rosalind M. de Cadiz of 3 Martello Terrace, Kingstown, who alleged that on 3 October 1924, when she was a patient in Monkstown Hospital suffering from severe spinal injury and fracture, Moorhead entered her room without her authority or consent, and despite her protests assaulted her, thereby seriously injuring her in her health.

The plaintiff's counsel said sarcastically, that three defences had been offered: first, that it had never happened; second that all that had happened was a reasonable and proper medical examination with the plaintiff's consent; third, that not merely did the thing never happen, not merely did the plaintiff consent to the examination made, but that Dr. Moorhead's professional position was so great that the whole thing was unthinkable.

Counsel's sarcasm was to no avail. It transpired that Moorhead, on behalf of the Ministry of Pensions, had examined Miss de Cadiz in consultation with her own doctor, in the presence of the matron and without undue protest from the patient. The plaintiff's hysterical temperament was stressed, and her action dismissed.

USA

Moorhead made an extensive tour of the United States and Canada in the summer of 1925. He visited medical clinics and research clinics in New York, Baltimore, Cleveland, Chicago, Rochester, Toronto and Montreal. He found the much-vaunted 'team system'—at any rate in private work—was not favoured so highly as he had expected, and there was considerable difference of opinion regarding the virtues of full-time professorships.

> Regarding equipment, one can only speak of the American and Canadian hospitals with awe. Money, especially in the States, seems obtainable for

---

[23] R. H. Micks, 'Notes on the Diagnosis and Treatment of Diabetes', *ibid*. (1923): 410–17.

the asking: in consequence there is not only no lack of appliances, but also no lack of personnel. Any number of assistants are available, with the result that laboratory work on the clinical problems which arise in the wards from day to day is being carried out on a most comprehensive scale by fully trained experts.[24]

He was brought up to date in diagnostic radiology, being greatly impressed by 'the new Graham-Cole method of demonstrating a normal gall-bladder', but remaining sceptical about the utility of bronchograms—'it is unlikely that this means of investigation will ever come into common use'.[25] At the Mayo Clinic his conservative attitude towards the surgical treatment of Graves' disease was altered. Regarding diabetes there was little to report, although innumerable investigations were in progress, and every hospital had its staff of trained dieticians

Blindness

Moorhead crossed to England in July 1926, to attend a meeting of the British Medical Association. Stepping down from the sleeper at Euston Station, he slipped and fell. Helped to his feet he was conscious but sightless. A bilateral retinal detachment had occurred when his head struck the platform. The accident, causing a permanent disability which would have terminated the career of a lesser man, was a prelude to Moorhead's greatness. Clinical work was necessarily curtailed (though with the assistance of a colleague to elicit certain clinical signs he still undertook consultations); he devoted more time to teaching, and was in demand as chairman of a multiplicity of committees. He continued to fill the role of examiner in medicine, and at finals candidates were inclined to complain at the prospect of a blind examiner.

Socially, he remained gregarious. He played bridge using braille playing-cards, and was a regular theatre-goer. Oliver St John Gogarty, poet and ear-nose-and-throat surgeon, expressed his admiration for Moorhead in a sonnet:

> *It takes us all our time with all our eyes*
> *To learn, to know, since knowledge comes from sight;*
> *And long before we give light back for light,*
> *The hour of sunset strikes and daylight flies:*
> *But you had swifter thought, your faculties*
> *Gathered more quickly, so the mind is bright*
> *That met, before the dial struck, the night;*
> *And that black darkness bids me moralise.*

---

[24] Moorhead, 'Some Experiences at American and Canadian Clinics in 1925', *ibid.* (1927): 61–9.
[25] *Ibid.*, p. 63.

> *When we old friends, old pupils have been sent*
> *Out of the brittle brightness of the air,*
> *If succour follow in such banishment,*
> *Gleams of your fortitude shall find us there*
> *Amidst the sudden vague beleaguerment*
> *Of that great darkness where you, living, are.*[26]

Despite his mordant wit, Gogarty was a kind man; he organized a 'panel' of friends who took it in turn to walk with 'T. G.' in the country on Saturday afternoons. One of these, Doolin, (the editor of the *Irish Journal of Medical Science* for which in the immediate aftermath of his accident, in a nursing-home with his head fixed between sandbags, Moorhead had dictated an already commissioned paper on medical education), has recalled how he came to know his former teacher during these outings, and to realize the man's courage and his determination to continue to use his mind as if nothing had happened. Doolin also remembered Moorhead's weekly dinner parties at the Royal Irish Yacht Club in Dún Laoghaire:

> One such nox ambrosiana in particular comes back to mind, when Robin Flower had been his invited guest; Dr E. H. Alton, William Fearon, 'Kirk' and Oliver Gogarty came to join them, and T. G. kept the ball rolling between all. Gogarty at one stage had told one of his more scabrous efforts, to which Flower, seated between T. G. and Alton, reminded the company present that there were still extant in the folklore of European literature the seven original naughty stories of which all present-day versions were derivatives; turning to the Provost, he appealed to him as a classical scholar for the original of Oliver's particular version![27]

As a keen but allegedly a somewhat uninspired dean of the school of physic, Moorhead was often in conflict with Joseph Warwick Bigger, the dynamic professor of bacteriology, who represented a group striving to make a place for research in an unambitious curriculum designed to turn out competent and resourceful general practitioners, and doctors suitable for the army and the colonial services. Moorhead's attitude is well illustrated by his earlier 'Remarks on the Teaching of Anatomy':

> Now, as a physician [Moorhead wrote] I am firmly convinced that the

---

[26] Oliver St John Gogarty, 'To Moorhead, Blind', *Wild Apples* (Dublin: Cuala Press, 1930), p. 19.
[27] Doolin, 'In Memoriam' (note 1), p. 439. Robin Flower (1881–1946), Celtic scholar, poet and translator; E. H. Alton (1873–1952), provost of TCD, 1942–52; Dr W. R. Fearon (1892–1959), biochemist and playwright; T. P. C. Kirkpatrick (1869–1954), physician and medical historian.

teaching of anatomy to the ordinary pass men in the medical schools should be invariably directed by a remembrance of the fact that a very large majority of those taught intend to enter into general medical practice. If this fact be remembered it at once becomes a matter of importance to limit the amount of anatomy taught...'[28]

He believed embryology to be 'too complex a subject for the average student'; clinical situations where detailed knowledge of embryology is required are uncommon, usually coming under the observation of specialists.

Moorhead's instincts were 'essentially conservative', but he 'ruled the school committee somewhat as an autocrat' and disliked indications of disrespect towards authority. Bigger has been described as a 'vigorous, plain-spoken Ulsterman' settled in Dublin, lacking suavity and the ability to compromise. When he became dean he 'very injudiciously (and unsuccessfully) tried to oust Moorhead from the chairmanship of the medical faculty which the latter held by tradition as regius professor of physic, and the ensuing bad blood only intensified Moorhead's suspicions of Bigger's reforms'.[29]

BMA in Ireland

When Dublin was the venue of the British Medical Association's 101st annual meeting in July 1933, Moorhead was president. He delivered a memorable address in the great hall of the RDS, speaking on 'The Work of the Association in Ireland', a subject which offered enormous scope for historical recall.

The BMA met first in Dublin in August 1867 under the presidency of William Stokes, and Moorhead had known three men who attended that meeting—the late Dr Walter Smith, the late Sir Hawtrey Benson, and the evergreen Sir John William Moore. Sir Dominic Corrigan had spoken on medical education, and Professor R. W. Smith delivered the address on surgery.

Since then the annual meeting of the BMA was held in Cork (1879) and attended by William Savory who opposed 'Listerism', but whose paper if read carefully, Moorhead said, revealed 'the germs of an aseptic system'; in Belfast (1884) where, at the insistence of Dr (later Sir William) Whitla, a section of pharmacology and therapeutics was inaugurated; in Dublin (1887) where the redoubtable Samuel Haughton (the triple doctor, DD, MD, D.Sc) demanded that Dublin's slums should be

---

[28] Moorhead, 'Remarks on the Teaching of Anatomy', *Dublin J. Med. Sc.* (1912); 133: 420–26.

[29] R. B. McDowell and D. A. Webb, *Trinity College Dublin 1592–1952 An academic history* (Cambridge University Press, 1982), p. 455.

wiped out, holding them responsible for the high death rate;[30] and in Belfast (1909). During the period of forty-two years covered by those five meetings, medicine had passed into the modern phase and the BMA played an important part in its evolution.

Andrew McCarthy, sometime president of the IMA, was present in 1933: he later recalled how 'A totally blind man stood alone on the platform addressing a crowded assembly . . . and, in common with the mass of his listeners, I was amazed at his courage and his triumphant disregard of his disability. His Presidential Address was masterly and inspiring, and I well remember the pride I felt in my fellow-countryman.'[31]

The late John Shanley has referred to Moorhead's fruitful engagement in medical politics:

> Those who worked in the 20's and early 30's of this century for the unity and consequent increase in the influence of the profession will well remember the invaluable help he gave them. It may be truly said that the unity and organisation which was sealed on New Year's Day, 1936, by the incorporation of the I.M.A., could not have been brought about but for his active assistance and wise counsel. There were too many qualms and fears rooted in national and sectarian differences, and too many vested interests to be dealt with to allow any hope of unification at the time. With his name in this connection must be linked that of Charles Macauley [surgeon to the Mater Hospital] whose influence in a different direction was the needed complement to Moorhead's in producing that symbiosis first known as the Irish Free State Medical Union and to-day as the Irish Medical Association.[32]

Honorifics

Mai Moorhead died in 1935. Three years later T. G. married Sheila Gwynn, at Brompton Oratory. The bride was given away by her father, the author, Stephen Gwynn,[33] and had as bridesmaid Miss Pamela Hinkson, a daughter of a poet, the late Katherine Tynan-Hinkson. The bestman was Moorhead's nephew, Dr Charles Moorhead.

Professor Moorhead was the recipient of many honours: he was consulting physician to the army in Ireland, an honorary FTCD and LL.D *honoris causa* of the NUI and of the Queen's University, Belfast. In 1952 (in which year a combined BMA/IMA meeting was held in Dublin) Moorhead was again president-elect of the two associations, but because

---

[30] For an account of Haughton see W. J. E. Jessop, 'Samuel Haughton: a Victorian Polymath', *Hermathena* (1973); 116: 5–26.
[31] Andrew McCarthy, 'In Memoriam Professor T. G. Moorhead', *J. IMA* (1960); 47: 77.
[32] John Shanley, *ibid.*, p. 77.
[33] Stephen Lucius Gwynn (1864–1950) nationalist MP for Galway city, 1906–18, served with the Connaught Rangers in the First World War; a journalist and prolific author, his books, more than fifty in number, included travel-books, biographies, essays and poems.

of his ill-health these offices were in the event filled by Dr P. T. O'Farrell, cardiologist to St Vincent's Hospital.

Moorhead endured great pain and depression in his declining years: death may have come as a friend on 3 August 1960. His remains were buried in Dean's Grange Cemetery.

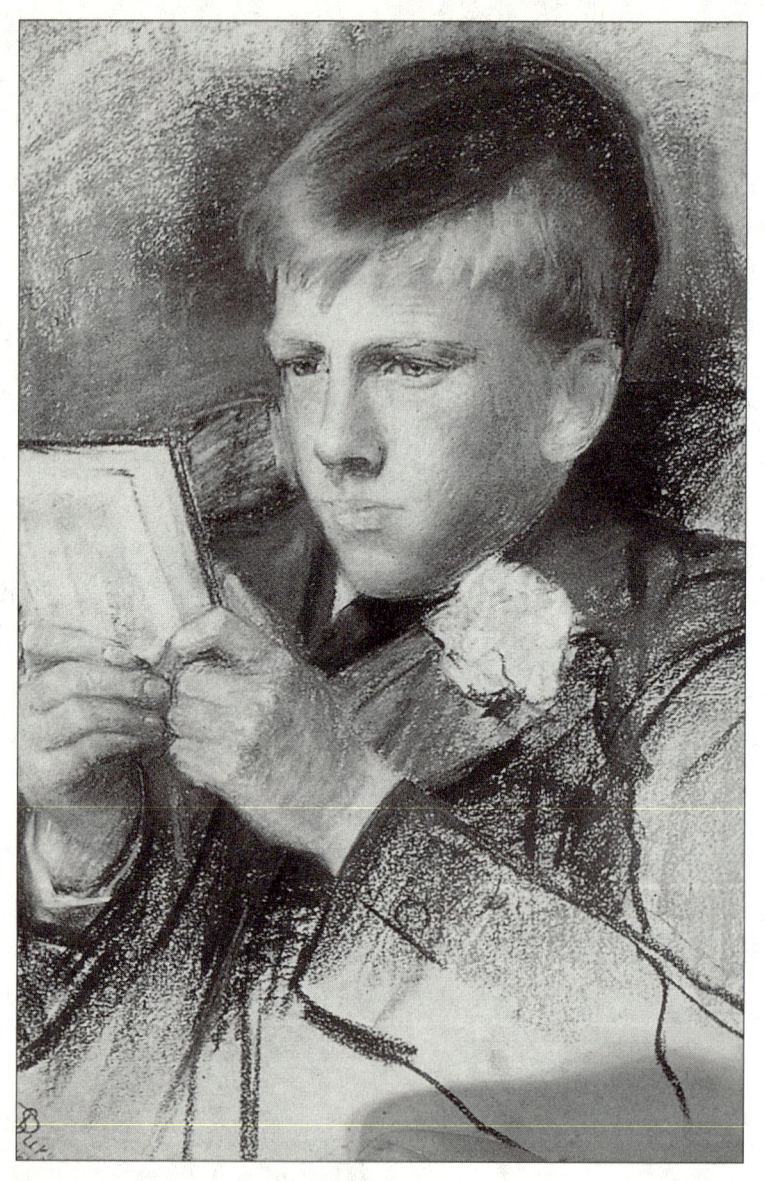

Francis Carmichael Purser, 1877–1934 Professor of Medicine 1917–26 (portrait by his aunt, Sarah Purser)

Chapter 11: Francis Carmichael Purser 1876–1934

By the nineteenth century the Pursers, a family with English roots, were well established in Dublin business circles. Benjamin Purser (1815–98) married Anne Mallet (1817–1901). Their ten children included two Trinity dons, and the distinguished artist Sarah Purser (1848–1943), the first woman RHA, who for many years held her famous salon at Mespil House.[1]

The fourth son, William Edward (b. 1845), married his cousin Elizabeth Geoghegan. Their son, Francis Carmichael Purser, was born on 16 September 1876 in India where his father held office in the civil service.[2] After the death of the little boy's mother from typhoid fever in 1877, it was decided to send him home to Ireland, to be circulated among his aunts. It was unfortunate, incidentally, that his vaccination did not take; he developed a disfiguring attack of smallpox during the voyage, and ever afterwards was sensitive about a pock-marked countenance.

Education

A maternal aunt was married to Dr Biggs, headmaster of Galway Grammar School, where Frank Purser was educated before entering TCD—his uncles, Louis Claude[3] and John Mallet Purser held chairs in classics and physiology respectively.[4] His academic success (MB 1899, MD 1901) was paralleled by prowess on the rugby field; he was capped for Trinity and Ireland.

In 1903 he married Mabel O'Brien. A grandaughter of William Smith O'Brien, the Young Ireland leader, Lucy Mabel O'Brien (b. 1873) supported the movement for women's suffrage, and served a prison sentence in 1913.

Early appointments

Purser was admitted MRCPI in 1901, and elected FRCPI three years later. After a short period as pathologist to Dr Steevens' Hospital he was appointed assistant physician to the Richmond, Whitworth and Hard-

---

[1] John O'Grady, *The Life and Work of Sarah Purser* (Dublin: Four Courts Press, 1996), *passim*. See also J. B. Lyons, *The Quality of Mercer's* (Dublin: Glendale Press, 1991), *passim*.
[2] According to O'Grady, (*ibid.* p. 172), W. E. Purser specialised in the languages of India. His linguistic expertise and habitual taciturnity led a relative to say he was silent in twelve languages.
[3] Louis Claude Purser was one of the editors of James Henry's posthumously-published *Aeneidea*.
[4] It is possible that John Mallet Purser may have fostered his nephew's interest in neurology.

wicke Hospitals (formerly the House of Industry Hospitals).

When the Hamburg publishers of an *Atlas of Pathological Anatomy* by Alfred Kast of Breslau and others, decided to republish the work in five European languages, Purser was invited to produce the English text. A notice in the *Dublin Journal of Medical Science* judged the way he had fulfilled his task to be above all praise. 'The English text reads so smoothly that it is hard to realize that it is a translation from the German.' One suspects that the anonymous reviewer was Sir John William Moore, in view of the following characteristic passage: 'By the way, in describing the fourth plate of the latter [eighth] fasiculus, Dr. Purser correctly translates the German word "lentescierende" (from the Latin "lentesco") by the word "healing"—not "softening"—for the ulcers are seen to be cicatrised to a considerable extent.'[5]

Mercer's Hospital

Purser's application for a post at the Meath Hospital in 1910 was unsuccessful,[6] but he joined the visiting staff at Mercer's Hospital as physician in 1913. This was Dublin's third-oldest voluntary hospital, founded in 1734 in a stone house built by a philanthropic spinster, Mary Mercer, as a shelter for poor girls, and later extended. Its first physician, Dr William Stephens, had studied under Boerhaave in Leyden, and published *Upon the Cure of Gout by Milk Diet* in 1732. Dr Samuel Clossy, author of *Observations on Some of the Diseases of the Parts of the Human Body*, joined the staff in 1762 but sailed for the New World in the following year and was one of the founders of New York City's first medical school. Mr Gustavus Hume, surgeon and builder, has a nearby street named for him; he published *Observations on the Origin and Treatment of Internal and External Diseases*. Dr Charles Lendrick published *Supplementary Observations on the Epidemic Cholera* in 1832. Dr Jonathan Osborne graced the staff for almost thirty years; he studied dropsy in 1835 confirming the presence of renal disease in nine autopsies, and the existence of Bright's disease.[7]

Purser's immediate colleagues at Mercer's included Dr (later Sir John) Lumsden, Mr Seton Sidney Pringle and the redoubtable Mr (later Sir) William Ireland de Courcy Wheeler.[8]

Clinical neurology

By the turn of the century clinical neurology was an established special-

---

[5] [Anon] *Dublin J. Med. Sc.* (1910); 130: 203–05.

[6] Peter Gatenby, *Dublin's Meath Hospital* (Dublin: Town House, 1996), p. 81.

[7] Lyons, *Mercer's*, (note 1), *passim*.

[8] For an account of Wheeler, see Lyons, *An Assembly of Irish Surgeons* (Dublin: Glendale Press, 1984), pp. 55–67.

ity, the outcome of the life's works of a scattered group of men (and women) dispersed over Europe, the United Kingdom and America. This group includes Romberg, Todd, Duchenne (de Boulogne), Lasègue, Charcot, Weir Mitchell, Erb, Gowers, Dejerine (and his wife Augusta Marie Klumpke), Henry Head and others. They were provided with the necessary anatomico-physiological substratum by predecessors and contemporaries whose names constitute another eponymic litany.[9]

Alcmaeon of Croton (fl. c. 500 BC) regarded the brain as the seat of the intelligence; Aristotle saw it as a gland secreting cold humours to prevent the body from overheating. Later it was accepted as the seat of 'the will', and early in the nineteenth century, as Purser puts it, the cerebrum 'was looked upon as a dish of macaroni, all parts alike in texture and function.' This was contested by Gall and Spurzheim, the phrenologists, who held 'that the hemispheres were a mosaic of special properties'.

Pierre Flourens demonstrated cerebellar function in co-ordination of movements, by ablation experiments on pigeons and dogs. The cell theory of Schleiden and Schwann was a forerunner of the neurone theory. The latter established the nerve cell as an anatomical entity supported by glial cells, and the inspired microscopist Ramon y Cajal confessed to his enthralment by the loveliness of the infinitely small.

Sir Charles Bell, who as we have seen was Cheyne's instructor in the technique of postmortem examinations, discovered that the anterior and posterior spinal nerve roots had separate functions, motor and sensory respectively. This was confirmed by Magendie, who was so ardent a vivisectionist that Richard ('Humanity') Martin challenged him to a duel, a contest wisely declined by the physiologist.

One of the many continental doctors impressed by Bell's work was Moritz Heinrich Romberg. He translated Bell's *The Nervous System of the Human Body* into German, and dedicated his own three-volume *Lehrbuch der Nervenkrankheiten des Menschen* (1840, 1843, 1846) to the great Scots anatomist. Romberg, known to generations of students through the eponymous sign he described in tabes dorsalis—'If he [the patient] is ordered to close his eyes while in the erect posture he at once commences to totter and swing from side to side'—was possibly Europe's first clinical neurologist. His appointment as lecturer in neurology at the University of Berlin in 1834 was the first official recognition of neurology as a special branch of medicine.

In London, according to the late Macdonald Critchley, 'the principal exponent of the lush but obscure symptomatology of nervous disease' was Dublin-born Robert Bentley Todd, who described the pathological anat-

---

[9] See Webb Haymaker and Francis Schiller (eds.) *The Founders of Neurology*, (Springfield: Thomas, 1970); Robert B. Aird *Foundations of Modern Neurology—A Century of Progress* (New York: Raven Press, 1994).

omy of tabes dorsalis and is still remembered for his account of postictal paralysis, 'Todd's paralysis'. James Parkinson had already issued *An Essay on the Shaking Palsy* in 1817 and contributions to the nosology were accumulating rapidly.

Eduard Hitzig and G. Fritsch in Berlin (1870), and David Ferrier (1873) in London, demonstrated the excitability of the cerebral cortex, and delineated a motor area which Hughlings Jackson had already postulated after studying seizures commencing unilaterally.

Hermann von Helmholtz's ophthalmoscope was presented to the Berlin Physical Society on 6 December 1850. The invention led Albrecht von Graefe to say: 'Helmholtz has opened a new world for us. How much there is to discover!' Swelling of the optic disc in cases of brain tumour was described by von Graefe as 'Stauungspapille' which Clifford Albutt translated as 'choked disc'. Hughlings Jackson recognised two kinds of 'optic neuritis', one with loss of vision and one without. Hermann Oppenheim was to say: 'He who does not understand how to use an ophthalmoscope is no neurologist.'[10]

Douglas Argyll Robertson drew attention in 1869 to pupillary abnormalities diagnostic of neurosyphilis. Heinrich Erb of Heidelberg (who simultaneously with Westphal reported in 1875 the value of tendon reflexes) used a reflex hammer in daily practice; he introduced a formidable system of examination that became generally accepted as a routine procedure. Joseph Francois Babinski introduced the toe reflex in 1896.

Aphasia

Purser practised as a general physician but was increasingly attracted to neurology, and studied the speciality in Germany before spending some time at the National Hospital, Queen Square, then the leading centre for nervous diseases in the English-speaking world. He established friendships with Gordon Holmes and F. M. R. Walshe. The former, a native of Castlebellingham, County Louth, was a graduate of TCD; Walshe, though a Londoner by birth had an Irish father and many Irish affinities. They both stayed with the Pursers in Dublin and the daughters of the house (like many generations of graduate students) were rather scared of Holmes, compared with whom Walshe was quite a charmer.[11]

'Current Theories of Aphasia' was the subject of Purser's presidential address to the Dublin University Biological Society in 1906.[12] The disorder was topical: Pierre Marie (whom Henry Head called 'the iconoclast')

---

[10] Thomas E. Keys, C. W. Rucker and H. W. Wolton, 'Helmholtz Commemoration Program'. *Proc. Staff Meetings Mayo Clinic* (1951); 26: 209–23.

[11] Hugh Staunton in E. O'Brien (ed.) *The Richmond Hospital: A Closing memoir* (Dublin: Anniversary Press, 1988), p. 121.

[12] Frank C. Purser, 'Current Theories of Aphasia', *Dublin J. Med. Sc.* (1907); 123: 260–78.

had attacked the accepted doctrine.

Hippocrates distinguished between loss of speech and loss of voice, though his contemporaries sometimes attributed the ailment to bewitchment, or possession of a devil. Jean-Baptiste Bouillaud (1786–1881), Marc Dax (1770–1836) and Paul Broca (1824–81) focussed attention respectively on the relevance of the frontal lobes, the left cerebral hemisphere and the third left frontal convolution. Broca's famous patient's vocabulary was reduced to the word 'tan' and a single oath; another patient articulated with difficulty, *oui, non, trois, toujours*, and made his needs known with those words. Surprisingly, Purser did not mention the important distinction between emotive and propositional speech made by Hughlings Jackson, but he recalled that Herodotus told how the mute son of Croesus spoke to save his endangered father at the siege of Sardis.

Both Wernicke and Kussmaul stressed the rôle of sensory centres in speech function; they introduced the terms 'word deafness' and 'word blindness', claiming focal significance for the posterior part of the first temporal gyrus (auditory word centre), the supramarginal convolution and the angular gyrus (perception of printed or written language). The trend was to parcel out the cortex, assigning particular aspects of speech to discrete areas depicted diagramatically.

When Pierre Marie examined brains with frontal lobe lesions deposited by Broca in the Musée Dupuytren, he saw that the pathology was far more extensive than Broca had appreciated. Marie's paper 'Revision de la question de l'aphasie: la troisième circonvolution frontale gauche ne joue acun rôle spécial dans la fonction du langage' (1906), sparked off a controversy. The precise systems of 'the diagram makers' were replaced by chaos. Marie reinterpreted 'Broca's aphasia' as equivalent to Wernicke's aphasia plus anarthria, postulating a deeper lesion in the neighbourhood of the lenticular nucleus.

Purser offered the theory to the students in his audience as an ingenious suggestion meriting careful consideration. 'It is an interesting and novel explanation of aphasia', he said, 'an explanation on clinical and anatomical evidence alone, sought out as one would seek the explanation of a cardiac or hepatic disease where psychology has no dominion, and it is pleasingly unprejudiced by any great regard for the preconceived opinions of other people.'

Being exclusively a human function, animal experiments cannot help in the investigation of speech. The 'experiments' of disease may be too diffuse, but trauma has been utilized. A modern study by Ritchie Russell and Espir of 255 penetrating wounds of the brain can be cited. Their observations confirm Dax's dictum that speech is a function of the left cerebral hemisphere. The relationship is almost invariable, even in sinistrals but the rare instances of right-sided speech centres occur in left-handed predominance.[13]

RAMC

It is hardly profitable to discuss Purser's right to be seen as Dublin's first neurologist, a title which elsewhere I have claimed for George Sigerson, who much earlier worked in Paris with Duchenne (de Boulogne) and J.-M. Charcot, and translated two volumes of the latter's *Leçons sur les maladies du système nerveux* for the New Sydenham Society. But Sigerson lacked a hospital appointment; his academic attachment was in botany and zoology, and he was deeply involved with history and literature.[14]

Purser quickly established himself as Dublin's leading authority on nervous diseases, and developed a busy consulting practice. During the First World War, he held the rank of major in the RAMC, and was consulting neurologist to the forces in Ireland. His services were rewarded with an OBE. He held the chair of medicine at the RCSI from 1917 to 1926, but caused disappointment in Mercer's in 1919 by resigning on becoming a senior physician in the Richmond, Whitworth and Hardwicke Hospitals.

Publications

His publications included reports of tabes dorsalis, amyotonia congenita and Friedrich's ataxia, and he discussed injuries to the peripheral nerves, and their surgical treatment, in the surgical section of the Academy on 7 April 1916. His instructions regarding sensory testing were meticulous, drawing attention to details frequently overlooked.

> The local condition of the part to be tested must also be considered; it should be comfortably supported and pleasantly warm. And the patient himself should be comfortable and as willing as possible to give help. The man

---

[13] The surface area of the speech centre delineated extended into the left frontal lobe a distance of about 2 cm in front of the central sulcus, and into the temporal lobe to within 2.5 cm of the temporal lobe; its upper limit, where wounds of the central sulcus were concerned, was about 5 cm to the left of the saggital line, inferiorly the lowest part of the temporal lobe seemed unrelated to speech; posteriorly it extended to within 1 cm of the tip of the occipital horn of the lateral ventricle, not reaching the occipital lobe. It included the lower half of the left precentral and postcentral gyri, the supramarginal and angular gyri, the inferior parietal gyrus, and a considerable part of the temporal lobe.

Ritchie Russell and Espir point out that 'The scaffolding on which speech is developed is built up in relation to hearing, vision, and the sensorimotor skills involved in uttering words. Injury to the central part of this structure disrupts all aspects of speech, but small wounds at the periphery of the scaffolding may lead to a special disorder of one or other speech function, such as motor aphasia, agraphia or alexia.' Thus to a considerable degree, without siding with the diagram makers, they vindicated the claims of Broca and others.

[14] Lyons, 'George Sigerson: Charcot's Translator'. *J. Hist. Neurosci.* (1997); 6: 50–60.

who wants his tea, or for some other reason resents your coming just when you do, will give much less accurate answers than he will give next day when the sun is shining and you are welcome. This reference to sunshine is not a mere pleasantry; there is no doubt that in any but crude testing a bright, fresh day conduces to answering quite appreciably more accurate than is obtainable on a damp gloomy one. It is always wise to have as few spectators as possible.[15]

No operation should be undertaken unless the wound be healed, or at least aseptic, but he believed the possibilities for surgical success to be increasing.

Shell-shock

Shell-shock—'a name covering a multitude of ideas'—constituted a major neuropsychiatric problem during the First World War, and Purser discussed it at the Academy on 11 May 1917. He recognised three groups—(1) Shell-shock proper; (2) traumatic neurosis; (3) mental alienation—and confined himself to the first. 'Most cases recover fairly quickly with rest, warmth, quiet and occupation.'[16]

English, Scotch and Irish soldiers were equally susceptible, younger men being more frequently affected.

> Many of the men know of the origin of their trouble only by hearsay: they remember, perhaps, an explosion, and then a blank, which may represent any length of time of unconsciousness. Some do not develop any symptoms until some days after the shock, this especially among the cases of traumatic neuroses . . . Others wake up to consciousness and misery, which as a rule become steadily less.[17]

Headache, vertigo, and insomnia were common symptoms. Bad dreams were constant. 'They are red, deafening and choking—nearly always about the war', or about family tragedies. Tremor, and a rapid pulse were present in most cases.

> There is through and through them all a something less tangible but quite definite. It is a *state of depression*, mental and physical; a state of silent hopeless inability. (And one must leave oneself open to feel this. It saves one from making harsh misjudgements, and it protects one from fraud. For sufferers from shell-shock have their imitators, and headache and bad dreams and dizziness are easy symptoms to feign. But the alert readiness to help, the energic muscles in the back, brisk standing to attention, and communica-

---

[15] Purser, 'On Injuries to Peripheral Nerves and their Surgical Treatment', *Medical Press* (1916); 152: 511–14.
[16] Purser, 'Shell-shock', *Dublin J. Med. Sc.* (1917); 144: 201–12.
[17] *Ibid*, p. 202.

tiveness are all foreign to the genuine sufferers.) They are not reminiscent. Nothing upsets them so much as being questioned about or reminded of their experiences. They hate a noise, they hate bustle, and they shun company. They also suffer greatly from the cold. They are happiest, and their condition improves most quickly in circumstances where they are warm and quiet and not bustled.[18]

The prognosis in general was good, but it was not possible at the outset to judge how any given case would do.

What is the pathology of shell-shock? Purser confessed his inability to answer this question. Most of the affected men escaped wounding. Its outward expression were classical signs of horror—'it seems as if the terror that flieth by night and also by day, to which all were exposed, has left greater or more enduring impressions on some nervous systems. . . than on others.' Yet he had seen genuine 'shell-shock' in men who had never been nearer the war than the south of England. He would not assert that shell-shocked men were wanting in courage. 'On the contrary, I know that many have behaved with conspicuous bravery.'[19]

Rat-bite fever

Purser did not restrict his practice exclusively to nervous diseases. His duties at the Hardwicke Hospital included the care of patients with a variety of fevers. He reported a case of typhoid meningitis[20] and published an account of the horrifying pain and suffering endured by a man who developed a diphteritic membrane on an appendicectomy wound (visiting relatives were the source of infection), followed by progressive, uncontrollable and lethal ulceration.[21]

The 'clinical trifle' Purser described with Dr Charles O'Connor of Celbridge was pyrexia affecting a little six-year-old. 'He was said to have been always lively and gay, but when he came under our observation he was pale, peevish and very ill.' The illness started with a swelling, thought to have resulted from an insect bite on the forehead but its course suggested rat-bite fever, an unlikely diagnosis, perhaps, but made more probable when the parents recalled the following incident.

> About three weeks before the swelling was first noticed, the boy, being perfectly well, had wakened his nurse at four in the morning saying his nose

---

[18] *Ibid.*, p. 204.
[19] Shell-shock is the theme of Pat Barker's sensitively-written *Regeneration Trilogy* (featuring W. H. R. Rivers and Sir Henry Head).
[20] J. O'Carroll and F. C. Purser, 'On a Case of Meningitis due to Bacillus Typhosus', *Dublin J. Med. Sc.* (1912); 134: 10–14.
[21] Purser, 'Widespread Ulceration following Appendectomy', *Irish J. Med. Sc.* (1932): 612–25.

was bleeding. This was found not to be so, but blood was noticed on his hand and the blanket under it was stained quite widely. Emulating Eleanor of Castile, his nurse licked the boy's finger and saw on it just distal to the middle knuckle a deep punctured wound. Realizing that there was no object near which could have caused such a wound had the boy knocked his hand against it she searched for a second puncture, but found only a scratch on the proximal side of the knuckle. The house they lived in, an old place, was 'full of rats.' The wound on the finger never festered.[22]

The little patient was given neoarsphenamine and soon recovered his wellbeing.

Medical textbook

Purser's colleagues on the RCSI's academic staff included William Boxwell (a grandson of William Stokes, and physician to the Meath Hospital), who held the chair of pathology (1918–43) and with whom he published a textbook of medicine. A glance at *An Introduction to the Practice of Medicine* (1924) reveals a very different situation from that reflected in, say, Clossy's or Lendrick's books. Clossy's endeavour to relate illnesses to diseased organs was realized by Jonathan Osborne in the single instance of renal pathology, but it was Boxwell and Purser's good fortune to practise at a time when the causes of most major diseases were broadly understood. Gout, for instance, was now seen as a disorder of uric acid metabolism, and instead of Stephen's milk diet Purser recommended the spas at Buxton, Aix-les-Bains and Contrexéville, conceding that 'it is open to question whether the local waters are of much more use than the equivelant amount of Vartry or Dodder, rivers of Ireland, with a morning dose of sulphate of magnesium.'[23]

Their opening pages establish prevention of disease as the medical profession's logical goal. There had been attainments already in this direction: 'It is hard to believe that less than eighty years ago the country was swept with epidemics of relapsing fever, small-pox, and typhus fever.'[24] Medical students were no longer obliged to harden themselves to the graphic examples of suffering *en masse* which, as we have seen, the pupils of Cheyne, Whitley Stokes and others were accustomed to witness.

Koch, as noted in Chapter 9, isolated the causative bacillus of tuberculosis in 1882; diphtheria was known to result from infection with the Klebs Löffler bacillus; insect vectors were incriminated in the transmission of malaria and yellow fever—these infections and others are outlined by Boxwell and Purser in a section followed by chapters detailing the

---

[22] Charles O'Connor and F. C. Purser, 'A Clinical Trifle', *ibid.* (1932): 78–9.
[23] W. Boxwell and F. C. Purser, *An Introduction to the Practice of Medicine* (Dublin: Talbot Press, 1924), p. 855.
[24] *Ibid.*, p. 1.

effects of disordered function of individual organs, including the recently-recognised endocrine system and the ill-effects of vitamin deficiency. Theirs is a fully modern medical textbook, even if certain salients in the landscape of pathology lack prominence.

The book is a watershed, presenting an excellent survey of medicine in the first quarter of the twentieth century, but without eradicating all the older ideas. Thus myocardial infarction is not yet recognised as a clinical entity; cancer of the lung is regarded as a rarity. Insulin was available, but leeches and Corrigan's button remained within the therapeutic armamentarium. The authors did not appreciate the full diagnostic potential of x-rays or electrocardiography. The noontime of 'high-tech' lay far ahead, and meanwhile Hippocratic principles were not forgotten:

> What 'Medical Etiquette' is, we confess we are not quite sure. It is certainly not medical ethics. Medical ethics is a question of honour, and the interest of patients is the foundation of its rules. It must govern all professional relations between doctor and patient. It can never be dispensed with.[25]

Leonard Abrahamson reviewed the book for the *Irish Journal of Medical Science*, praising the authors for offering adequate explanations while keeping classifications to a minimum. They could, he suggested, have omitted some of the rare diseases, giving more space to common conditions; saying more about diabetes, for instance, and less about yellow fever. Space could have been economized elsewhere, too; the authors had usefully drawn attention to the way the teaching of Stokes contributed to modern cardiology, but 'we think that the matter could have been dealt with more briefly, and perhaps more appropriately than by allotting to it a complete and somewhat controversial chapter.'[26]

The passage that understandably irritated Abrahamson, physician to the newly-opened ECG department at Mercer's Hospital, questioned the relevance of the polygraph and the electrocardiograph in the spheres of prognosis and treatment. 'What they have done must be appreciated by all [Boxwell and Purser stated]; but even experts do not always agree on the interpretation of records, and the dogmatism which has arisen among some cardiologists in recent years has not been tested by time, and need not be taken too seriously for the present.'[27]

Little wonder that young Dr Abrahamson bridled at these and other grudging comments, and to the following: 'The electro-cardiograph is very expensive and is not portable, so its applicability is necessarily limited.'

---

[25] *Ibid.*, p. 884
[26] L[eonard] A[brahamson], 'Book Review', *Irish J. Med Sc.* (1924): 44–5.
[27] Boxwell and Purser, *Introduction to Medicine*, (note 23), p. 399.

Professor of neurology

When John A. Scott, professor of physiology at the RCSI (1889–26), died on 2 March 1926, Purser's obituary notice recalled Scott's uneven temper: 'As a teacher he was indefatigable and patient provided he thought the pupil was a worker. To those of whom he thought otherwise, and to those who mouthed advanced physiology when they could not tell him the colour of blood he was ever impatient and often furiously scornful.'[28] Scott's avocation was photography; he was held in high regard by the Dublin Photographic Society.

Purser was appointed professor of neurology in Dublin University in 1926, the chair created 'for the present holder only'. He had no ambition to introduce special lectures on neurology into the curriculum, feeling that the course was wide enough already; the anatomy and physiology of the nervous system were taught satisfactorily in the appropriate departments and the principles of diagnosis of nervous diseases were adequately communicated in the hospitals.

> My impression of the Irish medical student as a whole [he said] is that he could not be kept too long in tutelage with profit to himself. He is an adventurous soul and needs the stimulus of sole responsibility to bring out all the good that is in him. On this account I feel that any extension of the undergraduate course would be an unsatisfactory investment.[29]

Sciatica

Purser's last and best neurological paper, 'On the Nature of Sciatica',[30] cast doubt on the then conventional acceptance of that common complaint as a 'neuritis'. It obviously bothered him—he puzzled over it endlessly, trying to make sense of the signs and symptoms. When his reasoning seemed about to lead him to the unavoidable conclusion that the nerve-root is involved, he was seduced by the attractive theory of a Copenhagen doctor who postulated a muscular lesion at the back of the leg.

That paper was published in 1931. Just two years later, at the annual meeting of the New England Surgical Society in Boston on 30 September, Jason Mixter and Joseph Barr drew attention to the frequency of neurological problems resulting from ruptured intervertebral discs. During the subsequent discussion Dr John Homans said: 'I should like to ask in my ignorance why protrusion of an intervertebral disc should cause pain upon one side?' Mixter replied: 'A tumour far out to the side of the intravertebral disc will compress the nerve roots as they leave the spinal

---

[28] *Irish J. Med. Sc.* (1926): 185.
[29] Purser, 'Discussion on the Teaching of Special Subjects: Neurology', *ibid.* (1932): 635–6.
[30] Purser, 'On the Nature of Sciatica', *ibid.* (1931): 583–99.

canal, causing severe root pain . . . Does that answer your question?'[31]

Calary

Frank and Mabel Purser lived at 32 Fitzwilliam Place. They had a son who held a post as assistant professor of English literature in Glasgow and two daughters, both of whom graduated in medicine. Frank had a powerful physique and a strong character; he disliked publicity, but from a sense of duty accepted important offices such as the presidency of the Irish Medical Association (IMA). An avid reader with a particular regard for Conrad, he would have relished more than most George Borrow's reference in *Lavengro* to 'the wind upon the heath.'

He loved the outdoor life, and when he could afford it he bought a smallholding at Calary, devoting what leisure he could spare to his hobby, reafforestation. He enjoyed the high skies, and the need to establish mastership over the obstinate earth. He was devoted to hill-walking, and had stood on the summits of most of Ireland's mountains.

His friend Boxwell, who thought him 'modest beyond understanding, sensitive and shy', conceded that at times he was dour and uncommunicative, a trait inherited perhaps from his taciturn father. A change of mood made Frank an ideal companion, a master of word-pictures. 'His descriptions of his climbs among the Reeks', Boxwell recalled, 'of being lost in a fog in the crater of Carrauntoohil, of being caught in a storm fishing for sharks in an open boat off Achill, or of herons keeping their twilight watch like grey ghosts by a stream in Galway—these are things to remember.'[32]

The autumn of 1933 was to be a busy period for the president of the IMA. In the Michaelmas term, Purser was appointed unopposed as King's Professor of the Practice of Medicine to Dublin University; on 18 October, St Luke's Day, he donned the ornate robe of the president of the Royal College of Physicians of Ireland. 'Life is sweet, brother, who would want to die?' Robust, vigorous, fifty-seven years old and at the summit of his career it may never have occurred to him to ponder Borrow's question. But he was to be the first PRCPI to die in office for more than two hundred years.

On Wednesday 28 February 1934, Purser lectured at the university in the afternoon and saw private patients in Fitzwilliam Place. Walking from his consulting room to the front door with his last patient, he experienced chest pain which he analysed with clinical detachment—certainly it was cardiac, *dolor cordis*, yet the sense of impending dissolution

---

[31] William Jason Mixter and Joseph S. Barr, 'Rupture of the Intervertebral Disc with involvement of the Spinal Canal', *New Eng. J. Med.* (1934); 211: 210–15.
[32] *Irish J. Med. Sc.* (1934): 134–6.

that may accompany angina pectoris was missing. An hour later he was dead.

St Stephen's Church, Upper Mount Street, was thronged at the funeral service but the interment upon lonely, windswept, Calary was private.

He shall not hear the bittern cry...

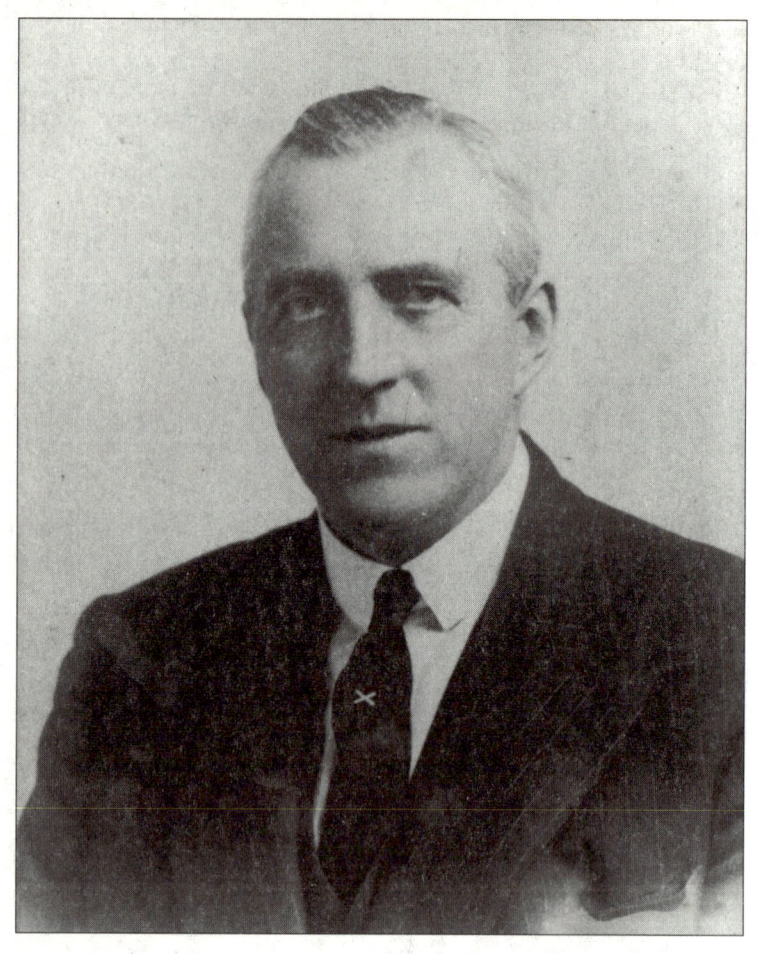

George Edward Nesbitt, 1882–1948 Professor of Medicine 1926–30

Chapter 12: George Edward Nesbitt 1882–1948

George Edward Nesbitt was one of the five sons of Alexander Nesbitt of Randalstown, County Antrim, a man who in his youth (1867) came to Dublin as an apprentice at Messers Arnotts of Henry Street, and forty years later was chairman of the board. George, the eldest son, was born in the capital in 1882, and educated at St Andrew's College and TCD.[1] Commencing BA 1904, he took the MB in 1907, proceeding MD in 1910. Admitted MRCPI 1910, he was elected FRCPI in the following year. Meanwhile, in 1908, he had joined the staff of the Richmond Hospital as assistant visiting physician, being promoted full physician in 1919. He was also on the staff of the National Children's Hospital, anaesthetist to the Dental Hospital and sometime specialist sanitary officer (he held the DPH) to the Dublin Military District. His appointment as medical officer to Arnotts (with a salary of £100) was a useful bonus.[2]

His avocations included sailing. When the Nesbitt boys were old enough to influence their parents, Alexander and Elizabeth were persuaded to move the family home to Dalkey. They lived at Breffni, Church Road, a short distance from Bullock Harbour where they had a boat. Later, George had a cruiser named *Charity* and was a member of the Royal Irish Yacht Club.

Modern developments

When elected to the presidency of the Dublin University Biological Society in 1923, Nesbitt, recalling that he had been awarded the society's medal in 1904, took 'Modern Developments of Medicine' as the theme of his inaugural address. Since 1904 he had witnessed a broadening of the clinical applications of x-rays, the introduction of radiotherapy, the discovery by Schaudin of the spirochaeta pallidum, the causative organism of syphilis in 1905, and the development of Wassermann's diagnostic test for that disease two years later. Ehrlich's 'Salvarsan' became available for the treatment of syphilis in 1910. The polygraph, electrocardiogram and sphygmomanometer had been invented.

> As the outstanding feature [he said] of the edifice which is being constructed so rapidly, I would draw your attention to the development of Biochemistry. The study of metabolism and the numerous tests by which the functional efficiency of our various organs can be ascertained; the elaborate methods of chemical analysis of our tissues and excretions, and the science of Dietetics—these are all new and they are blazing the trail of modern medicine. They have nearly torn away the veil

---

[1] Obituary notice, *The Irish Times*, 9 August 1948.
[2] Ronald Nesbitt, *At Arnotts of Dublin 1843–1993* (Dublin: A. & A. Farmar, 1993), p. 81.

that has shrouded diabetes since the time of Celsus and Aretaeus, and their latest triumph is the discovery of the world-famous 'Insulin'.[3]

Nesbitt was interested in metabolic disorders, and in what Sir Clifford Albutt designated 'Hyperpiesia', a term replaced by hypertension or high blood pressure.

> Of all the clinical apparatus at our disposal [Nesbitt said], I consider the sphygmomanometer about the simplest and the most valuable, and I would seriously suggest that all members of the community over, say, the age of 30, whose lives entail any kind of responsibility, should have occasional estimations of blood pressure, and a simple examination of the urine. Five minutes per annum would suffice.[4]

His earlier publications deal with this common disorder, and shall be referred to before considering Nesbitt's cautious acceptance of insulin.

Early papers

His first paper in the *Dublin Journal of Medical Science* discussed the clinical estimation of blood-pressure.[5] He recalled that almost a century elapsed between the classical experiments of Stephen Hales on blood-pressure, and the introduction of Poiseuille's mercurial manometer in 1828. Since then, factors concerned in the production of blood-pressure, its function and conditions determining its variations had been established. Physiologists were agreed as to the leading factors; these were published in every textbook, and had 'become so familiar that we regard them as physiological platitudes'.

Clinicians had tended to judge blood-pressure by 'feeling the pulse' until Vierordt in 1855, and von Basch more successfully in 1887, measured it instrumentally. Methods of sphygmomanometry inevitably multiplied, and Nesbitt pointed out that 'our zeal may, with faulty methods, lead us considerably astray in our diagnosis, treatment and result'. He had, himself, approached the procedure with excessive confidence:

> A very short practical experience, however, forcibly suggested to me that the sphygmomanometer was not the infallible judge presiding over clinical destinies that much current medical literature would have us believe. We read descriptions of cases, accompanied by charts of blood-pressure, stating the latter in mm. of Hg. as glibly as the record of temperature and pulse, and with no indication as to

---

[3] George E. Nesbitt, 'Modern Developments of Medicine', *Irish J. Med. Sc.* (1923): 349–70.
[4] *Ibid.*, p. 352.
[5] Nesbitt, 'The Clinical Estimation of Blood-Pressure', *Dublin J. Med. Sc.* (1912); 133: 323–36.

whether there is any doubt of their equal accuracy and reliability.[6]

Before long, he was aware of factors which could vitiate his conclusions. He discussed these under four headings:

> (1) *Instrumental:* he favoured the 'armlet method', pointing out that its faulty adjustment, or differences of cuff width, affected the readings.
> (2) *Personal:* related to the skill and experience of the examiner.
> (3) *Factors affecting the patient:* posture, recent exertion, emotional etc.
> (4) *Errors of deduction from correct observations:* e.g. variable interpretation of causation.

He believed high blood-pressure should never be diagnosed unless accompanied by additional signs such as forcibly acting heart, and an accentuated second sound. The tendency to resort to terms such as 'arteriosclerosis' or 'chronic interstitial nephritis' may console the examiner, while leaving the actual cause undetected. Of the many theories in vogue, Nesbitt mentioned a renal pressor substance postulated by H. Batty Shaw.

Laboratory tests

Aware of the laboratory investigation which regularly supplemented clinical examination at continental medical schools, Nesbitt complained that with the exception of an occasional case of special interest such methods were not used in Dublin hospitals. For his introduction to the application of laboratory tests he was indebted to Bauer of Vienna, and he presented a paper on tests of liver function to the Academy of Medicine's section of medicine on 16 May 1913.[7]

He described the laevulose and galactose tests, the amino-acid test and the aldehyde reaction. The last of these was simple to perform; it detected excess of urobilinogen in the urine, and Nesbitt believed it should be used routinely. The cases available to him, as an assistant physician, were insufficient to enable him to make an extended trial, but he believed other observers would find the tests 'of assistance in trying to illuminate a very dark corner of our complex organism'.[8]

Later, Nesbitt advocated the use of tests of renal function—the urea concentration test, estimation of blood urea and excretion of phenol-sulphonephthalein—which 'enable us to see a little further behind the scenes than even the soundest clinical examination will permit'.[9]

---

[6] *Ibid.*, p. 325–6.
[7] Nesbitt, 'Tests for Liver Function', *ibid.* (1913); 136: 327–35.
[8] *Ibid.*, p. 335.
[9] Nesbitt, 'Some Renal Efficiency Tests', *Irish J. Med. Sc.* (1923); 533–42.

Diabetes

Encouraged by the council of the section of medicine, Nesbitt spoke on the 'Allen treatment' of diabetes on 33 November 1916, and showed a patient who had benefitted from the regime. He explained that having obtained every grade of apparent diabetes in animals by removing portions of the pancreas, F. M. Allen of the Rockefeller Institute studied the dietary control.[10] The urines of the milder types were kept sugar-free by moderate restriction of carbohydrate and protein, but Allen's virtual starvation diet was enforced on severer grades for initial periods of varying length.

In the hospital setting the patient remained on his usual diet for two days after admission, permitting basic measurement of glycosuria. On the third day the patient remained in bed: absolutely nothing was given to him except black coffee, clear tea or meat extract every two hours, with water as required. 'If acidosis or coma threatens 1/2 to 1 oz. of whisky is given every 2–4 hours, or it may be given merely to relieve the strain of the fast, which is continued till the patient becomes sugar-free (2–10) days.'[11] The patient's tolerance of carbohydrate, protein and fat was then gradually ascertained.

The Allen diet had the support of Joslin of Boston, who told patients they would live longer if they followed the plan, but must live at a reduced rate. 'The problem', Nesbitt said, 'is of classical antiquity, and is not confined to diabetes.' His audience did not share his enthusiasm: Sir John William Moore objected to starvation, because of the fear of acidosis; Moorhead believed many cases got on very well on the old lines, and should not be subjected to such a severe treatment; Dr W. M. Crofton, who was himself seeking a pancreatic extract with which to control diabetes, referred to the use of hormonadin.[12]

Encephalitis

As a general physician Nesbitt would have been prepared to undertake the care of patients with a wide range of diseases. Thus in May 1915 he published 'Remarks on the recent Outbreak of Cerebrospinal Meningitis in the Dublin Military District'. It may be mentioned that he referred to stiffness of the neck as 'the soldered neck'. Examination of the CSF was undertaken and Gram-negative diplococci isolated.

With Joseph O'Carroll, his senior colleague at the House of Industry Hospitals, as co-author Nesbitt described four cases of encephalitis lethargica before the Royal Academy of Medicine in Ireland on 7 February 1919.[13] The

---

[10] Nesbitt, 'Remarks on the Allen Treatment of Diabetes', *Dublin J. Med. Sc.* (1916); 142: 379–85, 417–19.

[11] *Ibid.*, p. 381.

[12] *Ibid*, p. 418.

[13] J. O'Carroll and George Nesbitt, 'Some Recent Cases of Encephalitis Lethargica', *Dublin J. Med. Sc.* (1919); 148: 206–216.

purpose of their report was 'to draw attention to the existence of this remarkable disease' in Ireland. A relative newcomer to the nosology, it was first described by C. von Economo of Vienna in 1917.

Speaking as president of the section of medicine of the Royal Academy of Medicine in Ireland Nesbitt discussed 'the value of graphic methods' in the investigation of cardiac cases, illustrating his talk with a wide variety of electrocardiograms.[14]

He contributed to a series of articles on acute emergencies of practice, dealing with dyspnoea and covering a wide range of causes.

Blood transfusion

Although attempts to transfuse blood were made in the seventeenth century, the first successful transfusion in Ireland was not achieved until 22 February 1870. Then, in an emergency situation, Robert McDonnell gave blood to 'a very handsome, tall, well-made lady', exsanguinated by post-partum haemorrhage. Good fortune decreed that the donor (her husband) had compatible blood, for it was not until 1900 that the discovery of blood groups by Landsteiner of Vienna made transfusion a practicable procedure, soon facilitated by the use of sodium citrate as an anticoagulant.[15]

Nesbitt was one of the main speakers at a discussion on blood transfusion held by the section of surgery of the Academy of Medicine on 16 December 1921.[16] Being aware of the potential benefits, he regretted that 'the practice does not appear to have been widely accepted in this country up to the present.'[17] This resulted from the difficulty of providing a suitable range of donors, especially at short notice, for a number of small hospitals. He believed the procedure deserved a more extended trial.

The indications for transfusion were:

(1) Severe blood loss, or to improve a patient's condition preoperatively.
(2) To supply essential substances deemed to be missing, e.g. agglutinins, antibodies, etc.

It was with its use in the second connection, when dealing with anaemias, leukaemias and intractable haemorrhage that Nesbitt was most familiar. His practice was to test a drop of the patient's serum with a drop of the donor's blood. The result was usually unequivocal, but in severe anaemias indefinite reactions occurred. He used citrated blood in small quantities.

Henry Stokes, surgeon to the Meath Hospital had given twenty-nine

---

[14] Nesbitt, 'Some Cardiac Cases Illustrating the Value of Graphic Methods', *Irish J. Med. Sc.* (1927): 68–75.
[15] J. D. H. Widdess, 'Robert M'Donnell—a Pioneer of Blood Transfusion', *Irish J. Med. Sc.* (1952): 11–20.
[16] Widdess, 'Discussion on Blood Transfusion', *Irish J. Med. Sc.* (1922): 23–6.
[17] *Ibid.*, p. 23.

transfusions in 1920 and 1921. He had learned the necessary techniques in the RAMC during the First World War, and was attempting to grapple with the problems of transfusion in civil practice. 'How to have a group of donors available for emergencies is a puzzle I have not solved, but I suggest that it is the duty of all of us to have our bloods standardised so that time need not be wasted when the time arises.'[18]

Insulin

Returning to Nesbitt's address to the Biological Society in 1923 we find him discussing diabetes, and the dangers of acidosis. He emphasized that renal glycosuria and lactosuria could cause diagnostic confusion, and mentioned that Allen's 'somewhat drastic *régime*' had been replaced by the 'Basal Maintenance Diet', the object of which was to maintain nitrogenous equilibrium while supplying sufficient calories for a resting patient, and properly balanced in regard to ketogenic and antiketogenic substances. If successful in reducing glycosuria, the diet is gradually increased to permit activity.

Accustomed to a dietary approach, Nesbitt's acceptance of the role of insulin was extremely cautious:

> ... quite a small proportion of cases really require Insulin except as a luxury, but in acidosis and coma the drug is invaluable. In severe infections, in gangrene, or in the case of emergency operations in diabetes it will probably be life-saving. The Toronto Committee deprecates the indiscriminate use of Insulin as a real source of danger. Personally, I find that I have had to use it but seldom, though with uniformly satisfactory results. It is a trump card that I like to keep in my hand as long as possible. Its routine use would, I think, be justified only, if it transpires that there is a substantial gain in sugar tolerance after a course.
>
> The dose depends on the case—the patient should be rendered free from sugar and acidosis. Presumably the less that will do so the better.[19]

Nesbitt succeeded Frank Purser as professor of medicine at the RCSI in 1926 and held the chair until 1930. Details of his pedagogic years have not survived.

South Africa

Tall, handsome and powerfully built, Nesbitt was essentially a man's man (whom women admired), popular in rugby football circles. At the Richmond Hospital, where his colleagues included Drs Paul Murray and Morgan Crowe, he prepared members of the Irish team for their important matches.

He married Madeline Collins, a daughter of the manager of the Northern Bank's head-office in Dame Street. They had two daughters, Betty (b.

---

[18] See J. B. Lyons, *An Assembly of Irish Surgeons* (Dublin: Glendale, 1984), p. 103.
[19] Nesbitt, 'Modern Developments', *Irish J. Med. Sc.* (1923), p. 309.

circa 1915) and Dorothy (b. 1917); the former died of poliomyelitis in 1941.

Madeline Nesbitt was aware of her husband's attractiveness to many members of her own sex, and being intensely jealous of his women patients she often accompanied him in his car on professional visits. Personality problems disrupted the marriage and, of course, it is possible, indeed likely, that George did have a wandering eye. Eventually he developed an attachment to a young lady doctor, Molly Kiely. He resigned from the chair of medicine in 1930, and in the following year the couple went to South Africa and settled in East London where she took his name by deed poll.

Nesbitt remained active in his profession and Molly, too, had a successful practice. He was a member of the staff of the Frere Hospital, East London. He served on the federal council of the Medical Association of South Africa, and in 1947 was president of the South African Medical Congress. He was honorary physician to the members of the British royal family during their visit to South Africa. A keen golfer and yachtsman, he was president of East London's Kennel Club.

Nesbitt was district governor of Rotary for the area of Africa south of the Equator. He was very conscious of the existence of a colour bar in South Africa, and discussed the problem when speaking at a weekly luncheon of the Dublin Rotary Club on 10 August 1937. There was also, he told them, a division of the whites into British and Afrikaans. The natives, he believed, had picked up many of the white men's habits, and all of their vices. According to an *Irish Times* report, Nesbitt predicted that by a process of evolution the natives would become civilised—'as we know civilisation'—and a critical situation would precede a decision as to who was going to inhabit South Africa, the whites or the blacks.

He returned to Dublin in broken health in May 1948, and died from a bronchial carcinoma at his brother's house in Ailesbury Road on 7 August. There was no issue from the second relationship.

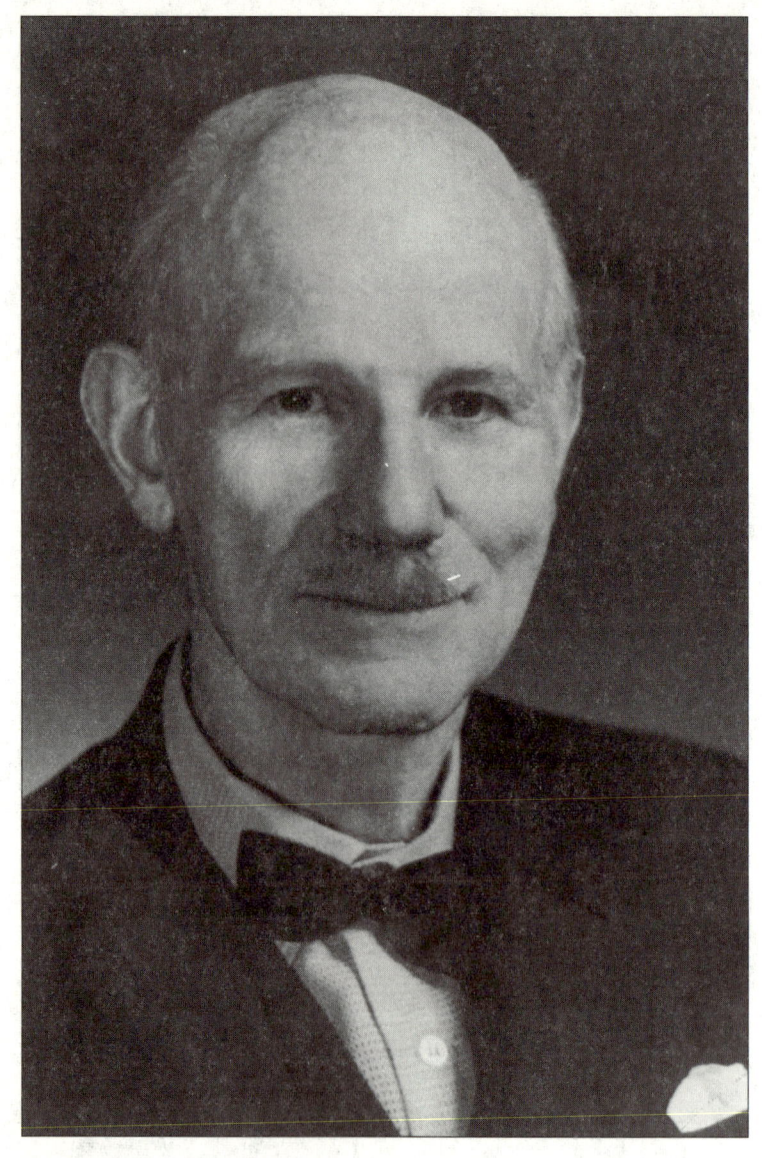

Victor Millington Synge, 1893–1976 Professor of Medicine 1930–34

Chapter 13: Victor Millington Synge, 1893-1976

The Synges were a County Dublin-based family, their best-known scion the playwright John Millington Synge (b. 1871), whose brother Samuel Synge graduated in medicine, took holy orders and sailed for China as a missionary.[1] Their father, John Hatch Synge, a barrister, died in 1872 from smallpox acquired while visiting a neighbour laid-up with a mild attack of the disease. A maternal grandfather, Dr Robert Traill, rector of Skull in County Cork, had perished from famine fever contracted from a parishioner in 1847. Through the Traills, the Synges were connected with Dr Antony Traill, TCD's only medically-qualified provost.

Victor Millington Synge, the playwright's nephew, was born at 15 Upper Leeson Street, Dublin, on 5 September 1893, the son of a land agent Edward Synge of Kingscourt, Cavan, and his wife Ellen Frances Pine. His secondary education was obtained at St Andrew's College. A foundation scholar of TCD, and Hudson scholar in the Adelaide Hospital, he enjoyed walking in the Dublin and Wicklow hills, an avocational pursuit that influenced his working methods—for he paced up and down endlessly as he studied, much to the irritation of John E. Coolican (future surgeon to Mercer's Hospital), whose room in Trinity was beneath Synge's.

Appointments

Victor Synge served in the Royal Navy as a surgeon-probationer, before graduating MB BCh BAO in 1918. He proceeded MD and took the DPH in the following year, spending some time in Paris, where dermatology was his particular interest. He was admitted MRCPI in 1920, and elected fellow in 1921.

Synge's qualifications included the LM of the Rotunda Hospital. This indicates that at first he may have had family practice in mind, but a brief period as pathologist to Sir Patrick Dun's Hospital was followed by an appointment in 1921 as visiting physician to the Royal City of Dublin Hospital, Baggot Street, and these posts determined the direction of his career. He practised as a general physician, and was elected to the chair of medical jurisprudence in the RCSI in 1923, moving in 1930 to the professorship of medicine, from which he resigned in 1934 on becoming King's Professor of the Practice of Medicine in TCD.

---

[1] Dr Samuel Synge wrote 'Notes on Chinese medicine', *Dublin J. Med. Sc.* (1905); 119: 184–9.

Publications

Victor Synge's contributions to medical literature were not numerous; according to his younger contemporary Dr Brendan O'Brien, he was reluctant to write unless he felt he had something of importance to say.[2] Diphtheria and rheumatic fever were major clinical problems of the time on which he did comment usefully, and he sent a note to the *Irish Journal of Medical Science* on a tumour of the spinal cord which he had diagnosed competently in Baggot Street in 1926. Physicians in the first half of the present century did not bow to the clinical superiority of neurologists.

His first clinical paper reported a gumma of the liver in a forty-nine-year-old man, admitted to Baggot Street Hospital on 27 September 1921 with ascites and hepato-spleno-megaly. His tentative diagnosis was 'Banti's disease', and the young physician must have been disconcerted when the autopsy revealed syphilitic aortitis and a nodular mass in the liver, 'obviously a gumma'. The Wassermann reaction had not been done, and presumably the purpose of publishing the case was to point to the diagnostic seriousness of the omission.[3]

Synge's tumour case, a thirty-nine-year-old married woman had developed a spastic paraplegia, with sensory loss below the epigastrium. The cerebrospinal fluid showed high protein and a yellow colour. The radiologist, Dr T. G. Hardman, localised the level of compression by myelgraphy; Seton Pringle and Adams McConnell (the latter Dublin's first neurosurgeon) removed the growth which unfortunately was a sarcoma.[4]

Diphtheria and rheumatic heart disease

'In 1925 in the Irish Free State 15 persons died from diphtheria.' The disease was a medical emergency, and the following is Synge's description of faucial diphtheria:

> The typical case, with the snowy white, raised, tough, adherent patch on one tonsil and invading the soft palate, the enlarged glands, the moderate pyrexia and rapid pulse, presents no diagnostic difficulties. The membrane may be yellowish or greenish, sometimes almost black and shrivelled in a case of long duration. Both tonsils are often involved. In an early case the membrane may not extend beyond the tonsil itself. If the membrane is only present on the medial, and not on the anterior, aspect of an enlarged tonsil, careful examination with good illumination is necessary in order to see it.[5]

---

[2] Brendan O'Brien, 'Obituary V. M. Synge, F.R.C.P., F.R.C.P.I.', *J. Irish Med. Assn.* (1976); 69: 132.
[3] V. M. Synge, 'Gumma of the Liver', *ibid.* (1922): 603–04.
[4] Synge 'Tumour of the Spinal Cord', *ibid.* (1926): 282.
[5] 'Acute Emergencies of Practice: Diphtheria', *ibid.* (1926): 29–30.

The laryngeal and nasal forms were duly described, and details of treatment given. Complications were likely to occur in the second or third week in mild untreated cases, and in severe cases in which treatment was delayed or inadequate. 'The commonest complication is paralysis of the soft palate, producing regurgitation of food through the nose.' Before serum treatment became available, sudden death from myocardial failure sometimes occurred in the third week.

He dealt, too, with the prophylaxis of diphtheria,[6] and in 1930 recorded a case of mumps meningitis, a comparative rarity in Dublin, he believed.[7]

The occasion for a formal lecture given at Baggot Street on 30 June 1939 is not stated, but his paper will recall for those who commenced practice in the first half of the twentieth century the gamut of signs in rheumatic valvular disease, and the importance of its complications.[8] 'Next to pulmonary tuberculosis mitral stenosis is certainly the commonest cause of haemoptysis in this country.' The epidemic of bronchial carcinoma had not yet manifested itself.

Unlike Charles Benson years before, Synge nursed no delusion as to the influence of medication on rheumatic myocarditis. 'Salicylates are useless. Digitalis is to be avoided. Once a person has had rheumatic fever he is liable to a recurrence of the disease. Prevention of recurrence is unsatisfactory.'

His account of the signs of mitral stenosis includes the following interesting passage:

> Usually, and sometimes even before there is any murmur, one hears what seems to be a reduplicated second sound, because in these cases when one listens at the pulmonary area the second sound is not reduplicated. What has occurred is that an extra sound has originated in close relationship to the normal second sound at the mitral area. The mechanism of this extra sound is not satisfactorily explained; possibly it is due to a powerful jet of blood coming through the stenosed mitral opening at the beginning of diastole and throwing a part of the wall of the left ventricle into a state of sudden tension. It is sometimes called Sansom's 'double-shock sound.' The name is awkward and the explanation is doubtful, but the sign is important.[9]

Surely this is what came to be called the 'opening snap'?

Presidential addresses

Election to the presidency of a student's medical society is an honour welcomed by consultants. The title of Synge's inaugural address as president of the Dublin University Biological Society on 7 November 1925 was 'A Criti-

---

[6] 'The Prophylaxis of Diphtheria', *ibid.* (1926): 131–4.
[7] 'Mumps Meningitis', *ibid.* (1930): 290.
[8] 'Rheumatic Heart Disease in Practice', *ibid.* (1939): 701–04.
[9] 'Rheumatic Heart Disease in Practice', *ibid.*, p. 702.

cism of Modern Medicine', and reading it today it is desirable that one attempts to recreate the atmosphere of the occasion—the solemn hall, the excitement generated by the event, the eager students from every year of the course, the VIPs and elders—nothing of which adheres to the printed page. And yet it is sufficiently peppered with aphoristic comments, to leave one in no doubt that young Dr Synge from Baggot Street held his audience's attention.

'The foundation of medical education is secondary education.' 'It is fatuous to spend 2½ years in the study of anatomy.' 'Two hemiplegias do not make a monoplegia.' 'Useless intellectual lumber often mars the free play of thought and reason.' 'We are too ready to apply unfinished biochemical research to clinical purposes.' 'The science of errors is, unfortunately, a neglected branch of study.' 'Money and equipment facilitate discoveries; it is brains alone which make them.'

Ten years later Synge's presidential address to the section of medicine, Royal Society of Medicine in Ireland was less aphoristic. He attempted, indeed, to express the practitioner's capacity for the care of his patients in a formula: $A + B + C + X$. Constant for each individual, 'A' depends on 'inherent mentality' and 'the mentality acquired during childhood and the school period'. 'B' is knowledge absorbed in medical school, and a few subsequent years—it diminishes gradually. 'C' is knowledge gained by practical experience. 'X' is the absorption of new medical knowledge and varies greatly in different individuals.

He divided specialists into three groups: (1) 'Those who know something about everything and a little more about something'—the old-fashioned specalist. (2) 'Those who know everything about something and nothing about anything else'—an increasing group. (3) 'Those who know something about everything and everything about something'—the most useful type.

He spoke caustically of research: 'There is a magic about the word "research." There is a feeling that anything which can be dubbed "research" puts the author in the seats of the mighty, and makes him feel that he is one of the elect who are advancing medicine.'[10] Money had little interest for Synge, who was notoriously slow to send out bills. He made no parade of his generosity but was known to have helped hard-up students. On an occasion that it came to his knowledge that a particularly bright boy had not entered for his finals Synge enquired why? Learning that the entrance fee was beyond the lad's present means the professor put up the money.

Participating in a discussion on 'The Irish Hospitals and the Public' in 1935, he attributed a bed shortage at certain times of the year to lack of convalescent homes, to which old and infirm patients could be transferred. And there was a small group who were starving rather than sick. 'They need food, not medicine.'

He complained that records were inadequately kept. Treatment of tuber-

---

[10] 'Tendencies in Medicine', *ibid.*, (1935): 653–7.

culosis was unsatisfactory—'We must have more large sanatoria with from 100 to 200 beds each, properly equipped with x-ray apparatus, operating theatres etc.'[11]

A disappointed candidate

Unsuited, perhaps, to high office, and particularly to the robust electoral procedures that lead to it, Synge agreed nevertheless to put his name in the hat in 1949, as a tentative candidate for the post of PRCPI. The ballot to elect three candidates was held at a college meeting on 30 September. Synge topped the poll with 24 votes. Professor Leonard Abrahamson came a not so close second with 19 votes. The third candidate selected was J. W. Bigger with 12 votes.

Sensing defeat, Bigger withdrew before the vital ballot on 7 October, leaving the contest for nomination between Synge and Abrahamson. The odds may have seemed to favour the former, if we are to judge from the earlier ballot. He was four years older than Abrahamson, highly respected and as Regius Professor of Physic in TCD he held the more prestigious chair. But being less the man-of-affairs than his worldy-wise opponent, he was unlikely to have canvassed the electorate (contemporary FRCPIs) with appropriate thoroughness, if at all.

Canvassing was frowned upon officially, but widely practised. It was not, Synge would have argued, playing the game, and the omission was possibly reflected in the voting: Abrahamson 27; Synge 22. Bitterly disappointed, Synge resolved to avoid future confrontations. Never again would he invite humiliation. This was rather to make a mountain out of a mole-hill, and the college elders fully expected to welcome him as president in due course.

When the years passed, and Synge failed to step forward to claim the presidency his years entitled him to, a younger fellow was deputed to speak a word in his ear. The young man did as he was bid—suggesting he should contest the coming election—and was answered in tones that did not brook argument.

'I certainly shall not', snapped Synge. 'I'm not a commercial doctor.'

Medical education

Commenting in *Studies* on an article, 'Medical Education in Ireland', by Dr Edward Freeman, PRCPI in 1954, Synge did not agree that all Irish medical schools were 'sadly deficient in both personnel and equipment'. Most of them had enough to instruct classes of sixty to eighty students in each medical year. 'It is not desirable, or indeed possible, to introduce knowledge into a student in the same way as a pigeon feeds her young.' He defended the capital's smaller hospitals. 'In Dublin the patient is still a patient—a human being of flesh and blood. In more advanced medical centres he has sometimes

---

[11] 'The Irish Hospitals and the Public', *ibid*. (1935): 209–10.

tended to become a case or just a number or sometimes even a numbered guinea pig or experimental mouse.' He opposed the plan to replace the small hospitals with one or two large ones and the prospect of specimens being sent from Baggot Street to the central laboratory at St James's made him shake with rage.

Synge thought Dublin too small for postgraduate teaching. 'Let foreigners come here to study midwifery and let our graduates go abroad to study medicine and surgery.' He had some words of praise for the way Americans had debunked spelling based on long-forgotten classical derivations. 'It is a delight to the orthographic dub to be able to leave the "o" out of oedema, to eliminate the middle "a" from anaemia, to interchange the positions of the "r" and the "e" in goitre and still be perfectly correct.'

Where Freeman expressed pessimism about what the future could offer Irish medical schools, Synge was more hopeful, and reiterated Provost Mahaffy's quip: 'Ireland is a country in which the unexpected always happens and the inevitable never comes off.'[12]

Victor Millington Synge was himself something of a polymath, a knowledgeable botanist, a linguist and well-read in German, Norwegian and Russian. He liked to talk to foreign patients in their own languages, and after conversing with a Ukranian sailor he remarked to the house-physician, 'that fellow speaks very bad Russian."[13] His brother, J. L. Synge, was a distinguished mathematician.

Alfie Parsons

Synge's contributions to the *Irish Journal of Medical Science* included three obituaries—those of Parsons, Pringle and Fearon, leading lights in their day but without eponyms, or major discoveries, to guide their names through the murk of oblivion. Senator Fearon (1892–1959) had represented Dublin University in Seanad Éireann since 1943; he held a chair of biochemistry, was the author of *Nutritional Factors in Disease* and a well-received standard textbook of biochemistry.

Synge recalled Fearon as both a scientist and an artist. 'He was an accomplished musician, he could write a play, he could compose charming verse. As a conversationalist he was supreme, he had a ready apposite, and always delightful wit—a wit which was never cruel, never wounded.' The biochemist's obituarist was kinder to him than TCD's academic historians McDowell and Webb who, while prepared to concede that Fearon was 'a remarkable man', and the best lecturer in the medical school, added some diminishing sentences:

---

[12] 'Medical Education in Ireland', *Studies* (1954); 43: 136–8.
[13] Davis Coakley *Baggot Street: A Short History of the Royal City of Dublin Hospital* (Board of Governors: Dublin, 1995), p. 59.

At an early age he fell, rather unfortunately, under the influence of Oliver Gogarty, and tried as Gogarty did with some success, to become a complete Renaissance man. But Fearon was shy and timid, and would not have lasted long in the world of Rabelais and Machiavelli. He would have been more at home in the seventeenth century with Sir Thomas Browne or the early members of the Royal Society.[14]

Seton Sidney Pringle (1879–1918) was a native of Clones, County Monaghan, and a graduate of TCD. With Mr Robert Maunsell and Mr William (later Sir William) Wheeler, he had formed a potent triumvirate at Mercer's Hospital, bringing it after a troubled period back to the forefront of Irish surgery. He moved to Baggot Street in 1918, and was also surgeon to Drumcondra Hospital.[15]

Students have a talent for nicknames, but the shifting of vowels that created 'Satan' Pringle was mere punning unless, somehow, it evokes a whiff of a Dantesque inferno where, amid ether fumes, a dauntless operator, unprepared to accept the word 'hopeless', essayed radical cures on advanced cancer cases. He was PRCSI in 1934–5.

Dr Alfred Parsons (1865–1952) had been Synge's closest colleague, his senior on the Baggot Street staff. According to Synge, his colleague never believed in telling patients much about their ailments, and few dared to question Parsons. 'He was beloved by them all, from the wheezy septuagenarian whom he was too kind-hearted to discharge from hospital in the cold winter months, to the small children in the nursery who greeted him every morning with shouts of joy.' Parsons was an octogenarian when the present writer attended his class; he was a most inspiring teacher.

His younger colleague, Dr Ethna MacCarthy,[16] physician to the children's dispensary, sent her valedictory lines to the *Irish Journal of Medical Science*:

---

[14] R. B. McDowell and D. A. Webb, *Trinity College Dublin 1592–1952 An Academic History* (Cambridge University Press, 1982), p. 452.
[15] J. B. Lyons, *The Quality of Mercer's* (Dublin: Glendale Press, 1991), p. 127.
[16] Dr Ethna MacCarthy, a grand-daughter of the Young Ireland poet, Denis Florence MacCarthy, was a poet in her own right and contributed verses and reviews to the *Dublin Magazine*. She has been described by James Knowlson as 'a feminist *avant la date*'. A foundation scholar in the early 1920s at TCD, where before studying medicine in the 1930s (MB, 1941; MD, 1948) she specialized with great success in French and Spanish; she was physically attractive, and had many male admirers including the future playwrights, Denis Johnston and Samuel Beckett. She is featured as 'the Alba' in the latter's *Dream of Fair to Middling Women*. She entered a long term relationship with Con Leventhal; they married in 1956 after the death of his wife. Ethna died from cancer on 25 May 1959. See James Knowlson, *Damned to Fame—the Life of Samuel Beckett* (London: Bloomsbury, 1996).

> *His was the green old age of the god*
> *that sadly watched a world decay*
> *Now the dark ferry paddles him away,*
> *but as black Charon dips his blade*
> *the god will say:*
> *'He is the immortal*
> *I the shade.'*

Despite the proverbial odiousness of comparisons, it must be said that beside 'Alfie', Victor Synge was inevitably at a disadvantage. Many students will remember him as a tall, lean and colourless person of ascetic mien, if one excepts the invariable cigarette with its ash about to fall. As a teacher he was much less dramatic than Parsons (an actor *manqué*), but a former pupil, Dr Harry Hitchcock, speaks well of him: 'His teaching method was quite the opposite of Alfie Parsons. No histrionics, calm and quiet and very polite. Even when one gave him a ridiculous answer to one of his searching questions, he did not try to ridicule one but just quietly said, "No, I do not think that is correct", whereas many another teacher would deride one. And yet his quiet approach was quite as effective in teaching as Alfie's flamboyance; it just lacked the entertainment value of the latter's method.'[17]

Holistic medicine

Unlike Parsons, who was so opposed to alcohol that he refused nomination for the presidency of the RCPI, which would necessitate presiding over a dinner at which drinks were served, Synge enjoyed a party, and was known to unbend sufficiently to sing rebel songs. Accompanied by a favourite student he attended a certain garden party in the 1950s, and seemed determined that his *savoir faire* should impress his young companion. He tipped the wine waiter lavishly, and explained in a whisper that this was 'so that he will look after us'.

He despatched the first glass of champagne in a matter of seconds, indicating that his student should do likewise. He drank a second glass almost as quickly, accepted a third—and gestured that now they were ready to circulate. As they moved off, the excessively long ash fell from the drooping cigarette. 'Oh, dear!' the professor said a little tipsily, 'that can't be good for the—er—carpet.'

'It won't harm the—er—grass', the student assured him soberly.

Long before 'holistic' medicine became a buzzword, Victor Synge treated the whole person, and not the disease. His effectiveness in consulting practice was reduced by the difficulty in extracting a clear-cut opinion from him. He was unlike a rival of whom he said: 'He was never in doubt but often wrong.'

---

[17] Harry Hitchcock, *TB or not TB?* (Galway: Centre for Health Promotion Studies, 1995), p. 10.

Dr Brendan O'Brien recalled Synge's dry sense of humour, and how he 'took a delight in leading one up the garden path of discussion and tipping one into the pond of deflation at the end of it'.

Synge wrote a foreword for Liam Price's memoir of his wife *Dr. Dorothy Price* (1957), an account of pioneer work in St Ultan's Hospital, of Dr Price's stimulating visit to Vienna in 1931, and her introduction of BCG to Ireland as a preventive measure against tuberculosis. Prior to her disabling illness, Dorothy Price (neé Stopford) held a post as paediatrician to Baggot Street Hospital.[18]

With a candour uncommon in obituarists, Brendan O'Brien wrote of Synge: 'Many of the younger men of today would probably regard him as out of date.'[19] Examination candidates found him unsettling. 'He looked at me over his glasses', one of them recalled a lifetime later. 'Then he looked at me through his glasses, before taking off his glasses and looking at me once again.' Students credited the professor with 'a Mona Lisa smile'—this indicated failure for a student when displayed.

Peter Gatenby offers a more sympathetic assessment, recalling the personal attention Synge gave to his patients, and his ability (as already mentioned) to converse with most foreign patients in their vernaculars. 'Those who were his students will remember his particular style of clinical teaching. Like a detective he would carefully extract the significant signs and symptoms, each being noted on the blackboard, and from these clues he would draw from the students, by question and answer, the differential diagnosis and eventually the final diagnosis.'[20]

His hospital patients in the 1960s included Brendan Behan, sent in by Dr Rory Childers who while in a bar with Brendan, realized that the playwright's thirst was not explained fully by alcoholism. Childers suspected diabetes. The diagnosis was confirmed by Synge who stabilized the disorder with insulin, and gave the customary warnings about hypoglycaemia. Synge told Behan to keep a few lumps of sugar in his pocket in a matchbox whenever he went out. 'I suppose that's in case I meet a horse', said Behan dryly.[21]

Victor Synge resigned in 1974, after a connection with Baggot Street Hospital of more than fifty years. Like his famous uncle, he loved the Irish countryside and had a cottage at Killakee Mountain where he lived in his retirement. His wife predeceased him, and he was survived by two sons at his death on 25 February 1976.

---

[18] See also 'Dorothy Stopford Price' in J. B. Lyons, *Brief Lives of Irish Doctors* (Dublin: Blackwater Press, 1978), pp. 161–2.
[19] O'Brien, 'Obituary, (note 2).
[20] PBBG [Peter Gatenby] 'Obituary V. M. Synge', *Brit. Med. J.* (1976); 2; 118.
[21] Coakley, *Baggot Street*, (note 13), p. 83.

253

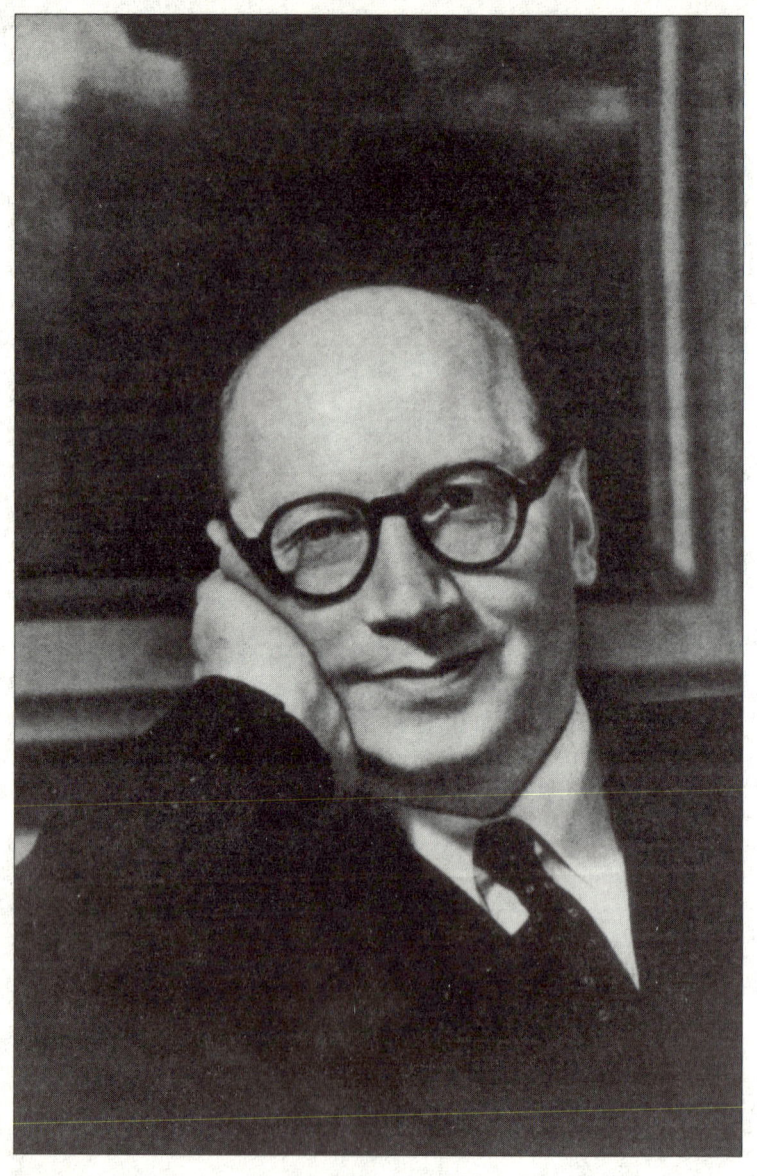

Leonard Abrahamson, 1897–1961 Professor of Medicine 1934–61

Chapter 14: Leonard Abrahamson 1897–1961

Though below average height, Leonard Abrahamson—known to generations of students as 'the Abe', and to his colleagues as 'Abie'—was metaphorically a towering figure in Irish medicine in his prime. He was born in Newry, County Down, in 1897, the second of the four children of Jewish Russian immigrants. His siblings were Esther, Bessie and Mervyn Saul. The latter also was to have a career in medicine, graduating from UCD and settling in London.[1]

Leonard Abrahamson was educated at the local Christian Brothers school, and entered TCD with a sizarship in Gaelic and Hebrew. Later he gained a scholarship in modern languages, and was awarded the Dompierre Chaufepie Prize for French. He then transferred to the school of physic graduating MB in 1919 with first-class honours in medicine, surgery and obstetrics.

During his years at Trinity, he was an active member of the Gaelic Society, and its honorary librarian. In 1915, despite the provost's opposition, the Gaelic Society invited 'a man named Pearse' to address them. Abrahamson's closest friend at Trinity was Max Nurock, a brilliant classical scholar, whose sister Tillie he married in 1920. Dr Abrahamson and his bride spent a protracted honeymoon in Paris, funded by a travelling scholarship that enabled him to work for a year as a graduate student in Paris and London.

At the Academy of Medicine on his return to Dublin, the ambitious young man discussed his impressions of the French school of medicine, so prolific of new ideas. 'Some of these [he said] are fantastic, and deservedly still-born; others reach a successful culmination, and form a valuable addition to medical science; others, again, disappear, returning after a longer or shorter interval to the horizon of the discoverer, who finds with exasperation that they are labelled with the name of another—often a German—worker, who was able to bring them to a practical issue.'[2]

He had visited the laboratories of Widal, Brulé and others, and found the French classifications of chronic nephritis and jaundice useful. Four types of nephritis were recognised: (1) simple albuminuria (2) dropsical (3) hypertensive (4) azotemic. Cases of jaundice were placed in three groups: (a) hepatic insufficiency (b) obstructive (c) haemolytic, according

---

[1] Mervyn Saul Abrahamson (1900–86) graduated MB (NUI) in 1922; having worked as house surgeon and RMO in Mercer's Hospital he settled in London as a general practitioner. He was medical adviser to Organon Laboratories Ltd.
[2] L. Abrahamson, 'Some Impressions of the French School of Medicine', *Dublin J. Med. Sc.* (1921); 14: 208–16.

to cause. He was impressed by Pierre Marie's use of a double tartrate—the 'tartrate borico-potassique'—which was less toxic than bromides in the treatment of epilepsy.

Abrahamson's major interest was in the cardiovascular system, and his attention was attracted by 'the great, perhaps overweening, stress laid on the estimation of blood-pressure, both systolic and diastolic—chiefly, perhaps, the latter, and the number of patients under treatment for high blood-pressure alone'.[3] The blood-pressure was recorded routinely by students, and new methods of estimating it 'spring up like mushrooms'; some of them a tribute to ingenuity rather than to commonsense. 'Two instruments are in common use—the first, discovered by Pachon, affords blood-pressure readings by the oscillatory method; the other, which is in universal use in Paris, is that of Vaquez and Laubry, which I have brought with me to-night.'

The polygraph was used extensively in Paris but the electrocardiograph 'is represented by a solitary instrument in the Vaquez clinic'. And what astonished young Abrahamson most of all, was to find that in Paris, the city where the stethoscope had been invented, immediate auscultation was the rule, and few students possessed the instrument. He conceded that he heard the 'bruit de galop' better when he discarded his own stethoscope and placed his ear on the chest. He was pleased that Stokes was well known, but to his disgust he learned that French students thought he was English or American. Aortic incompetence was divided into two types: Corrigan's disease and Hodgson's disease; the latter term applied when syphilis was accountable, and the x-rays (which were widely used) showed dilatation of the aorta.

The young Jewish doctor, uncertain as to where his future lay, had already taken a licentiate in midwifery at the Rotunda Hospital, probably with the intention of entering general practice. Now he proceeded MD, was admitted MRCPI (1921) and elected FRCPI (1922). He aspired to achieve recognition as an expert in the treatment of heart diseases. He was not, as is sometimes stated, a founder member (1922) of the Cardiac Club (its only Irish founder member was John E. McIlwaine of Belfast), but was elected in 1934 to that elite body, the forerunner of the Cardiac Society which held its first annual meeting in Edinburgh on 15 April 1937.

Cardiology

William Harvey's discovery of the circulation of the blood (*De Motu Cordis*, 1628) made no immediate clinical impact and, as Peter Fleming points out in *A Short History of Cardiology*, the word cardiology was not used prior to 1847. Meanwhile accretions of knowledge are credited to

---

[3] *Ibid.*, p. 211.

Raymond Vieussens of Montpellier who described death from mitral stenosis in 1715; to Lancisi of Rome who stressed the importance of pulsation of the jugular veins; to Albertini of Bologna who detected cardiac enlargement by palpation of the chest; to Stephen Hales, a Teddington clergyman, who measured blood-pressure in horses.

Copious information on heart diseases was contained in Albrecht von Haller's *Primae Lineae Physiologiae* (1947), Jean-Baptiste de Senac's *Traité de la structure du coeur, de son action et de ses maladies* (1749), and Morgagni's *De sedibus et causis morborum* (1761). William Heberden lectured on what he said might 'not improperly be called Angina pectoris' in 1768; but J. B. Herrick's clarifying paper on 'Clinical Features of Sudden Obstruction of the Coronary Arteries' was not published until 1912.

David Pitcairn discussed the association of heart disease with rheumatism at St Bartholomew's Hospital in the 1780s. Benjamin Rush of Philadelphia mentioned (1794) a letter received from an unnamed correspondent in Dublin who had referred to involvement of the heart 'as a muscle' in association with acute rheumatism.

Mediate auscultation was introduced by Laennec on 13 September 1816, at the Necker Hospital in Paris, and before long the diagnostic value of percussion was also widely appreciated. The wealth of eponymic terminology increased with the multiplication of clinical signs.

William Senouse Kirkes published an influential description of infective endocarditis from St Bartholomew's in 1852. Thomas Tufnell contributed an account of what became known as mycotic aneurysm to the *Dublin Quarterly Journal of Medical Science* in the following year. The lesions known as Osler's nodes were described in 1893 and 1909.

Authors of significant books in Victorian Dublin were William Stokes, *Diseases of the Heart and Aorta* (1854); O'Bryen Bellingham, *A Treatise on Diseases of the Heart* (1857); Thomas Hayden, *Diseases of the Heart and the Aorta* (1875).

Varieties of congenital cardiac disorders were gradually separated. Henri Roger described interventricular septal defect in 1879. A. Fallot's 1888 analysis of *la maladie bleue*—described by Farre (1814), Gintrac (1824), Peacock (1858)—created the term 'tetralogy of Fallot'. Maude Abbott's important publications began to appear early in the 1900s

Sir James Mackenzie (1853–1925) stressed the harmlessness of extra-systoles: 'I have watched individuals for twenty-five years who have presented extra-systoles . . . and these people have lived laborious lives, and have never shown the slightest symptoms of heart failure, or any other evidence of heart impairment.'

Mercer's Hospital

Leonard Abrahamson joined the staff at Mercer's Hospital in 1920, as honorary anaesthetist and assistant physician. He was promoted visiting physician in 1927, being then professor of materia medica and therapeutics in the RCSI, and a recognised expert in electrocardiography.

He presented 'An Introduction to Electrocardiography' to the Academy of Medicine in December 1921. The machine he used, as Sir John Lumsden explained, had been presented by the Red Cross and the Order of St John, and installed at Mercer's, as being a suitable central situation with the understanding 'that it should be available free for the examination of cases from any of the hospitals'.

The diagnosis of arrhythmias was facilitated by electrocardiography, and Abrahamson published a series of papers on this theme based on presentations to the Academy, where on 26 May 1922 he described a case of heart-block, and another with auricular fibrillation. The latter patient (admitted to Mercer's under the care of Sir John Lumsden), was probably an old soldier, as his previous illnesses included malaria and dysentery. Quinidine was prescribed by Abrahamson and on the third day the patient complained of dizziness and malaise. 'These symptoms yielded with suspicious rapidity to a dose of alcohol administered in general principle by the sister-in-charge and were disregarded.' A normal rhythm was satisfactorily restored. 'An electro-cardiogram showed a definite "P" wave, complete regularity, absence of fibrillation waves.'[4] Paroxysmal tachycardia[5] was discussed by Abrahamson at the Academy in 1923, and in 1930 he gave a paper on a patient with an atrioventricular nodal rhythm.[6]

Abrahamson was a member of the Association of Physicians of Great Britain and Ireland. He described four cases of congenital dextra-cardia in the *Quarterly Journal of Medicine* (1925) but his publications were by no means confined to cardiology. Thus he contributed papers to the *Irish Journal of Medical Science* on Frolich's syndrome, diabetes insipidus and achrestic anaemia; his account of thrombophlebitis migrans appeared in the *British Medical Journal* in 1928, with Moorhead as co-author. This migratory thrombophlebitis is now known as an occasional precursor of neoplasia.

The Biological Society

He was elected president of the undergraduates' Biological Society in Trinity College in 1930, and his inaugural address on 25 October (later

---

[4] 'Two Cardiac Cases', *Irish J. Med. Sc.* (1922): 271–3.
[5] 'Two Cases of Paroxysmal Tachycardia', *ibid.* (1923): 58–66.
[6] 'Atrioventricular Nodal Rhythm with Bigeminy', *ibid.* (1930): 64–5.

published in the *Irish Journal of Medical Science*) took the form of a major review of recent advances in cardiology.⁷ The diagnostic problems of the arrhythmias he held to be largely solved, permitting attention to be directed to the assessment of the condition of the myocardium, and evaluating the significance in that respect of bundle-branch block.

Changes in the ECG following coronary obstruction were first demonstrated experimentally in dogs, and in 1920 H. E. B. Pardee recorded a similar curve in man. John Parkinson and D. E. Bedford demonstrated 'sequential alterations of the R-T segment and of the T waves occurring in the course of a short space of time' as strong presumptive evidence of myocardial infarction. Inverted T waves in Leads I and II may be associated with coronary sclerosis. 'The importance of serial tracings is receiving increasing recognition.'⁸

Signe Toksvig

In 1927 Abrahamson had made the first report to the Academy of a case of coronary thrombosis in which the diagnosis was made in Dublin during life and verified by autopsy. The disease was comparatively new to Irish clinicians, and the caution required in prognosis may not yet have been fully realised when towards the end of June 1933 'the Abe' was called to Cooldrinagh, Foxrock, to see an overweight, but physically active quantity surveyor, Bill Beckett, who had had a sudden heart attack. Or, perhaps, he felt nothing was to be lost by optimism? Be that as it may, the consultant predicted the patient's recovery, to the delight of all at Cooldrinagh.

Abrahamson called again in the forenoon of 26 June, a beautiful summer day, and said Beckett was much improved. When later in the morning Samuel Beckett dropped into his father's bedroom, the latter remarked, *'What a morning!'* These were almost the last words he spoke; there was a sudden setback and he died at about 4 p.m.

The slings and arrows of outrageous fortune may be invoked to explain errors of prognosis, but a rare instance in which 'the Abe's' renowned ability to handle patients let him down has also been recorded. The place was the Portobello Nursing Home—'Room with brown snakeskin wall-paper where the close-stool was by the bedside and I slew a cockroach in the breakfast tray'—the patient Signe Toksvig, a Danish writer who was married to the Kilkenny-born author Francis Hackett. Their marriage was voluntarily childless, a vital piece of information deliberately withheld from the doctor by Signe, who subsequently complained in her diary:

---

⁷ 'Recent Advances in Diseases of the Heart', *ibid.* (1930): 594–606.
⁸ *Ibid.*, p. 597.

Well, I was in Portobello 4 days, then home and ordered to stay in bed all morning and go in 3 times a week for arsenic treatments. I liked Dr A. at first, then he had to make the idiotic break of asking in that melting way 'why don't you have a child?' This panacea for all ills, apparently. Sentimental ass!⁹

The credit for her improvement—'less feverish, fatter, sleep better, less harassed'—went to Mr Oliver St John Gogarty, who had discovered that the cause of her 'fever, ache, anaemia', was an infection in the stump of a tonsil. When Gogarty came to the nursing-home to investigate her antra, he did so 'expertly, delicately, and magnetically'. Immediately she felt quite in love with him—'partly because he had given me a lot of cocaine which made me go quite faint and want to cling to his hand. All my dislike of him suddenly went. He was so perfect in his art.'[10]

Abrahamson, incidentally, was one of the owners of the Portobello Nursing Home, an investment which facilitated his vast private practice.

Professor of medicine

Abrahamson left Mercer's in 1930, attracted by the larger clinical opportunity offered by the Richmond Hospital where he was appointed physician. Four years later he succeeded Victor Millington Synge in the chair of medicine in the RCSI, and held this position until his death in 1961. A former pupil, Alan B. Eppel, recalled him as 'a legendary clinician and teacher . . . an extraordinary individual [who] epitomized the best in Irish medicine by his human clinical approach and the clarity of his teaching style.' He was the third president of the Biological Society of the RCSI (1933–4) founded in the early 1930s by Drs Joe Lewis and J. D. H. Widdess.[11]

Describing Abrahamson as 'a man of short stature' the late Adrian Cowan added: *'small* is a word that could never be applied to him in any aspect'.[12] Paddy Bofin, 'the Abe's' student and house-physician (and later professor of forensic medicine in the RCSI and Dublin coroner), recalled his magnetic personality, with eyes glittering behind horn-rimmed glasses. 'He was flamboyant, with the ever-present cigar, not always lit.

---

[9] Lis Phil, ed., *Signe Toksvig's Irish Diaries 1926–1937* (Dublin: Lilliput Press, 1994), p. 67.
[10] *Ibid.*, p. 67.
[11] The RCSI had a students' medical society in the 1790s of which little is known. The Junior Surgical Society of Ireland was mentioned in Chapter 6. The Biological Society of the Royal Colleges of Physicians and Surgeons in Ireland was founded in 1931 and held its first ordinary meeting on 17 February 1932. See J. D. H. Widdess *The Royal College of Surgeons in Ireland and its Medical School 1784–1984*, 3rd ed. (Dublin: RCSI, 1984), p. 83.
[12] A. Cowan, 'Leonard Abrahamson—The Man', *J. Irish Colls. Phys. & Surgs.* (1983); 12: 158–63.

He was always ready with a riposte, though his wit could be acerbic.'

Professor Abrahamson's Thursday morning 'clinics' (bedside instruction) were attended by a large number of students from the three Dublin medical schools.

> He was a controlled, disciplined teacher, who spoke with the relaxed ease that comes when the material is very well prepared. He was of a generation when laboratory back-up was minimal and clinical expertise was paramount. 'Look at the face lad'—the facies of Parkinson's, myxoedema, the Dresden china skin of aortic regurgitation, capillary pulsation on the forehead, tabetic facies, pellagra face, and sadly the Hippocratic facies of cachexia; one saw them all working with the old Abe.[13]

He peppered his talk with sardonic comments on Dublin medicine and its votaries. Referring to two brothers on the staff of a Catholic teaching-hospital he said, 'I call them the Badminton Brothers', implying that cases were shuttled from one to the other. Concerning Dr X—at the Meath Hospital, who was known to have submitted to intracranial surgery, he said, 'Mr McConnell didn't remove Dr X—'s tumour. He took out his brain instead.'

> After his class the professor retired to the staffroom to drink tea, eat buttered toast and enjoy a cigar. Standing with his back to the coal fire he discussed the problems of the day. But when Dr Bofin, who had his eye on a job in a Belfast pathology laboratory, asked if he could use his name as a referee the Abe smiled and said: 'Don't be a bloody fool, lad. What hope would you have? A Roman Catholic recommended by a Newry Jew!'

His formal lectures in the college started at five o'clock exactly. Students said he arrived in the lecture theatre at four seconds to the hour, to allow for the time it took to walk from the door to the podium. He spoke without notes for forty-five minutes at a moderated speed that facilitated note-taking; he had the invaluable gift of introducing amusing anecdotes certain to evoke laughter.

Charles Dupont, now a Dublin dermatologist, remembered his professor as small and very bright. 'He spoke with a slight lisp and took a mischievous delight in referring to syphilis—which he pronounced "thyphilith"—as a very common Oirish disease.' He said the perfect textbook hadn't been written, because he hadn't the time to write it. Students swapped stories about the Abe. He was reputed to have told a famous surgeon whom he accompanied to the races that he hoped the surgeon gave better advice to his patients about surgery than he had given

---

[13] P. Bofin in Eoin O'Brien, Lorna Browne and Kevin O'Malley (eds.) *The House of Industry Hospitals, 1772–1987* (Dublin: Anniversary Press, 1988), p. 110.

to him (Abrahamson) about horses.

When an admiring house-physician complemented him on his new high-powered Armstrong-Siddley, saying, 'I bet it'll pass everything on the road', the Abe replied drily: ' yes, everything except the petrol pumps.'

At a time when lady doctors were uncommon, a female house-physician phoned in the night to discuss a problem. Telling his students next morning how he had reassured her, the Abe smirked and said, 'we then went back to bed—individually.'

Amused by a rival Jewish physician's enthusiasm for naso-gastric milk drips as a treatment for duodenal ulcers, Abrahamson asked his students if they had been to Mercer's to see Dr Lewis's milk-bar.

His swipe at the British National Health Service was to advise prospective Irish candidates for jobs in English general practice to buy a very good pen, which would be more necessary than a stethoscope.

He could be a formidable opponent at the Academy of Medicine, where leading specialists tussled over clinical problems. Having presented to the section of medicine a complicated case of rheumatoid arthritis, to whom over a number of years he had given courses of gold, but who had finally died, he was confronted by Mr J. C. Flood who asked *had the physician recovered the gold?* Flood, an able surgeon, had degrees in arts, medicine, commerce and law—he possessed a mordant wit and posed his question as if addressing a Shylock. The Academy audience was pleased, feeling that for once, somebody had the better of 'the Abe', and hardly expecting the latter's devastating reply: 'Mr Flood has more degrees than a thermometer, but without the same capacity for registering warmth.'

Family man

Leonard and Tillie Abrahamson had four sons and a daughter. Mrs Abrahamson, according to her nephew Adrian Cowan, was small, plump and as dark as a gypsy. 'A completely natural person, she had a transparently gentle way with her.' He was a devoted father, prepared to put family matters before all else. 'He always had time to stop whatever he was doing and give his complete attention to a problem of one of his children, treating it with full adult importance no matter how trivial the incident; a natural genuine thoughtfulness which gained him the equally natural respect of all his children.'[14]

Like Oliver St John Gogarty, who was said to have driven himself into practice in a buttercup-coloured car, the Abe favoured ostentatious motors, progressing from a Swift to a de Dion, and on to a Hupmobile, the petrol-guzzling machine mentioned above, a Bently and finally a chaffeur-driven Rolls Royce. As an art collector he owned paintings by

---

[14] Cowan, 'Abrahamson' (note 12), p. 160.

Jack B. Yeats and a valuable piece, 'the Ragamuffin' by Epstein. Unathletic, he enjoyed poker and racing, and was eventually a race-horse owner. According to Cowan his horses won some important races, and he 'could sometimes be seen wreathed in smiles in the winner's enclosure but the vast number of friends he had among the racing fraternity respected him as a physician rather than as a judge of horseflesh.'

When offered a horse in lieu of a fee by a farmer he went down to the country to see the animal, bringing along a trusted expert. 'What do you think?' he asked his companion when they had inspected the horse. 'Could I race him?' 'Indeed you could, doctor,' the expert replied, 'and what's more, you'd probably beat him.'[15]

Two of his sons joined the medical profession; in some of the Abe's later papers Mervyn Leonard Abrahamson (who attained a chair of therapeutics at the RCSI) was his co-author. Mervyn (1921–93) eventually succeeded his father on the staff of the Richmond Hospital, but finally left Dublin to take an appointment at the Rebecca Sieff Government Hospital at Safed in Israel. David Abrahamson embarked on a career in veterinary surgery but in due course became a psychiatrist.

President Royal College of Physicians of Ireland

Professor Leonard Abrahamson's election to the presidency of the RCPI 1949–51 has been described in the previous chapter. Throughout the 1950s he played an active part in the Irish Medical Association, as William Doolin recalled:

> I saw much of him in his active service to his colleagues through the country in the ranks of the Irish Medical Association from 1950 onwards. There his service to both the city hospitals and the body of general practitioners was unstinted. There as a member of council and as chairman of our executive committee, through the initial ... difficulties with the Ministry of Health his loyalty to the Hippocratic code was unshakable through those unhappy and difficult years, and his generosity to the Association's funds and time was immense. His even temper, his level headed common sense, and his administrative ability were always there to help in moments of discomfort; his words of criticism were never *cassants*; his shrewd judgement of men and things always helpful.[16]

The present author recalls an occasion in the late 1950s when, at the end of a long meeting, it fell to Abrahamson, as chairman, to sum-up. He did so, without reference to notes, offering with masterly recall an absolutely fair summary of all the arguments presented. Such a moderating intellect was a valuable asset in those clouded times.

---

[15] *Ibid.*
[16] William Doolin, 'Obituary: Leonard Abrahamson', *Brit. Med. J.* (1961); 2: 1295–6.

The 'difficulties' to which Doolin alludes were of medico-political origin. The creation of the British National Health Service in 1948 had prompted Irish legislators to draw up plans for similar, though necessarily more modest developments in this country. Before long the relationship between the IMA and the recently-established Department of Health became contentious. The 'Mother and Child' débacle in 1951 was a victory for the profession, whose storm troopers in that imbroglio were the bishops. The late Dr Noel Browne is generally featured in the struggle as a defeated (but morally uplifted) David, overcome by wily and reprehensible medical Goliaths. Those who were close to the scene of action, however, saw the young minister for health as 'inexperienced, arrogant and fanatical'.[17]

Dr Browne's autobiography, *Against the Tide*, has stigmatised articles written by medical critics as 'tendentious and misleading'. He added: 'It was a measure of the resourcefulness of our opponents that they were able to mobilise a wealthy Jewish specialist named Abrahamson and a Protestant paediatrician named Colles [sic] in support of the bishops' opposition to the mother and infant health service.'[18] Dr Robert Collis, it is relevant to explain, had used the royalties accruing from his successful play, *Marrowbone Lane*, to establish a fund for tuberculous children. Browne's animus towards 'the Abe' and Collis, incidentally, arose from an occasion in 1948 when as guest-speaker at the RCSI's Biological Society's inaugural meeting he laid aside the speech written for him, and made a blistering attack on doctors. Abrahamson and Collis, present in the audience, defended the profession with equal vehemence.

The minister's resignation was demanded by the leader of his party in 1951. The officials in the Custom House (headquarters of the health ministry) regrouped; 'state medicine' was seen to be alive, well and intent on annexing what the doctors liked to believe was a free profession. Historians have not adequately explained why an altruistic profession should have so often found itself in dispute with a well-intentioned Department of Health. J. J. Lee ascribes it to *greed*, picturing 'those who worship at the altar of Croesus, while demurely draped in the robes of Hippocrates'.[19] A more sympathetic metaphor might visualize the IMA as a resentful Laocoön struggling against the encircling coils of bureaucracy. The profession's concern certainly was not entirely financial. The doctors sincerely believed that 'state medicine' would lower standards, and for that reason must be opposed.

---

[17] Malachy Powell, 'Noel Browne—a hero or a villain?', *Irish Medical News* (1997): 7 July, p. 21; see also Harry O'Flanagan, 'The Health Services in Ireland: A perspective on origins', *Irish Medical Journal* (1987); 80: 217–18.
[18] Noel Browne, *Against the Tide* (Dublin: Gill and Macmillan, 1986), p. 215.
[19] J. J. Lee, *Ireland 1913–1985* (Cambridge University Press, 1989), p. 315.

The IMA has been spoken of pejoratively as 'the most successful trade union of all'. Actually its negotiators were at a disadvantage in discussions with trained civil servants who had time on their side, but it took Mr Seán MacEntee (minister for health 1957–65) to assert that the association had no right whatsoever to negotiate under the Trades Union Act, 1941. This situation came about when a quarrel with the Department of Health over professional secrecy (which the civil servants wished to transgress) caused the IMA to insert an 'Important Notice' in its journal. In effect this 'banned' (a much-disputed word) applications for certain public appointments. The outraged, and dictatorial minister embarked on a campaign 'punctuated with moments of heated passion and high comedy'. The description is Ruth Barrington's (*Health Medicine and Politics in Ireland 1900–1970*) and relates particularly to an occasion in 1959 when the minister was scolded by William Doolin, who had added the journal of the Irish Medical Association to his editorial responsibilities, for pointed discourtesy in sending the association a cheque for £5 to pay for a dinner in Killarney at which MacEntee and his wife (a very large person) were guests. The editor when referring to the minister 'and his formidable escort', may have had the accompanying civil servants in mind, but the minister interpreted it as an insult to Mrs MacEntee. 'The incident was followed by a complete disruption of communications between the Custom House and the profession.'[20]

Jewish community

Apart from Abrahamson's professional activities, he was active in the Jewish community, and was honorary president of the Jewish National Fund.[21] He was said to preside over a local 'court' that settled minor disputes, and his work for the State of Israel led to a forest being dedicated in his name by the community in 1951.

Physician, heal thyself! Leonard Abrahamson died at his home from a coronary thrombosis on 28 October 1961.

---

[20] Ruth Barrington, *Health, Medicine and Politics in Ireland 1900–1970* (Dublin: Institute of Public Administration, 1987), p. 256.
[21] Eoin O'Brien, 'From the Waters of Sion to Liffeyside—the Jewish Contribution: Medical and Cultural', *J. Irish Colls. Phys. & Surgs.* (1981); 10: 107–119.

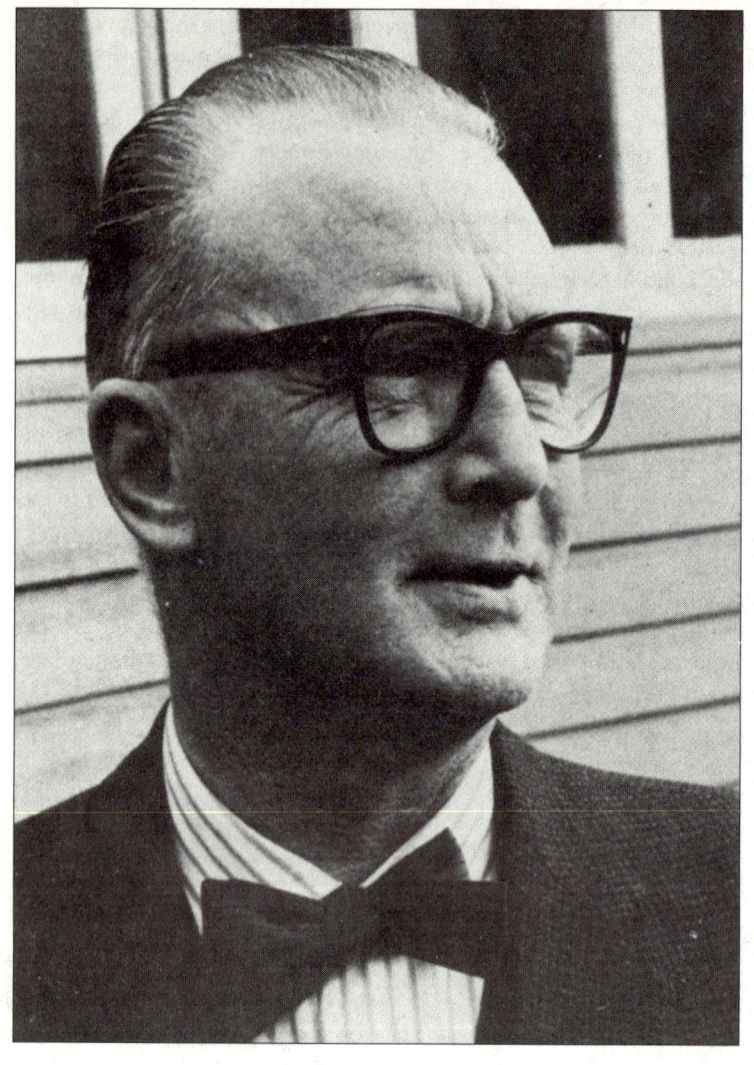

Alan Thompson, 1906–74 Professor of Medicine 1962–74

Chapter 15: Alan Herbert Thompson, 1906–74

Alan Thompson's students are unlikely to forget him. One of them, Pierce Grace, recalled how he taught them to think while amusing them with witty comments such as 'Like the Egyptian mummy, we are pressed for time', or 'To err is human but to eh! while speaking in public is unforgivable.' 'There seems to be a lot of shifting dullness about this hospital', was another characteristic Thompson comment, as was the somewhat pedantic assertion that it would be better to break a wrist than to split an infinitive.[1]

Born into a Quaker family in County Wexford in 1906, Alan Herbert Thompson attended the Tate and Newtown schools before moving with his elder brother Geoffrey to Portora School in Enniskillen, where he developed a love of cricket, an interest in English literature, and became a close friend of Samuel Beckett. At TCD, where Geoffrey Thompson had graduated MB in 1928, Alan took the BA (1928) with moderatorship and gold medal; in the School of Physic he won many prizes, graduating MSc (by thesis) and MB in 1930. From 1930–32 he was lecturer in bacteriology at TCD. He availed of a travelling scholarship to visit European medical centres, and having taken the MRCPI (1932) became assistant physician to the Whitworth Hospital in 1932.[2]

Thompson also served the Richmond and Rotunda Hospitals as pathologist from 1934 to 1937, but on becoming MRCP (London) in 1937 he withdrew from laboratory work and confined himself to clinical practice. He was elected FRCP (London) in 1967.

He certainly had a brilliant mind, but his colleagues sometimes felt he lacked either the energy, or the ambition and direction required to reap the full potential of his gifts.

Publications

At the Rotunda, to which he was consultant, he spent a great deal of time following the progress of the late toxaemias of pregnancy. His publications in the 1930s included a review article on the epidemiology and laboratory diagnosis of undulant fever; an account of an Addisonian crisis; a case report of achrestic anaemia, with Leonard Abrahamson as co-author.

Between 1942 and January 1944, eighty-seven cases of nephritis were admitted to St Laurence's Hospital under Alan Thompson's care. He

---

[1] Pierce Grace, 'Sic Transit Gloria Mundi', *J. Irish Colls. Phys. and Surgs.* (1993); 22: 204–5.
[2] P. J. Bofin, 'Obituary: Alan H. Thompson', *ibid.* (1974); 3: 131–2.

published a clinical study of acute nephritis in 1950, having meanwhile taken 'Bright's disease' as the theme of his presidential address to the RCSI's Biological Society on 6 November 1943.

Brucellosis The disease which became known as Mediterranean fever, Malta fever, or gastric fever, was commonly observed among the troops in the Crimean War, but was mentioned centuries before in the Hippocratic Collection.[3] Bruce discovered the causative organism, which he called Micrococcus Melitensis. Later it was found to be identical with 'Bang's bacillus' (Brucella abortus), accountable for contagious abortion in cattle. As the Maltese resented the slur inherent in the term Malta fever, the disease was renamed undulant fever or brucellosis. The raw milk of goats and cows was a major source of infection and in the 1930s pasteurization was not yet practised widely in Ireland.

Serum testing of apparently healthy persons against brucella abortus suspensions was carried out by J. W. Bigger and by Alan Thompson. It was found that many individuals showed agglutinins for Brucella abortus in their blood in low titre. This was interpreted as implying that there had been a localised invasion of lymph nodes of the intestine, or in the mesenteric glands. 'Infection, as distinct from invasion, can be considered to have occurrred only when the symptoms characteristic of undulant fever are definitely manifested.'[4]

Thompson condemned 'the lamentable readiness' with which some clinicians attached the label brucellosis to febrile patients with agglutinins for Brucella abortus in their blood. Diagnostic criteria must be strict; ideally they should include definite bacteriological confirmation. He conceded that because of the inherent difficulties of isolating the organism, culture was of limited value as a diagnostic procedure, yet he said: 'We should be loath to diagnose undulant fever in Ireland in the absence of a positive culture from the blood or urine.' He expressed both conservatism and scepticism by closing the article with the affirmation 'that undulant fever is as yet unknown in Ireland'.[5] Events were to prove this opinion untenable. Before long, brucellosis was firmly established as a not unlikely contender in the differential diagnosis of 'PUO', and with the establishment of meat factories it became an important industrial hazard. The concept of 'chronic brucellosis' was to introduce further therapeutic and medicolegal challenges.

Addison's disease Speaking to the South London Medical Society in 1849, Thomas Addison (1793–1860), physician to Guy's Hospital, described 'The Constitutional and Local effects of Disease of the Supra-Renal Cap-

---

[3] Folke Henschen, *The History of Diseases* (London: Longmans, 1966), p. 86.
[4] A. H. Thompson, 'Recent Work on Undulant Fever and Brucella Abortus', *Irish J. Med. Sc.* (1931): 655–62.
[5] *Ibid,*. p. 622.

sules', and created the eponym 'Addison's disease'. As a preface to his paper, he offered an account of 'a very remarkable form of general anaemia'; the latter became known as the Addisonian anaemia, or pernicious anaemia. 'It makes its appproach [Addison wrote] in so slow and insidious a manner that the patient can hardly fix a date to his earliest feeling of that languor which is shortly to become so extreme.'[6]

Addison's disease, characterised by 'anaemia, general languor and debility, remarkable feebleness of the heart's action, irritability of the stomach, and a peculiar change of colour in the skin'[7] can nowadays be controlled satisfactorily with cortisone and a mineralocorticoid. The Whitworth Hospital where a ten-year-old girl was admitted, already in the dreaded state of an Addisonian crisis, had little enough to offer in 1935. 'Glucose in saline was given intramuscularly . . . a supply of suprarenal cortical extract was not obtainable at the time.'[8] Postmortem examination showed tuberculous destruction of the supra-renal glands.

By the 1930s the Addisonian anaemia was known to be megalocytic in type, accompanied by histamine-fast achylia gastrica, and quickly responsive to treatment with potent liver extracts which induced a typical 'reticulocyte crisis'. Wilkinson and Israëls in a large series of patients investigated at the Manchester Royal Infirmary encountered three anomalous cases. They had normal gastric acidity, failed to respond to medication with liver and were labelled 'achrestic' anaemia. An account of a nineteen-year-old youth whose ailment 'agrees in all essentials with the description of achrestic anaemia by Wilkinson and Israëls' was presented by Leonard Abrahamson and Alan Thompson in 1937.[9]

Nephritis The unexpectedly large number of patients with nephritis who came under Thompson's care in the early 1940s sent him back to the early literature on the disease, and to Bright's classical account (1827) published in the first volume of his *Reports of Medical Cases, selected with a view of illustrating the Symptoms and Cure of Diseases by a Reference to Morbid Anatomy*. Richard Bright, like Addison, was physician to Guy's Hospital, but unlike his colleague who was born in humble circumstances, Bright belonged to an affluent family.

St Lô and Samuel Beckett

Alan Thompson was among those who in 1945 established an Irish Red Cross hospital in France, at St Lô in Normandy which was almost di-

---

[6] R. H. Major, *Classic Descriptions of Disease* (Springfield: Thomas, 1945), p. 291.
[7] *Ibid.*, p. 292.
[8] Thompson, 'Addison's Disease in a Young Girl', *Irish J. Med. Sc.* (1935): 606.
[9] Leonard Abrahamson and Alan Thompson, 'Achrestic Anaemia', *ibid.* (1937): 66–9. With a fuller understanding of the causes of megaloblastic anaemias achrestic anaemia has been eliminated from the nosology.

rectly south of the D-Day invasion beaches, and had been devastated by bombing. It was he who invited Samuel Beckett, with whom he had maintained his friendship, to join the staff as interpreter and storekeeper. Before doing so he had availed of an opportunity to examine Beckett (who from time to time had called on both Alan and Geoffrey Thompson professionally), to assure himself there was nothing physically amiss that rest and proper diet could not remedy.[10]

Beckett had been Alan's patient in 1935 with pleurisy, and in January 1938 the writer had survived a knife attack in a Paris street sustaining a pneumothorax. Beckett also suffered ill-health of a pyschoneurotic nature, in which connection, as well as its relation to his writing, he sought advice from Alan Thompson and his brother Geoffrey. The latter, who trained in psychiatry, was among Beckett's closest confidants; he diagnosed an anxiety-depressive disorder and sent his friend to the Tavistock Clinic for analysis. Beckett derived benefits from his sessions there, but remained convinced that he had angina pectoris (from which his father had suffered as related in Chapter 14), and would die suddenly. When he mentioned these fears to Geoffrey Thompson, he received only an enigmatic smile and a polite assurance that they were groundless.

During the writing of *Murphy* (in which Murphy takes a job in a mental institution) Beckett had obtained background information by making frequent calls on Geoffrey Thompson (who in 1935 was working at Bethlehem Royal Hospital), and secretly availed of the opportunity to study the grounds and the wards.

It may be added that after many long conversations over the years with Beckett, in London and elsewhere, about his work and his creativity, Geoffrey Thompson could not avoid seeing the plays as the outcome of depression verging on the psychotic. The doctor did his best to avoid discussing them, and the playwright was offended when Geoffrey admitted he disliked *Endgame*. But Beckett continued to send his friend theatre tickets and signed first editions.

Alan Thompson was relieved to find Beckett's physical condition satisfactory. The physician left Dublin on 7 August 1945 with the director, Colonel Thomas J. McKinney, and Beckett. The advance party went to Normandy through London, and spent a few days in Paris to confer with the French Red Cross. The scene that greeted them on their arrival at St-Lô was described by Beckett:

> St-Lô is just a heap of rubble, la Capitale des Ruines as they call it in France. Of 2600 buildings 2000 completely wiped out, 400 badly damaged and 200 'only' slightly. It all happened in the night of the 5th to 6th June. It has been raining hard the last few days and the place is a sea of mud. What it

---

[10] See Deirdre Bair, *Samuel Beckett* (London: Cape, 1978), *passim*.

will be like in winter is hard to imagine. No lodging of course of any kind. We stayed just with the chatelain of Tancry, about 4 miles out, in a huge castle with a 12th century half wing still standing. But since last Wednesday we have been with a local doctor in the town, quite near the hospital site, all 3 in one small room and Alan and I sharing a bed!'[11]

In order to make their way about, Thompson and his companions were obliged to step 'from one pile of loose bricks to another or from a rusty girder onto the end of a buried bedstead'.[12]

The *Hôpital de la Croix-Rouge Irlandaise* had an abundance of supplies, including penicillin and an aluminium-lined operating theatre. Thompson was joined later in the month by his colleagues, Mr Freddie Gill, FRCSI, Drs Arthur Darley and Jim Gaffney (assistant physician and pathologist respectively) and others. Their first impressions of the area are recorded in Eoin O'Brien's *The Beckett Country*.[13] McKinney believed it imperative 'that Ireland help France, her neighbour and friend';[14] Gaffney found that one street of ruins looked very much like another —'There are still about 5,000 people in it, but you would wonder where they live; mostly in boarded up cellars and mattresses...'[15]

The French erected huts for the advance team, but electricity, running water and sanitation were lacking. They were assisted by German prisoners of war in the heavy task of sorting and stacking their supplies, and occasionally enjoyed the luxury of hot showers at an American base thirty miles away. Thompson submitted a confidential progress report in September 1945, a resume of which is included in *The Beckett Country*:

> It was necessary to find a temporary store in Saint-Lô. We were fortunate in getting a large granary in a Stud Farm near the hospital. When the ship arrived we saw the stores off the ship to railway wagons, and returned to St. Lô. After a few days railway wagons commenced to arrive at St. Lô. We had to move the stores by lorry 1½ miles to our store. Everything had to be taken upstairs. Some packets weighed over 2 cwts. Stores came in for days and days. All are stored safely now. It was a considerable task... The present position is that stores are safely housed under lock and key and well protected from the rain. The *Storekeeper* (Samuel Beckett) and assistant are making out stock cards for all material... We borrowed beds and camped

---

[11] James Knowlson, *Damned to Fame: the Life of Samuel Beckett* (London: Bloomsbury, 1996), p. 345.
[12] Anthony Cronin, *Samuel Beckett: the Last Modernist* (London: Harper Collins, 1996), p. 349.
[13] Eoin O'Brien, *The Beckett Country* (Dublin: Black Cat Press,1986), pp. 315–42.
[14] *Ibid.*, p 384.
[15] *Ibid.*, p. 324.

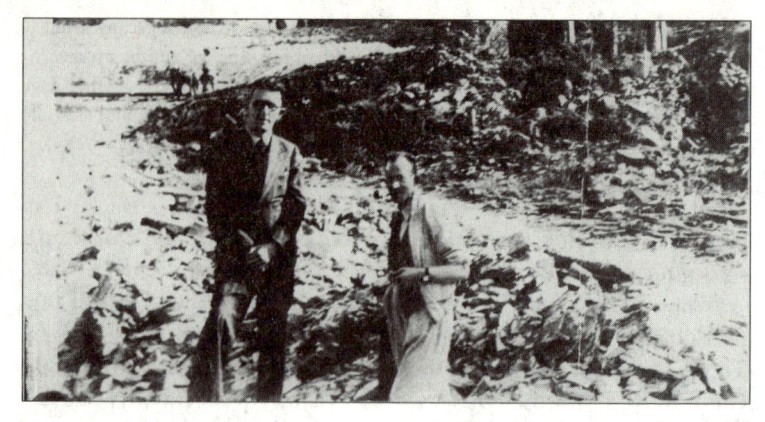

Members of the Irish hospital team at St Lô (P. Gaffney Humanity Amid the Ruins*)*

out in the hut. No running water—no sanitation of any kind. The water had to be carried in buckets . . . Sanitation was held up due to lack of pipes and still consists of a hole in the ground with sacking around it. It is impossible while sanitation is so primitive, to contemplate bringing out any additional staff . . .The climate is very wet and muddy. Facilities for amusement are virtually nil . . . the people seem to be very anxious for us to work there. They are asking all the time when the hospital will be open and taking in patients. The Mayor is very keen on the hospital functioning...[16]

Thompson and Beckett filled many of their evenings with bridge or chess; with others of the Irish group they mingled socially among the local people. Eleven of them were given a seven-course dinner by the Reverend Mother of a nearby convent, followed by a convivial evening around the piano, and the physician and the writer felt obliged to say 'they hadn't thought that convents were such nice places'.[17] The full hospital staff had arrived by Christmas, and by March 1946 in-patients were being treated while outpatients approached 200 daily. When the formal opening of *l'Hôpital Irlandais de Saint-Lô* took place on 7 April 1946, Irish whiskey proved too strong for some of the French guests. The hospital flourished and was handed over to the French Red Cross on 31 December 1946 as a fully going concern.

Beckett, still an obscure writer, described its achievement sensitively for Radio Éireann:

> And yet the whole enterprise turned from the beginning on the establishing of a relation in the light of which the therapeutic relation faded to the merest of pretexts. What was important was not our having penicillin when they had none, nor the unregarding munificence of the French Ministry of

---

[16] *Ibid.*, p. 384.
[17] *Ibid.*, p. 326.

Reconstruction (as it was then called), but the occasional glimpse obtained, by us in them and, who knows, by them in us (for they are an imaginative people), of that smile at the human condition as little to be extinguished by bombs as to be broadened by the elixirs of Burroughes and Welcome [sic], the smile deriding, among other things, the having and not having, the giving and the taking, sickness and health.[18]

Like other members of the hospital staff, Thompson was awarded the *Medaille de la Reconaissance Française* when he returned to Dublin where he resumed private practice and his work at the Richmond Hospital and the Rotunda.

When Samuel Beckett consulted Alan Thompson again in 1947 the prescription, as before, was rest and an adequate diet. This advice failed to impress the patient, who felt that homoeopathy, or no doctor at all, would suit him best. He did, however, arrange for Thompson to give his mother a new experimental tonic for Parkinson's disease, which had incapacitated Mrs Beckett.[19]

Alan and Sylvia, his wife, were visited in 1949 by Beckett who came to Dublin with decreasing frequency. The men played chess, at which they had achieved a high standard, and for hours they enjoyed surprising each other with unexpected moves. Once, Beckett's move was so subtle that he did not appear to understand it himself, and while puzzling over it he kept repeating softly, 'Ah, yes, ah, yes . . .' He then said that music and chess 'had the same intellectual beauty—the unfolding of one was much the same as the other', a remark that seemed to please him greatly.[20]

Cybernetics supplied a congenial theme for Thompson's presidential address to the section of medicine of the Royal Academy of Medicine in Ireland on 9 February 1951.[21]

Chair of medicine

Thompson succeeded 'the Abe' in the chair of medicine at the RCSI in 1962, accepting without demur a new decree that established the professorship of medicine as a fulltime appointment, excluding private practice.

> He proceeded to modify the curriculum [a colleague recalled] with characteristic efficiency and a minimum of disturbance. He maintained that the merely well-informed mind is in danger of becoming the closed mind and he regretted that the crowded undergraduate courses . . . left little time for discussion and criticism. 'Information becomes knowledge', he said, 'by the

---

[18] Samuel Beckett, cited by O'Brien, (note 13), p. 335.
[19] Bair, *Beckett*, (note 10), pp. 365–6.
[20] *Ibid.*, p. 397.
[21] Thompson, 'Cybernetics and Animal Integration', *Irish J. Med. Sc.* (1951): 297–303.

process of inward digestion and through integration with existing knowledge and personal experience.' To his students he was a benevolent and respected figure; ever receptive to their problems. Alan Thompson's joy was to see his students emerge from their undergraduate training with that maturity of mind, knowledge and common sense so essential for the practice of medicine.[22]

He was by now a widely experienced general physician, particularly skilled at bedside teaching, and determined that basic principles should be given the same attention that some teachers reserve for the arcane and the dramatic. He reached a wider audience through his attachment to Radio Éireann as 'Radio Doctor', a post he held for many years. Even doctors made a point of listening to his broadcasts, enjoying excellent descriptions of something so commonplace as, say, measles.

Alan Thompson was elected president of the Royal College of Physicians of Ireland in 1966, and still held office in the following year when the college celebrated its tercentenary. 'This was seemly', the late Paddy Bofin has remarked, 'as the exertions of an ancestor of his, the 1st Duke of Ormonde, were largely responsible for the procurement of the College Charter from Charles II in 1667.'[23]

His avocations included music (he was an accomplished pianist), golf and fly fishing, and nothing pleased him more than to introduce younger colleagues to these sports. 'He harnesssed the brash enthusiasm of the novice [Bofin recalled] with patience and gently guided our early clumsy attempts. When we landed a fish or holed a chip shot he was as overjoyed as we.'[24] He played golf with left-handed clubs.

Alan Thompson was of average build, a good-looking man with a full head of hair swept back smoothly from an impressive brow; he dressed immaculately but, an uncompromising chain-smoker, he was rarely without a cigarette in his mouth. Endowed with a whimsical sense of humour, his stories against himself featured instances of verbal abuse in the Dublin demotic. He liked to recall the busdriver whose space he invaded, only to find their vehicles drawn up at the lights two minutes later, enabling the driver to roll down a window, view him with professional contempt, and call him 'a melon-headed fucker'. There was, too, the occasion after a consultation with Dr Billy Chapman in Amiens Street when, while washing his hands in the tiny bathroom, he overheard his patient's unimpressed husband on the landing asking the GP, 'an' what'll I have to pay that pale-faced Protestant whore?'

Thompson bought an old rectory at Tinahely, County Wicklow,

---

[22] 'Obituary' (note 2), p. 132.
[23] *Ibid.*
[24] Bofin, in Eoin O'Brien, Lorna Browne and Kevin O'Malley (eds.) *The House of Industry Hospitals 1772–1987: A Closing Memoir*, (Dublin: The Anniversary Press, 1988), p. 109.

which he intended to renovate on the DIY principle, but did not live to see its completion. He died from coronary heart disease after some weeks' illness on 23 March 1974, survived by Sylvia and their sons, Jeremy, Piers and Marcus. He was buried under a beech tree in the Quaker cemetery at Blackrock, County Dublin.

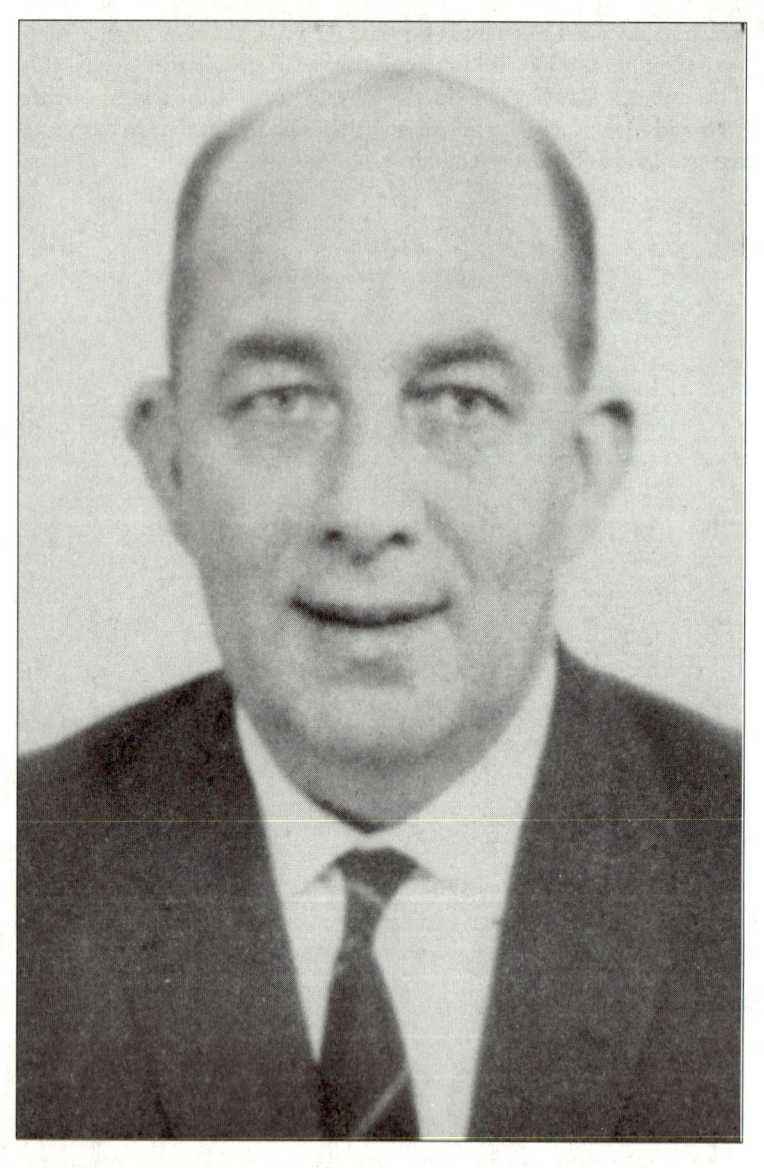

William Francis O'Dwyer, 1916–99 Professor of Medicine 1975–85

Chapter 16: William Francis O'Dwyer, 1916–99

William Francis (known universally as 'Billy') O'Dwyer was born in Dublin on 22 September 1916. His primary schools were Sion Hill Convent and Blackrock College, from which he went to Belvedere and Clongowes before entering the medical school at UCD. He attended clinics at St Vincent's Hospital, and played rugby for its cup-winning team in the keen inter-hospitals competition. He had the good fortune to be clinical clerk to D. K. O'Donovan, a brilliant clinical scientist recently returned from postgraduate study in Canada, but whether he availed fully of this opportunity is open to question. 'It was summertime', he later recalled with the insight of maturity, 'and I was very fond of tennis.'

The professor of medicine in the 1930s was James N. Meenan 'who taught us by example as much as by precept'. Professor Meenan was not an 'academic' in the modern sense, nor did he possess the 'flamboyance' underlying many of his colleagues' success. 'He was a good man and we all benefited incalculably from his goodness.'[1]

Another who could not fail to influence him (Billy had a gift for expression and was to speak eloquently in his prime from many public platforms) was William Doolin, surgeon to St Vincent's and Temple Street Hospitals, and editor of the *Irish Journal of Medical Science*.

> I think it was at a bedside clinic in Temple Streeet Children's Hospital [O'Dwyer recalled in his Doolin Lecture in 1978] that William Doolin really captured my imagination. He was talking to us about a little child on whom he had operated the previous day for acute intussusception and he said 'Looking into the little laddie's abdomen was like gazing down on a pit of writhing snakes.' This almost poetic vision of the wild and desparate peristalsis of acute intestinal obstruction has lived with me in a way that no audiovisual aid could ever have inspired.[2]

O'Dwyer graduated MB (NUI) with honours in 1940, and was appointed house-surgeon to Mr Doolin. 'No moment passed with him was a wasted one, and I am as grateful for those spent in drinking coffee and listening to his brilliant conversation, as I am for the hours we spent together in the operating theatre, and in the wards.' In those distant days every tyro, within days of taking up his first appointment, was expected to be a competent anaesthetist, administering ether with the Clover in-

---

[1] W. F. O'Dwyer, 'Nephrology 1980—Twenty Years a Growing', *J. Irish Colls. Phys. & Surgs.* (1981); 11: 15–20.
[2] O'Dwyer, 'The Making of a Consultant', *Irish Medical Journal* (1978); 71: 282–8.

haler, or with a rag and bottle, and young Dr O'Dwyer had a mortifying, but not uncommon experience, when attempting to put a policeman to sleep while the surgeon waited, scalpel in hand. Eventually the restive patient sat erect on the operating-table swearing loudly. Unperturbed, Doolin waited without a rebuke until the house-surgeon eventually obtained control.

O'Dwyer proceeded MD in 1945. Meanwhile, during the 'Emergency' (as the wartime period was called in neutral Ireland) he was commissioned in the Irish army medical corps. Back in civilian life and with a wife to support—he married Dr Fanty FitzGerald from County Mayo in 1943—he held a temporary post in Jervis Street Hospital, and in 1946 was appointed to its staff as honorary visiting physician.

The Charitable Infirmary

The Charitable Infirmary, to give the institution its proper name, was Dublin's oldest voluntary hospital. Founded by six surgeons in a little house in Cooks' Street in 1718, it accommodated at first only four patients.[3] Six years later its trustees took a house in Anderson's Court, on the north side of the Liffey where the Charitable Infirmary of Dublin was opened on 12 August 1728. A larger premises on the Inns Quay was secured in 1736, and the Infirmary moved finally to Jervis Street in 1786. Down the years it attracted many distinguished doctors to its wards; Robert Adams contributed the account of heart-block in 1827 that earned him an eponym, the 'Stokes-Adams syndrome'; his contemporary Dr (later Sir) Dominic Corrigan described aortic incompetence in 1832; William Wallace introduced potassium iodide as a therapy for syphilis in 1836 and proved that the secondary stage of the disease was infective.

This tradition of excellence was largely forgotten by the 1940s, by which time Jervis Street Hospital had become rather a lack-lustre place, kept busy because its central situation in the city was favoured by ambulance drivers with accident cases. Towards the end of the 1950s it was suddenly re-invigorated, and the Charitable Infirmary's doctors stood again on the frontiers of clinical science.

What had happened was this: the late Arthur Barry, a gynaecologist, greatly concerned by the plight of women suffering from kidney failure as a result of obstetrical complications, discussed the problem with a few colleagues. It was a dramatic and tragic situation. Women dying after childbirth might be saved by dialysis therapy—but dialysis was not available in Dublin. Rather than appeal to the Department of Health, slow to

---

[3] The six surgeons were Francis and George Duany, Patrick Kelly, Nathanial Handson, John Dowdall and Peter Brenan. See J. D. H. Widdess (ed.), *The Charitable Infirmary, Jervis Street, Dublin, 1718–1968* (Dublin: Thom, 1968).

respond to such demands, Barry and four others—Billy O'Dwyer, Gerry Doyle (pathologist), the late Anthony Walsh (urologist), the late Joe Woodcock (anaesthetist)—decided to buy a Kolff twin-coil artificial kidney for the hospital, and to pay for it with their own money.

As a preparatory step they underwent what Michael Carmody has called 'a four-day crash course' in Leeds in the techniques of dialysis, under the direction of Dr Frank Patterson. 'The Dublin novices were instructed in the mysteries of connecting the patient's circulation to dialysis, the complexities of making up dialysis fluids, and the principles of transfer across semi-permeable dialysis membranes.'[4]

Renal dialysis

Renal dialysis at the Charitable Infirmary began in May 1958, and in the first year the procedure usually was done at night, each session lasting about nine hours. Cases of renal failure in obstetrics were given precedence, but with improvements in obstetrical management, and the availability of family planning for women at risk, these emergencies became uncommon. The management by dialysis of 300 cases of uraemia (of which fifty-nine had obstetrical or gynaecological causes) was described in the *Journal of Obstetrics and Gynaecology* in December 1964.

Like other units they encountered the teething problems of a developing art, the most sinister being wastage of blood vessels caused by the numerous canulations needed to gain repeated access to the circulation, a difficulty overcome in 1960 when Dillard and Scribner of Seattle introduced an exteriorised shunt composed of teflon and silastic. This permited repeated access, and led to the development of regular dialysis treatment (RDT).

The concept developed six years later by Cimino and Brescia at the Veterans Administration Hospital in the Bronx, consisted of the surgical creation of an arterio-venous fistula in the arm which provided large veins distended by shunted, partially arterialised blood. 'These were easily accessible to puncture with needles of sufficiently wide bore, allowing double access to the circulation for the removal and return of blood. Adopted tentatively at first, this ingenious manoeuvre confounded the Cassandra-like prognostications of those who foretold disaster, and eventually it became accepted practice throughout the world.'[5] The well-constructed fistula is amazingly stable and it facilitated the development of dialysis in patients' homes.

---

[4] Michael Carmody in Eoin O'Brien (ed.) *The Charitable Infirmary Jervis Street 1718–1987*, (Dublin: The Anniversary Press, 1987), p. 182.
[5] O'Dwyer, 'Nephrology' (note 1), p. 18.

Nephrology

Galen's *On the Natural Faculties* describes how experiments on animals showed that urine is formed by the kidneys, and transmitted by the ureters to the bladder. Andreas Vesalius envisaged the production of urine as a straining off from the blood by the kidneys, of some but not all of its serosity. The process was difficult to understand, for the renal substance was dense and firm, nothing being then known of its microscopic structure. This knowledge was offered by Bellini (tubules), Malpighi (glomeruli), Bowman (capsule) and others. Carl Ludwig suggested in 1844 that from the arterial blood supplied to the glomeruli a protein-free filtrate is separated; as it passes along the tubule, the filtrate is reabsorbed, except for urea and other waste products.

Richard Bright's *Report on Medical Cases* (1827), which has been referred to in the previous chapter, contained what R. H. Major has called an 'epochal account' of renal disease. It was not by any means the first treatise on renal pathology, but Bright 'not only pointed out the association between dropsy, albuminuria, and hardened kidneys, but also found that there was an excess of urea in the blood of these patients'.[6] He had made an important contribution to nosology. The eponym 'Bright's disease' passed into common parlance, but before long it was applied to almost any and every renal disorder.

Dr O'Dwyer's interesting essay, 'Nephrology 1980—Twenty Years a Growing', reminds us of the 'futile semantics leading to fresh and evermore confusing classifications of Bright's Disease'.[7] Students at UCD had to know both Professor Meenan's classification and another favoured by Professor Moore, his counterpart at the Mater Hospital. Ellis's simpler classification was helpful, and the increasing frequency of acute renal failure as typified by the 'crush syndrome' was directing attention to the management of acute renal shut-down. The 'Bull regime' (following the protocols of Dr Graham Bull and his colleagues) could be life-saving. O'Dwyer calls it 'a historic landmark, the first real contribution by physicians to the treatment of kidney disease. Hitherto the only person to provide any positive help was the surgeon urologist dealing with obstructive lesions in the outflow tract.'[8]

Dialysis

Meanwhile, at Gröningen's University Hospital in the late 1930s, Willem Kolff, a young Dutch doctor, unable to forget his sense of helplessness when called upon to treat a farmer of about his own age dying of

---

[6] R. H. Major, *Classic Descriptions of Disease* (Springfield: Thomas, 1945), p. 535.
[7] O'Dwyer, 'Nephrology' (note 1), p. 16.
[8] *Ibid.* p. 16.

uraemia, had turned his mind to the salutary project of inventing a machine capable of replacing renal function. A local biochemist explained to him the suitability of cellophane in the process of dialysis.

When the German armies invaded the Low Countries, Kolff's teaching-hospital was taken over; a Dutch Nazi replaced the Jewish professor of medicine who was reported to have committed suicide. Dr Kolff moved to a hospital in Kampen, where he continued with his work.

> Three years later [O'Dwyer tells us], in February 1943, his machine completed he dialysed his first patient. This was an old gentleman in end stage failure due to neglected prostatic obstruction. The effort failed. His second patient, a young woman of 20 also in end stage irreversible failure with malignant hypertension lived for 26 days. He now knew that it was possible to replace renal function. It was to be another two years before his 17th dialysed patient became his first survivor. In September 1945, the Netherlands, now liberated, a 67-year-old female collaborator imprisoned in the local barracks, developed acute renal failure in association with acute cholecystitis and jaundice. As she was unconscious and anuric for upwards of a week before diuresis, there is no doubt that without dialysis her subsequent recovery with normal renal function would not have been possible.[9]

After the Second World War Kolff presented some of the machines he had built to medical centres abroad; one went to London to the Hammersmith Hospital, others to the Royal Victoria Hospital, Montreal, to the Mount Sinai Hospital, New York City, to Amsterdam and to Cracow. Copies and modifications were made, and from the Necker Hospital in Paris a machine was sent to the Leeds General Infirmary.

It was to Leeds, as mentioned above, that the Jervis Street group went for instruction. Billy O'Dwyer described them romantically as 'naive wandering scholars in search of the new learning.' Whatever else they were—and they had much to learn—they were not naive. They had a solemn purpose, and were to supply a clamant need. The Department of Health did not bless them for leaping into action to initiate a costly service without prior consultation. They were, however, obeying an irrefutable maxim—*Salus populi, suprema lex*—and in 1964 the Department relented, giving the unit some financial support.[10] By then, however, nephrology was well established in Dublin, and Dr O'Dwyer's expertise was recognised by his appointment as consultant to the Coombe Lying-in Hospital.

Renal unit

The treatment of acute renal failure was the primary object of the Jervis Street Hospital renal unit, but O'Dwyer and Michael Carmody reporting in 1968 on RDT for patients in end-stage renal failure, opened their

---

[9] *Ibid.* p. 17.
[10] Carmody in *Jervis Street* (note 4), p 175.

paper on a note of caution: 'Regular Dialysis Treatment from its beginnings has been bedevilled by an aura of prestige, glamour and emotion leading all too frequently to its application where in retrospect all would admit there never was any real hope of success.'[11]

Frequency of dialysis was the single most important factor in achieving success, and between November 1964 and December 1965 when thirteen patients were given only one haemodialysis weekly, ten patients died. In January 1966 it was possible to increase dialysis frequency to three every two weeks, and seven of the ten patients admitted to the programme survived.

> Since February 1967 [they wrote], twenty-one patients have been treated with two dialyses per week and though one patient died (unexpectedly) as a result of an error in Dialysis Technique, the twenty survivors have given no cause for significant apprehension while on Regular Dialysis Treatment and all who were more than three months on treatment have returned to work. On inadequate dialysis a high mortality from cardiovascular causes must be expected in the first year . . . It should be added that the morbidity rate is high also in such circumstances and experience would suggest that inadequate Regular Dialysis Treatment is now ethically indefensible.[12]

During the period under review they were using three twin-coil dialysing machines, and their facilities were greatly improved by the addition of five new machines. Peritoneal dialysis was used increasingly for the treatment of acute renal failure.

Seven patients with end-stage renal failure received cadaveric transplants between October and December 1967. 'It is now our definite policy that patients accepted on the Regular Dialysis Programme should be considered as potential candidates for transplantation.'[13]

O'Dwyer spoke on pregnancy and the kidney at a renal symposium in Dublin in 1971, mentioning the normal modifications of renal function in pregnancy and discussing hazards to which the normal kidney may be subjected as a result of pregnancy, and those which may occur when pregnancy is superimposed on primary renal disease or hypertension. A series of emergency admissions to the renal unit in Jervis Street Hospital, when compared with a similar series at the Hôpital Necker in Paris, had shown that the incidence of post-partum renal failure was higher in the Irish patients, as were parity and

---

[11] O'Dwyer and M. Carmody, 'Regular Dialysis Treatment', *J. Irish Med. Assn.*, (1968); 61: 189–194.

[12] *Ibid.*, p. 190.

[13] The first renal tranplant at the Charitable Infirmary was performed on 31 January 1964 by W. A. L. MacGowan, Anthony Walsh (d. 1997) and Peter McLean. The donated (cadaveric) kidney ceased to function after a few hours; the patient died next day. Success was not attained until the fourth attempt. Tissue typing was introduced in the early 1970s.

age. Among the means of redressing this situation was a realistic family planning service—'an essential requirement for future protection against premature death and chronic ill-health.'[14]

In the *British Medical Journal* he suggested that the depression and loss of libido reported in association with oral contraceptives, were 'psychological rather than pharmacological in origin'. They did not occur in the patients under his care, for whom oral contraceptives were then the only available method of birth-control. They were motivated by bad obstetrical histories, and an absolute need to avoid further pregnancies.[15]

O'Dwyer was angry 'to find himself prevented by the law from giving his patients life-saving advice'.[16] He became a member of the Fertility Guidance Company (later re-named the Irish Family Planning Association) established by Dr Michael Solomons and others. This group encouraged Mrs Mary McGee to take a legal action against the state for interfering with her rights as a citizen.

Mrs McGee, the twenty-nine-year-old mother of four, had suffered from hypertension during her pregnancies; she used a diaphragm (fitted by a member of the Guidance Company), but the spermicide she ordered from England was confiscated by customs as illegal. Her case against the Attorney General and the Revenue Commissioners was dismissed by the High Court, a judgement reversed by the Supreme Court in December 1973.

The availability of contraceptives soon became a political issue: the first move to legalize their sale was defeated in 1974, when in a free vote situation the taoiseach of the day (Liam Cosgrave) voted against his government's bill; the Family Planning Act 1979—Charles J. Haughey's celebrated 'Irish solution for an Irish problem'—a medium-term strategy, permitted contraceptives to be sold to married couples with a doctor's prescription; the amendment of a later Minister for Health freed conditions of vending.

The nephrologist and his staff, in the course of their daily work, face an increased risk of hepatitis B infection, a risk to which their patients are exposed in greater degree. O'Dwyer (1976) reported freedom from this infection in both patients and staff at the Jervis Street renal service.[17]

The chair of medicine

Appointed associate professor in the RCSI in 1962, O'Dwyer was elected in 1975 to the chair of medicine which he held for ten years, becoming

---

[14] 'Pregnancy and the Kidney', *J. Irish Med. Assn.* (1971); 64: 460–62.
[15] 'Oral Contraceptives, Depression, and Libido', *Brit. Med. J.* (1971); 3: 702.
[16] Michael Solomons, *Pro Life? The Irish Question* (Dublin: Lilliput Press, 1992), p. 34.
[17] O'Dwyer, 'Nephrologists at Risk?', *Proc. Conjoint Ann. Gen. Meeting, 1976*. Dublin: IMA, (1976), pp. 109–13.

emeritus professor in 1985. Billy obviously enjoyed the academic life and all it entailed, the company of young people and their instruction, the febrile contention of committee meetings, the excitement and competitiveness of examination days. He was a painstaking examiner, going almost to extremes to get the best out of a weak candidate, or to test a brilliant boy (or girl)—especially if dealing with a Jervis Street pupil who might be in the running for honours. If he had a fault (and who has not?) it was in his rather obvious loyalty to his own hospital.

As a teacher he was held in high regard and a former pupil has referred recently to his 'humane and gentle ward rounds'. He talked in a kind and personal way to his patients, and a delicate hand on the shoulder, or a little extra pressure on a hand established a bond that seemed special to that individual.

> We had a particular habit [a former intern recalled] of breaking the ward round half-way through for coffee made with milk, and chocolate biscuits. One noticed how the ladies in the kitchen, and the cleaners on the floor were treated by the Prof with the same respect and concern that he reserved for his hospital colleagues. And they in turn displayed an obvious fondness for Billy O'Dwyer.
>
> Not, indeed that all was sweetness and light in those days at meetings of the medical board, occasions which generated such heat that a wit from the Richmond Hospital labelled the Jervis Street staff 'the Lavender Hill Mob'.

Professor O'Dwyer acted as extern examiner for a number of Irish schools, and for the University of Glasgow and the University of Garyounis, Benghazi, Libya. He was visiting lecturer in Benghazi from 1978–80, and visiting professor at the University of Natal in 1986.

Medical politics

A gregarious person, Billy was a 'natural' for societies, a member of the Clinical Club, the Corrigan Club, the Association of Physicians of Great Britain and Ireland (council member 1975–7), a fellow of the Royal Academy of Medicine in Ireland, a member of the European Dialysis and Transplant Association, the Irish Society of Nephrology, the Renal Association, etc., not to mention purely social clubs.

He was also a member of the Irish Medical Association (IMA), and when after a long spell on its central council he was elected president in 1963, he was determined to put an end to the state of 'cold war' then existing between the IMA and the Department of Health, and restore harmony to the field of medical politics. It was a task for which his emollient personality made him particularly suited. If there were hawks and doves in the IMA, Billy was a dove, seeing little virtue in what he referred to as 'a constant stream of uncritical and emotional invective'.

When elected to presidential office, Billy O'Dwyer's ambition was to break the silence sundering the IMA and Department of Health referred to in Chapter 14. He was helped to do so when, fortuitously, a parliamentary secretary came under his professional care. He availed of the opportunity to discuss the absurd situation with the civil servant, who offered to act as intermediary between the IMA president and the minister.

'I told him gently to allow the Minister to know my desire', O'Dwyer recalled. 'My new found patient and helper, at my request, persuaded Mr MacEntee to accept our invitation to the dinner which in 1963 was held in Drogheda.'[18] In the course of his placatory presidential address, Billy announced that 'the cold frustrating silence between the IMA and the Department has ended'[19]; in his after-dinner speech MacEntee reciprocated this cordiality saying the occasion 'was the harbinger of a happier relationship between the Minister for Health, whomsoever he may happen to be, and the great and learned and so necessary profession upon whose willing co-operation the Minister must lean.'[20]

The president canvassed those on the central council who favoured mending fences, and assured himself of the necessary two thirds majority that enabled the withdrawl from the journal of the 'Important Notice'. Certain modifications were agreed, to circumvent the problem of professional confidentiality mentioned in Chapter 14. The next important event was Billy's secret meeting with MacEntee.

> One night at the house of a friend common to both of us [he wrote], I turned up, was ushered into a drawing room, and invited to sit down opposite to another chair with a coffee table between on which a bottle of Napoleon Brandy (the Minister's favourite drink) had been placed. In due course a black limousine pulled up and the great man appeared and sat opposite me. He asked what were the conditions the IMA would accept, and I told him about the conclusions of the recent Council meeting. He said that that would be satisfactory, but was I quite sure that this would be satisfactory to the body as a whole? Feeling a little nervous I answered that I was sure it would ... It was then decided that we would each get our henchmen to organise an official and formal meeting.[21]

That meeting took place in the Custom House, early in December 1963 and was the beginning of the resumption of a normal relationship. O'Dwyer saw the IMA's practice of engaging in 'belated criticism of *faits accomplis* in the development of the Health Service' as of little avail. 'It is

---

[18] Personal communication WFO'D/JBL.
[19] O'Dwyer, 'Time and Tide', *J. Irish Med. Assn,*, (1963) 53: 32–6.
[20] Seán MacEntee, 'Address by Minister for Health', *ibid.*, p. 36–8.
[21] Letter WFO'D/JBL.

for us to anticipate new requirements and provide a continuing stream of fresh concepts and ideas, many of which must eventually be incorporated in the plans of the state and Local Authorities.'

It is relevant to say that Seán MacEntee's machinations harmed the medical profession by achieving a desired effect, 'divide and rule'. Some doctors, who regarded the IMA as an organisation dominated by Dublin consultants, argued that if it lacked legal rights (as MacEntee asserted) it should be replaced by a de facto trade union. They took the logical step of forming the Irish Medical Union (IMU). This introduced 'an element of potential conflict' which O'Dwyer and others reduced by setting up a liaison committee to ensure discussion between the IMA and the IMU—'once again the simple process of sitting down at a table with one's apparent adversaries has paid handsome dividends'. A later generation has reunited the opposed groups in the Irish Medical Organisation (IMO) which, regrettably, was not joined in appropriate strength by consultants. In due course the latter formed the Irish Hospital Consultants Association, diminishing the influence of the IMO. At the individual level, Seán MacEntee became 'almost a personal friend' of Professor O'Dwyer, and made him president of An Bord Altranais, the Nursing Board.

Looking to the future of 'this brave new world of increasing longevity and affluence', Billy O'Dwyer predicted in 1963 the emergence of new patterns of ill-health. 'Affluence removes the spectre of want but it creates a new restlessness. Increasing leisure [the enforced leisure of unemployment was not then so evident] can be a dangerous gift . . .' Medicine is likely to have to deal with psychological disorders in greater numbers.

More than thirty years later O'Dwyer's predictions are fulfilled. One is obliged, however, to question the desirability of his wish to preserve 'the image of the doctor as a father figure'; not only are fathers frequently disregarded but they are often, albeit kindly, rather puzzled and inept. Paternalistic is used increasingly as a pejorative term, and besides he/she (the doctor) is always so obviously pressed for time. Understandably, the lay counsellor, the chat-show and the herbalist have become challenging alternatives. The doctor's image needs a more radical change.

Medical education

O'Dwyer's presidential address to the Biological Society discussed the choices relating to his future the newly-qualified doctor must make, and cautioned him against the 'inconsequential drift'—the danger of moving from one hospital post to the next without a career plan in mind—and the 'pre-mature decision' in selecting a particular speciality without adequate consideration of all it involves.[22] 'Surgery clad in her romantic trappings—not excluding the aseptic yashmak of the theatre staff—is in

---

[22] 'The Young Doctor on the Threshold', *J. Irish Med Assn.*, (1964); 54: 1–8.

my opinion a clear winner among the sirens which threaten the early Odyssey of the young doctor.'

Psychiatry was 'undoubtedly the Cinderella' of the specialities, but before graduation few had a true appreciation of its overwhelming importance. 'Neither scientific knowledge nor technical skill will prevent the doctor of the future who has no knowledge of or interest in this aspect of disease from becoming a professional anachronism.'

General practice is in itself a specific speciality 'to be entered only when the basic training in its essentials is complete'. He rejected the concept developing in some countries 'of a different kind of education for intending G.P.s on the one hand and hospital specialists and research workers on the other.'

Facilities for postgraduate education were meagre in Ireland in the first half of the present century, a problem Billy O'Dwyer discussed when president of the IMA:

> We live in what is undoubtedly the most rapidly progressive period in the history of medicine, and all over the world there is apparent an increasing volume of thought and organised energy directed towards the continuing education of the doctor. Even in the newly emerged nations, faced often with appalling circumstances of malnutrition and epidemic disease and in which the shortage of medical personnel is pathetic, there is an awareness that postgraduate education is not a luxury that can await a happier future for consideration... That we in Ireland have attempted little in this direction is in part due to our propinquity to Britain and, with improving communications, to the United States of America. It is always possible for a proportion of our young doctors to go to these countries for postgraduate experience and teaching. That this should continue is desirable, but it cannot exempt this country from the obligation of providing facilities at home.[23]

An annual refresher course for fifty or so general practitioners was insufficient. Facilities should be established throughout the country, using hospitals as focal points. Small discussion groups could be easily organised, supplemented by more formal lectures and demonstrations, but this 'should be sustained and regionalised.'

Improvements were not delayed, and when fifteen years later O'Dwyer discussed the training of specialists in his Doolin Lecture it seems as if profusion and complexities were creating the problems. Departments had evolved in which the consultant formed the apex of a pyramid supported by registrars, senior house officers and interns. The aspirant consultant faced an intolerably long period of 'professional adolescence'.

O'Dwyer confessed 'a healthy agnosticism' as to the best training

---

[23] 'Time and Tide', *J. Irish Med. Assn.*, (1963) 53: p. 34.

schemes, and enumerated those who now had a finger in the pie.

Already there is a truly formidable collection of academic institutions and committees, councils, faculties, hospital groups and health boards involved in the structuring of these programmes. The Department of Health and three major statutory bodies—Comhairle na nOspidéal, the new Irish Medical Council and the Council for Postgraduate Medical and Dental Education will have their separate and powerful influences. It is easy to imagine that such an accumulation of vested interests, which once having been indulged and satisfied, may well render impossible any significant change in the future, were such seen to be desirable. We may be, even now, in the process of winding a skein of such complexity that it can never be untangled.[24]

Research

The 25th anniversary of the foundation of the department of renal medicine and transplantation was celebrated in the RCSI on 3 December 1983. This almost fortuitous development had brought the Charitable Infirmary into the limelight, and kept it there offering new goals and fostering the spirit of investigation and research. Professor O'Dwyer's numerous research papers were related to renal medicine, and most were co-authored. With G. D. Doyle, Michael Carmody and Brian Keogh he published in 1967 a review of forty-one cases of the nephrotic syndrome, in all of whom percutaneous renal biopsies were performed. The histological diagnoses were: normal or minimal change lesions, 5; basement membrane thickening, 12; epithelial proliferation, 14; DLE, 2; diabetic neuropathy, 3; amyloid disease, 5. 'It appears from our series and others published since 1958 that approximately 16 per cent of patients with the nephrotic syndrome have little or no histological abnormality and may be expected either to undergo spontaneous remission, or to respond to steroid therapy.'[25]

Dialysis was not achieved without occasional complications, some puzzling and untoward. Fifteen cases of 'dialysis dementia' occurred in the Jervis Street renal unit between 1972 and 1976, an incidence of five per cent. 'This encephalopathy . . . remains an unsolved mystery in its aetiology, pathology and biochemistry [,] it dramatically appeared at the beginnng of this decade [1970] and seems now to be almost as suddenly on the wane.'[26]

A series of forty-one cases of acute renal failure in pregnancy treated in the Jervis Street Hospital unit between 1969 and 1978 was reported in

---

[24] 'The Making of a Consultant', *Irish Med. J.* (1978); 71: 285.
[25] O'Dwyer, G. D. Doyle, M. Carmody, B. Keogh, 'The Nephrotic Syndrome', *J. Irish Med. Assn.* (1967); 60: 409–16.
[26] B. Silke, G. R. Fitzgerald, S. Hanson, M. Carmody, W. F. O'Dwyer, 'Clinical Aspects of Dialysis Dementia', *Irish Med. J.* (1978); 71: 10–12.

1980. Management was by alternate day haemodialysis: five patients had cortical necrosis, thirty-six had tubular necrosis; foetal and maternal mortality were 73 per cent and 10 per cent respectively. 'The contrast with the previous decade is marked—the overall [maternal] mortality was then 28% but, whereas no deaths occurred from cortical necrosis in the current review period, the mortality in the previous decade approached 80%.'[27]

From a family viewpoint (and from that of reproductive medicine), pregnancy after a successful renal transplant must appear to be a notable event. Fourteen of 142 women in the childbearing age (9.9 per cent) given renal transplants in the Jervis Street transplant unit had subsequent pregnancies.[28] There were twelve live births, two sets of twins and nine foetal deaths. Experience had shown that pregnancy is not contraindicated in women with satisfactory renal function, but there was a melancholy prognostic shadow to temper their counselling—the reduced life-expectancy of the group as a whole. Three of the twelve children born were motherless within six years of birth.

The Charitable Infirmary closed its doors in 1987 and its staff joined that of St Laurence's Hospital at the newly-opened Beaumont Hospital.

R. I. P.

In the course of production of this book, the sudden death of Billy O'Dwyer, on 8 March 1999, was announced. He is survived by his wife, a son and a daughter.

---

[27] B. Silke et al., 'Acute Renal Failure in Pregnancy—a Decade of Change', *Irish Med J.*, (1980); 73: 191–3.
[28] D. Mulcahy, P. Garrett, S. Hanson, J. Donohoe, W. F. O'Dwyer, and M. Carmody, 'Pregnancy following Renal Transplantation', *Irish Med. J.* (1986); 79: 69–74.

Selected Sources

Abrahamson, L. 'Book Review', *Irish J. Med. Sc.* (1924): 44–5.
Adams, R. 'Cases of Disease of the Heart Accompanied by PathologicalObservations', *Dublin Hosp. Reps.* (1827); 4: 396.
Aird, R. B. *Foundations of Modern Neurology—A Century of Progress* (New York: Raven Press, 1994).
Bair, D. *Samuel Beckett* (London: Cape, 1978).
Barrington, R. *Health Medicine and Politics in Ireland—1900–1970* (Dublin: Institute of Public Administration, 1987).
Beatty, W. 'A Case of Myxoedema successfully treated by Massage and Hypodermic Injections of the Thyroid Gland of a Sheep', *Brit. Med. J.* (1882); 2: 544–5.
Bigger, J. W. *Man Against Microbe* (London: English Universities Press, 1939).
Bofin, P. 'Obituary: Alan H. Thompson', *J. Irish Colls. Phys. & Surgs.* (1974); 3: 131–2.
——in E. O'Brien, Lorna Browne and Kevin O'Malley (eds.) *The House of Industry Hospitals, 1772–1987* (Dublin: Anniversary Press, 1988).
Boxwell, W. and Purser, F. C. *An Introduction to the Practice of Medicine* (Dublin: Talbot Press, 1924).
——'Obituary Francis Carmichael Purser', *Irish J. Med. Sc.* (1934): 134–46.
Breathnach, C. S. 'Sir John William Moore', *Irish J. Med. Sc.* (1983); 152: 69–72.
Brennan, C., 'Architectural History (1805–1997) of the RCSI.' MA thesis UCD; Dublin, November 1997.
Brock, W. H., N. D. McMillan and R. C. Mollan, (eds.) *John Tyndall: Essays of a Natural Philosopher* (Dublin: RDS, 1981).
Browne, A. D. H. and B. Doran 'The external statuary of the RCSI', *J. Irish Colls. Phys. & Surgs.* (1988); 17: 177–9.
Browne, N. *Against the Tide* (Dublin: Gill and Macmillan, 1986).
Cameron, Sir Charles *History of the Royal College of Surgeons in Ireland*, 2nd ed. (Dublin: Fannin, 1916).
Carmody, M. and P. A. McLean 'The Department of Nephrology and the Development of Kidney Transplantation' (pp.171–188) in Eoin O'Brien (ed.) *The Charitable Infirmary Jervis Street 1718–1987*, ed. (Dublin: The Anniversary Press, 1987).
Cheyne, J. *Cases of Apoplexy and Lethargy with Observations upon the Comatose Diseases* (London: Underwood, 1812).
——'Autobiographical Sketch' in *Essays on Partial Derangement of the*

Mind (Dublin: Curry, 1843).

Coakley, D. *Masters of Irish Medicine* (Dublin: Town House, 1992).

Collis, R. *To Be a Pilgrim* (London: Secker & Warburg, 1975).

Cowan, A. 'Leonard Abrahamson—The Man', *J. Irish Colls. Phys. & Surgs.* (1983); 12: 158–63.

Critchley, M. *Sir William Gowers 1845-1915* (London: Heinemann, 1949).

Cronin, A. *Samuel Beckett: The Last Modernist* (London: HarperCollins, 1996).

Doolin, W. 'Sir John William Moore', *Irish J. Med. Sc.* (1937): 654.

——'In Memoriam T. G. Moorhead', *ibid.*, (1960): 438.

——'Obituary: Leonard Abrahamson', *Brit. Med. J.* (1961); 2: 1295–6.

Foot, A. W. 'Reminiscences of the Dublin Biological Club', *Dublin J. Med. Sc.* (1892); 93: 421–41.

Gatenby, P. B. 'Obituary V. M. Synge', *Brit. Med. J.* (1976); 2: 118.

——*Dublin's Meath Hospital* (Dublin: Town House, 1996).

Gogarty, O. St. J. *Wild Apples* (Dublin: Cuala Press, 1930).

Grace, P. 'Sic Transit Gloria Mundi', *J. Irish Colls. Phys. & Surgs.* (1993); 22: 204–5.

Graves, R. J. in William Stokes (ed.) *Studies in Physiology and Medicine*, (London: Churchill, 1863).

Grimshaw, T. W. 'The Intimate Nature of Infection and Contagion', *Dublin J. Med. Sc.* (1878); 66: 1–15.

Haymaker, W. and F. Schiller, (eds.) *The Founders of Neurology* (Springfield: Thomas, 1970).

Henschen, F. *The History of Diseases* (London: Longmans, 1966).

Hitchcock, H. *TB or not TB?* (Galway: Centre for Health Promotion Studies, 1995).

Jessop, W. J. E. 'Samuel Haughton: a Victorian Polymath', *Hermathena* (1973); 116: 5–26.

Keys, T. E., C. W. Rucker, and H. W. Wolton 'Helmholtz Commemoration Program', *Proc. Staff Meetings Mayo Clinic* (1951); 26: 209–23.

Kirkpatrick, T. P. C. *An Account of the Irish Medical Periodicals* (Dublin: Falconer, 1916).

——*History of the Medical Teaching in Trinity College Dublin and of the School of Physic in Ireland* (Dublin: Hanna & Neale, 1912).

Knowlson, J. *Damned to Fame—the Life of Samuel Beckett* (London: Bloomsbury, 1996).

Lectures on Public Health delivered in the Lecture Hall of the Royal Dublin Society (Dublin: Hodges, Foster & Co., 1874).

Lee, J. J. *Ireland 1913–1985* (Cambridge University Press, 1989).

Lindeman, G. A., *Herman Boerhaave* (London: Methuen, 1968).

Little, J. 'Life and work of the late Dr. Hudson', *Dublin J. Med. Sc.* (1882); 74: 1–9.

Lyons, J.B. 'Sylvester O'Halloran (1728–1807)', *Irish J. Med. Sc.*, (1963): 217–32, 279–88.

——*Brief Lives of Irish Doctors* (Dublin: Blackwater Press, 1978).

——*An Assembly of Irish Surgeons* (Dublin: Glendale Press, 1984).

——'John Cheyne's classic monographs', *J. Hist. Neurosci.* (1995); 4: 27–35.

——*The Quality of Mercer's* (Dublin: Glendale Press, 1991).

——'George Sigerson: Charcot's Translator', *J. Hist. Neurosci.* (1997); 6: 50–60.

McCarthy, A. 'In Memoriam Professor T. G. Moorhead', *J. IMA* (1960); 47: 77.

McCollum, S. 'The roots of the Royal College of Surgeons in Ireland: the barber/chirurgeons of Dublin', *J. Irish Colls. Phys. & Surgs.* (1994); 23: 53–59.

McDowell, R. B. and D. A. Webb *Trinity College Dublin 1592–1952 An academic history* (Cambridge University Press, 1982).

MacEntee, S. 'Address to IMA by Minister for Health', *J. Irish Med. Assn.* (1963); 53: 36–8.

McHenry, L. C. *Garrison's History of Neurology* (Springfield: Thomas, 1969).

Mackenzie, H. 'A Case of Myxoedema Treated with Great Benefit by Feeding with Fresh Thyroid Glands', *Brit. Med. J.* (1892); 2: 940–41.

Major R. H. *Classic Descriptions of Disease* (Springfield: Thomas, 1945).

Maunsell, H. *Political Medicine* (Dublin: Fannin, 1839).

Maxwell, C. *Dublin Under the Georges* (London: Faber, 1956).

Micks, R. H. 'Notes on the Diagnosis and Treatment of Diabetes', *Irish J. Med. Sci.* (1923): 396–405.

Mitchell, D. *A Peculiar Place* (Dublin: Blackwater Press, 1989).

Mixter, W. J. and J. S. Barr 'Rupture of the Intervertebral Disc with involvement of the Spinal Canal', *New Eng. J. Med.* (1934); 211: 210–15.

Moore, Sir J. *Text-Book of Eruptive and Continued Fevers* (Dublin: Fannin, 1892).

——'In Memoriam: James Little', *ibid.*, 1917; 143: 73–9.

Murray, G. R. 'Note on the Treatment of Myxoedema by Hypodermic Injections of an extract of the Thyroid Gland of a Sheep', *Brit. Med. J.* (1891); 2: 796–7.

Nesbitt, R. *At Arnotts of Dublin 1843–1993* (Dublin: A. & A. Farmar, 1993).

O'Brien, B. 'Obituary V. M. Synge, F.R.C.P., F.R.C.P.I.', *J. Irish Med.*

Assn. (1976); 69: 132.

O'Brien, E. 'John Cheyne (1777–1836)', *J. Irish Colls. Phys and Surgs.*, 1974; 3: 91–3.

—— 'From the Waters of Sion to Liffeyside—the Jewish Contribution: Medical and Cultural', *J. Irish Colls. Phys. & Surgs.* (1981); 10: 107–19.

—— *The Beckett Country* (Dublin: Black Cat Press, 1986).

O'Dwyer, W. F. 'Time and Tide', *J. Irish Med. Assn.* (1963); 53: 32–6.

—— G. D. Doyle, M. Carmody and B. Keogh 'The Nephrotic Syndrome', *ibid.,* (1967); 60: 409–16.

—— 'Nephrology 1880—Twenty Years a Growing', *J. Irish Colls. Phys. & Surgs.* (1981); 11: 15–20.

O'Flanagan, H. 'The Health Services in Ireland: A perspective on origins', *Irish Medical Journal* (1987); 80: 217–18.

O'Grady, J. *The Life and Work of Sarah Purser* (Dublin: Four Courts Press, 1996).

Ormsby, Sir L. H. *History of the Meath Hospital* (1888).

Osler, Sir W. *The Principles and Practice of Medicine*, 7th ed. (London: Appleton, 1909).

Powell, M. 'Noel Browne—a hero or a villain?' *Irish Medical News* (1997): 7 July.

Shanley, J. 'Obituary notice T. G. Moorhead', *J. IMA* (1960); 47: 77.

Silke, B., Fitzgerald, S., Hanson, S., Carmody, M. and W. F. O'Dwyer, 'Clinical Aspects of Dialysis Dementia', *Irish Med. J.* (1978); 71: 10–12.

—— 'Acute Renal Failure in Pregnancy—a Decade of Change', *ibid.,* (1980); 73: 191–3.

Solomons, M. *Pro Life? The Irish Question* (Dublin: Lilliput Press, 1992).

Stelfox, A.W. 'Arthur Wynne Foot, M.D., Irish Naturalist', *The Irish Naturalist's Journal* (1931); 3: 260–61.

Toksvig, Signe *Signe Toksvig's Irish Diaries 1926–1937*, Lis Phil (ed.) (Dublin: Lilliput Press, 1994).

Wheeler, W. J. 'A Record of Cases Treated Antiseptically, and of Cases According to Lister's Method', *Med. Press & Circ.* (1881); 82: 155–9.

Widdess, J. D. H. 'Robert M'Donnell—a Pioneer of Blood Transfusion', *Irish J. Med. Sc.* (1952): 11–20.

—— *The Royal College of Surgeons in Ireland and its Medical School 1784–1984*, 3rd ed. (Dublin: RCSI, 1984).

—— *A History of the Royal College of Physicians of Ireland* (Edinburgh: Livingstone, 1963).

Whytt, R. *Observations on the Dropsy in the Brain* (Edinburgh: Balfour, 1768).

[Wilde, W.] 'The Editor's Preface', *Dublin J. Med. Sc.*, 1846; 1: xxxvii.

Index

Abbott, Maude, 257
Abercrombie, John, 27
Abrahamson, David, 263
Abrahamson, Leonard, 232, 249, 255–65, 267, 269
  Biological Society, 258–9
  cardiology, 256–7
  family of, 262–3
  in Jewish community, 265
  Mercer's Hospital, 258
  president, RCPI, 263–5
  professor of medicine, 260–2
Abrahamson, Mervyn Leonard, 263
Abrahamson, Mervyn Saul, 255
Academy of Medicine in Ireland, Royal, 160–1, 165, 170, 187, 190, 193, 204, 207, 239, 240–1, 284
  Abrahamson, 255, 258, 262
  Moore, 197, 206
  Moorhead, 212–13
  Thompson, 273
  centenary, 179
Act of Union, 14–16
Adams, Robert, 19, 108, 278
Addison, Thomas, 115, 135, 176, 268–9
Addison's disease, 268–9
Adelaide Hospital, 152, 154, 162, 245
Adrien, Mr, 105
Albertini, 257
Albutt, Sir Clifford, 184–5, 226, 238
Alcmaeon of Croton, 225
Alcock, 112
Allen, F. M., 240, 242
Andral, Dr, 142
Andrews, Maria, 149
antisepsis. *see* germ theory
aphasia, 42–3, 226–8
Apjohn, Dr, 143
apoplexy, 21–4
Apothecaries Hall, 1, 180
Archer, Clement, 6
Aristotle, 225
Armagh County Infirmary, 151
Armagh Fever Hospital, 151
Armstrong, Louisa Emma, 187

Arnotts, 237
Arthur, Mrs Mary Henrietta, 96–7
Association of Physicians of Great Britain and Ireland, 164, 187, 258, 284
Astwood, E. B., 173

Babinski, Joseph François, 226
Baggot St Hospital. *see* Royal City of Dublin Hospital
Baillie, Matthew, 21
Banks, Dr, 97
Banting, Sir F. G., 214–15
Barker, Francis, 32, 65
Barr, Joseph, 233
Barrington, Ruth, 265
Barry, Arthur, 278–9
Bauer, 239
Beatty, Thomas, 129
Beatty, Wallace, 162
Beaumont Hospital, 8, 289
Beckett, Bill, 259
Beckett, Samuel, 259, 267, 269–73
Beddoes, T., 29
Bedford, D. E., 259
Bedford Asylum, 16
Behan, Brendan, 253
Belfast General Hospital, 146
Bell, Benjamin, 11–12
Bell, John, 13
Bell, Sir Charles, 12–13, 44–5, 225
Bellingham, O'Bryen, 257
Bellini, 280
Bennett, Edward Halloran, 158
Benson, Arthur, 149
Benson, Charles, 112, 114, 119, 131–49, 155, 247
  acute rheumatism, 148
  asiatic cholera, 140–4
  chair of medicine, 133–6
  examination for fellowship, 144
  gastrointestinal tract, 137–9
  germ theory, 144–6
  introductory address, 146–7
  last years, 148–9
  PRCSI, 147–8
  preliminary appraisal, 136–7

INDEX

venous pulsation, 132–3
Benson, George Vere, 149
Benson, Sir John Hawtrey, 149, 152, 219
Bernard, Claude, 141, 172
Best, C. H., 214–15
Bigger, Joseph W., 157–8, 218–19, 249, 268
biochemistry, 237–8
Biological Club, Dublin, 78, 173–5
Biological Society, RCSI, 211, 260, 264, 286
Biological Society, TCD, 226, 237, 242, 258–9
   presidential address, 1925, 247–8
birth control, 283
Black, Joseph, 11
Blacker, Lt Colonel William, 52
blood transfusion, 164, 241–2
blood-letting, 23, 28–9
Boate, Dr Gerard, 196, 197
Boerhaave, Herman, 1
Bofin, Paddy, 260–1, 274
Bord Altranais, An, 286
Bouillaud, Jean-Baptiste, 227
Bowman, 280
Boxwell, William, 231–2, 234
Breathnach, C. S., 179, 205
Brenan, Dr, 72
Brescia, 279
Bright, Richard, 115, 135, 176, 269, 280
Bright's disease, 280
British Association for the Advancement of Science, 196
British Medical Association, 128, 145–6, 173, 190, 217, 219
British Medical Journal, 258, 283
Broca, Paul, 42, 227
Browne, Dr Noel, 264–5
Brown-Sequard, Dr C. E., 170, 174–5
brucellosis, 267–8
Brule, 255
Bull, Dr Graham, 280
Burrowes, Peter, 66
Bushe, Charles Kendal, 66
Byrne, Dr, Archbishop of Dublin, 38

Cajal, Ramon y, 225
Cameron, Sir Charles, 5, 99, 133–4, 148, 157, 175, 197, 203
Cardiac Society, 256
cardiology, 256–7
Carmichael, Richard, 75–6, 111–12

Carmichael School, 5, 173, 179
Carmody, Michael, 279, 281, 288
Catholic University Medical School, 4
central board of health, 94
Chapman, Dr Billy, 274–5
Charcot, J.-M., 171, 225, 228
Charitable Infirmary, Jervis St, 14, 108–9, 284
   O'Dwyer, 278–9
   renal unit, 281–3, 289
Cheyne, John, 7, 11–45, 47, 85, 115, 120, 121, 138, 225, 232 ambition, 13–14
   apprenticeship, 11–12
   army surgeon, 12–13
   Cases of Apoplexy and Lethargy, 21–3
   contagion, 145
   depression and retirement, 39–43
   in Dublin, 14–16
   Dublin Hospital Reports, 19–20
   dysentery, 33–4
   eponym, 18–19
   Essays on the Diseases of Children, 20–1
   Hardwicke Hospital reports, 28–33
   Henry on, 44–5
   House of Industry Hospitals, 16–18
   hydrocephalus acutus, 24–8
   malingering, 34–7
   Prince of Hohenlohe, 37–9
Cheyne-Stokes breathing, 18–19, 152–3
Childers, Dr Rory, 253
Children's Hospital, Belfast, 180
cholera, 94, 116, 201–2
   Benson on, 139–44
   spread of, 155–6
Churchill, Dr, 116
Cimino, 279
City Bridewell, 30
Clare, Lord, 51–4, 77
Cleghorn, James, 15
Cleghorn, Thomas, 67–8
climatic change, 196–7
Clinical Club, 284
Clossy, Samuel, 224, 231
Cobbe, Thomas, 62–3
Colles, Abraham, 15, 19, 82, 100–5, 109, 131, 132
Collins, Madeline, 242–3
Collis, Maurice H., 73, 168
Collis, Robert, 179, 264
Colvan, John, 140–1, 151
Comhairle na nÓspidéal, 288
Commissioners of Lunacy for Scotland, 151

295

Connellan, Thaddaeus, 59
consumption, 40
contraception, 283
Coolican, John E., 245
Coombe Lying-in Hospital, 109–11, 181, 205, 281
Corbet, Bertie, 205
Cork Street Fever Hospital, 14, 29, 32, 69, 181, 182–3, 192, 202
   smallpox, 192–3
Corrigan, Sir Dominic, 94, 191, 219, 278
Corrigan Club, 284
Costello, Thomas, 5
Council for Postgraduate Medical and Dental Education, 288
County Down Hospital, 146
Cowan, Adrian, 260, 262, 263
Cowper, William, 137
Crampton, John, 15, 82, 84
Crampton, Sir Philip, 15, 38, 65, 73, 82, 87, 94, 119, 120
Cranfield, Dr, 140, 143
Crawford, Rev. Mr, 99
Critchley, Macdonald, 225
Crofton, W. M., 240
Croly, Henry Gray, 158
Crookshank, Professor Anne, 47
croup, 20, 115–16
Crowe, Morgan, 242
Cullen, 136–7
Cullen, William, 12
Cuming, Thomas, 151, 154, 161
Curran, John Philpot, 66
Cusack, James William, 73, 97, 124

Daniel, Michael, 105, 109
Darby, T., 158
Darley, Arthur, 271
Darwin, Charles, 125–8
Davaine, Casimir Joseph, 145
Dax, Marc, 227
de Cadiz, Miss R. M., 216
de Courcy Wheeler, Sir William Ireland, 224
de Senac, Jean-Baptiste, 257
Dease, Richard, 15, 65, 100–1, 131, 132
Dease, William, 6
Dejerine, 225
Demours, 172
Dental Hospital, 237
diabetes, 83–4, 214–16, 240
dialysis, 279, 280–1, 288

Dickens, Charles, 90, 146
Dillard and Scribner, 279
diphtheria, 246–7
dissection
   deaths from, 131–2
   grave-robbing, 104
Dixon, Kit, 141
Dr Steevens' Hospital, 14, 69, 82, 84, 94, 158, 223
Doolin, William, 179, 204, 207, 212, 218, 263–5, 277–8
Doyle, Dr J., Bishop of Kildare and Leighlin, 38
Doyle, G. D., 279, 288
Doyle, J. Stephen, 8
Drennan, Dr William, 50
Drumcondra Hospital, 187, 251
Drury, M. I., 93
Dublin Association for Discountenancing Vice, 58
Dublin Corporation, 203
Dublin Hospital Reports, 18, 19–20, 138
Dublin Journal of Medical and Chemical Science, 120
Dublin Journal of Medical Science, 121, 126, 153, 157, 179, 224
   Kirby in, 115–16
   Little editor, 152
   Moore editor, 181, 185, 186, 187, 203–4
   Moorhead co-editor, 209
   Nesbitt in, 238–9
Dublin Medical Press, 122, 126, 134
Dublin Natural History Society, 167
Dublin Pharmacopia, 122
Dublin Photographic Society, 233
Dublin Quarterly Journal of Medical Science, 152, 257
Dublin Society of Surgeons, 2
Dublin Rotary Club, 243
Duchenne, G. B. A., 225, 228
Duggan, James, 108
Duigenan, Paddy, 51–4
Duncan, Andrew, 11
Dupont, Charles, 261–2
Dupuytren, Baron, 142, 143
dysentery, 33–4

Eames, Henry, 168
Edward VII, King, 164, 186
Egan, Dr Thomas, 66

INDEX

Ehrlich, P., 213, 237
electrocardiograph, 232–3, 256, 258
Ellis, 280
emphyema, 94–5
emphysema, 95–6
encephalitis, 240–1
epidemiology, 29–33, 201–3
Eppel, Alan B., 260
Erb, Heinrich, 225, 226
'Erinensis,' 71–2, 73, 75, 119
   on Kirby, 99, 102, 103, 104
eugenics, 215
European Dialysis and Transplant Association, 284
Evanson, Richard Tonson, 97, 112, 114, 119–29, 133
   chair of medicine, 119
   evolution, 125–8
   marriages, 128–9
   paediatrics, 120–2
   preventive medicine, 122–3
   verses, 123–5
evolution, 125–8
exophthalmic goitre, 90–4, 170–3

Fallot, A., 257
Farre, 257
Fearon, Senator, 250–1
Ferrier, David, 226
fevers, 84–7, 182–3, 195
   famine fevers, 94
   infectious diseases, 187–8, 191
   Moore on, 191–4
Fielding, John, 8
First World War, 79, 210–11, 228, 242
   shell-shock, 229–30
FitzGerald, Dr Fanty, 278
Flajani, 172
Fleetwood, John F., 111
Fleming, Peter, 256
Flood, J. C., 262
Flourens, Pierre, 225
Foley, John H., 97
Foot, Arthur Wynne, 167–77, 179, 181
   Biological Club, 173–5
   birth and ancestry, 167–8
   chair of medicine, 173
   Ledwich School, 168–9
   literary stylist, 175–7
   neurology, 169–70
Forbes, John, 95
Fothergill, John, 23

Four Courts Marshalsea, 147
Freeman, Edward, 249, 250
Freeman's Journal Sanitary Commission, 205
Fritsch, G., 226

Gaelic Society, TCD, 255
Gaffney, Jim, 271
Galen, 280
Gall, P. J., 225
gastric ulcer, 163–4
gastrointestinal tract, 137–9
Gatenby, Peter, 253
Gelineau, M., 170
General Medical Council, 164, 187, 194
Geological Society of Dublin, 126
George V, King, 164
Gerhard, W. W., 27, 121
germ theory, 2, 132, 144–6
   discussion on, 157–60
   Moore, 188–90
Gilborne, 6
Gill, Freddie, 271
Gintrac, 257
Glasgow Royal Infirmary, 146
Gmelin, L., 139
Gogarty, Oliver St John, 217–18, 260, 262–3
Goldsmith, Oliver, 26
Gowers, Sir William, 193, 225
Grace, Pierce, 267
Grangegorman Cholera Hospital, 140
grave-robbing, 104
Graves, Richard, 53
Graves, Robert J., 19, 39, 40, 73, 82, 89, 94, 115, 191
   infection, 188–9
   on Kirby, 105
   Meath Hospital, 72–3, 77
   Park St School, 87
Graves' disease, 93, 170–3, 213–14, 217
Gray, Sir John, 202–3
Greene, 112
Greenfield, William Smith, 172
Gregory, James, 12, 13
Gregory, Richard, 109
Grey, Charles, 47, 77
Grimshaw, Thomas, 157–8, 197
Guersant, 27
Gull, Sir William Withey, 172–3
gunshot wounds, 104–5
Gwynn, Sheila, 220

Hackett, Francis, 259
Halahan, John, 5, 100, 105
Hales, Stephen, 238, 257
Hall, Marshall, 146
Hamilton, Alexander, 11
Hamilton, E., 158
Hamilton, Mr, 105
Hamilton, Professor James, 12
Hardman, T. G., 246
Hardwicke Hospital, 14, 16, 30, 131, 223, 228, 230
  reports from, 28–33
Hargrave, William, 112, 139
Harkans, Dr, 72
Harrison, Professor, 114
Hart, Dr, 143
Harvey, Joshua, 93
Harvey, Reuben J., 182
Harvey, William, 2, 15, 256
Haughey, Charles J., 283
Haughton, Rev. Samuel, 126–8, 159, 219–20
Hayden, Thomas, 257
Head, Henry H., 162, 225, 226
Health, Department of, 264–5, 279, 281, 285–6, 288
Healy, Colonel, 210
Heberden, William, 194, 257
Helmholtz, Herman von, 226
Hennen, John, 104–5
Henry, Arnold K., 187, 204
Henry, James, 38, 44–5
Herodotus, 227
Herrick, J. B., 257
Hill, Edward, 14–15, 77
Hippocrates, 2, 194, 227
Hitchcock, Harry, 252
Hitzig, Eduard, 226
Hodgkin, T., 135
Hohenlohe, Prince of, 38–9
Holmes, Gordon, 226
Homans, John, 233
Home, Francis, 28–9
Hooker, Joseph D., 126
Hopkins, Francis, 15
House of Industry, 69
House of Industry Hospitals, 16–17, 82, 151, 224, 240
Houston, John, 19
Hudson, Alfred, 151, 161, 164, 180–1
Hughes, James Stannus, 94

Hume, Gustavus, 224
Hunt, Edward, 175
Hunter, John, 145
hydrocephalus, 24–8
hyperthyroidism, 172–3, 213–14

infectious diseases, 187–203, 205, 231–2.
  see also cholera; typhus
  legislation, 200–1
insulin, 204–5, 238
  Nesbitt, 242
Irish Ecclesiastical Record, 128
Irish Family Planning Association, 283
Irish Journal of Medical Science, 179, 232, 246, 258, 259
  Doolin editor, 218, 277
  Moore in, 185, 193–4
  obituaries, 250–2
Irish language, 58–9
Irish Medical Association, 220, 234, 263–5, 284–6, 287
Irish Medical Council, 8, 288
Irish Medical Organisation, 286
Irish Medical Union, 286
Irish Society of Nephrology, 284
Irish Times, 243
Israels, 269

Jackson, Hughlings, 226, 227
Jacob, Arthur, 8, 85, 87, 89, 119, 122, 131, 145
Jameson, Robert, 49–50
jaundice, 95–6, 211
Jebb, Sir Henry, 6
Jenner, E., 146
Jervis Street Hospital. *see* Charitable Infirmary
Jewish National Fund, 265
Johnson, Charles, 87
Johnson, Dr, 134, 135
Joly, Professor John, 185
Joslin, 240
Journal of Obstetrics and Gynaecology, 279
Joyce, James, 149
Joynt, Richard Lane, 185
Junior Surgical Society, 148

Kane, Robert, 94
Kast, Alfred, 224
Kelly, Thomas, 100
Kemmis, Mrs Mary H., 96
Kendall, Edward Calvin, 173

INDEX

Keogh, Brian, 288
Kidd, G. H., 152
Kiely, Molly, 243
King and Queen's College of Physicians, 5, 96
King's College Hospital, 39
Kirby, John Timothy, 75, 99–117
  chair of medicine, 111–13
  Charitable Infirmary, 108–9
  Coombe Hospital, 109–11
  demonstratorship, 100–1
  national surgical hospital, 106–8
  publications, 115–17
  resignation, 113–15
  Theatre of Anatomy, 82, 101–5, 110–11, 112
Kirkes, William S., 257
Kirkpatrick, T.P.C., 19–20, 53
Kirwan, Richard, 49–50
Klebs, 188
Klumpke, Augusta Marie, 225
Knott, Dr John, 191
Koch, Robert, 2, 144–5, 156, 188, 190, 200, 205, 231
Kocher, 172
Kolff, Willem, 280–1
Kussmaul, 227

Laennec, R. T. H., 95, 257
Lalor, Maria, 38–9
Lamarck, Chevalier de, 126
Lancet, The, 71–2, 73, 75, 89, 99, 103, 146, 205. *see also* 'Erinensis'
  on Kirby, 111–12, 113–14
  on RCSI, 119
Lancisi, 257
Landsteiner, Karl, 164, 241
Lasègue, 225
Laubry, 256
Lavelle, Nurse, 75
Law, Dr, 90
Leahy, James, 104
Lecky, W. E. H., 56
Ledwich School of Medicine, 5, 152, 153, 168–9, 173, 175, 179
Lee, J. J., 264–5
Leeds General Infirmary, 281
Lehman, Dr, 115
Lendrick, Charles, 224, 231
Lentaigne, Benjamin, 105
Lewis, Joe, 260
Lindsay, Dr, 140

Lister, Sir Joseph, 144–6, 158, 160, 206
Little, James, 151–65, 168, 187
  Cheyne-Stokes breathing, 152–3
  College of Physicians, 164–5
  in Dublin, 151–2
  gastric ulcer, 163–4
  geographical distribution of disease, 155–6
  migraine, 161–2
  myxoedema, 162–3
  practical therapeutics, 160–1
  typhoid fever, 153–5
Local Government Board, 201
Lock Hospital, 14
locomotor ataxy, 169–70
London Medical & Surgical Journal, 172
Ludwig, Carl, 280
Lumsden, Sir John, 224, 258
Lyell, Sir Charles, 126
Lynch, Patrick, 58

Macartney, 103
Macartney, Rev. Dr George, 14
Macauley, Charles, 220
McCarthy, Andrew, 220
MacCarthy, Ethna, 251–2
McConnell, Adams, 246
MacCormac, Sir William, 146
Macdowell, Mr, 31
McDowell, Mr, 109
McDowell, R. B., 54–5, 250–1
MacEntee, Seán, 265, 285–6
McElvaney, Gerard, 8–9
MacGowan, W. A., 5
McGee, Mrs Mary, 283
McHenry, L. C., 21, 22–3
Machonchy, John, 146
McIlwaine, John E., 256
Mackenzie, Hector, 162–3
Mackenzie, Sir James, 257
McKinney, Colonel Thomas J., 270
Macnamara, Rawdon, 75, 109, 158–9, 181
McTier, Samuel, 50
Magee, William, 66
Magendie, F., 225
Major, R. H., 280
malingering, 34–7
Malpighi, 280
Malthus, Robert, 54, 60–1, 70
Manchester Royal Infirmary, 269
Mapother, Edward, 156, 159
Mareschal, Georges, 2

299

Marie, Pierre, 226, 256
Marine, David, 173
Marsh, Rev. Digby, 81
Marsh, Sir Henry, 77, 81–97, 112, 119, 121, 124, 138, 145
    ancestry, 81–3
    chair of medicine, 87–9
    clinical lectures, 94–6
    death of, 96–7
    diabetes, 83–4
    exophthalmic goitre, 90–4
    fevers, 84–7, 94
    phosphorescence, 89–90
Marsh, Rev. Robert, 81
Martin, Richard 'Humanity,' 225
Mater Hospital, 146, 204, 215, 280
Maunsell, Henry, 119, 121–2, 197–8, 212
Maunsell, Robert, 251
Mayo, Charles, 172
M'Coy, Simon, 140, 143
M'Donnell, James, 67–8, 70
M'Donnell, Robert, 158, 185, 174, 241
Meath Hospital, 14, 76, 82, 95, 158, 224, 231, 261
    blood transfusion, 241–2
    Cheyne, 15, 17, 39
    cholera, 201
    Evanson, 119, 120
    Foot, 167, 168, 175
    Graves' disease, 170–2
    lectures, 65
    Marsh, 90
    Moore, 179, 180, 181, 184, 188, 204–5, 206, 207
    smallpox, 192
    Stokes family, 66, 72–5, 77, 79
    tuberculosis, 191
Medical Association of Ireland, 147–8
Medical Benevolent Fund, 147
medical education, 249–50, 286–8
Medical Press & Circular, 181
Medical Research Council, 204
Meenan, James N., 277, 280
meningitis, 27–8
Mens Medica, 184–5
Mercer's Hospital, 3, 14, 102, 168, 245, 251
    Abrahamson, 258, 260
    ECG, 232–3
    Purser, 224, 228
Merle, William, 196
Mersburg Triad, 171

meteorology, 193–7
Micks, R. H., 215–16
migraine, 161–2
Mills, Dr, 29
Mitchell, George, 50
Mitchell, Silas Weir, 225
Mixter, Jason, 233
Moebius, Paul Julius, 172
Molyneux Asylum for Blind Females, 181
Monro, Alexander, 11, 13
Montpellier, 257
Moore, Henry, 204, 215
Moore, Sir John William, 152, 160, 162, 164, 165, 168, 173, 179–207, 219, 224, 240
    birth and education, 179–81
    climatic change, 196–7
    fever, 182–3
    Foot obituary, 177
    hospital appointments, 181
    infectious diseases, 187–90
    insulin, 204–5
    last years, 206–7
    marriages, 186–7
    Mens Medica, 184–5
    meteorology, 194–6
    private hospitals, 183–4
    publications, 185–6, 191–4
    state medicine, 197–203
    treatment of children, 205–6
    tuberculosis, 190–1
Moore, Surgeon-Commander M. S., 187
Moore, Norman, 88
Moore, Professor, 280
Moore, William Daniel, 179–80
Moore, William Edmund, 205
Moorhead, Charles, 220
Moorhead, James Herbert, 209
Moorhead, T. G., 185, 209–21, 240, 258
    Academy of Medicine, 212–13
    blindness, 217–19
    BMA in Dublin, 219–20
    chair of medicine, 212
    diabetes mellitus, 214–16
    early career, 209–10
    honorifics, 220–1
    hyperthyroidism, 213–14
    sued for assault, 216
    in USA, 216–17
    war service, 210–11
Moorhead, William Robert, 209
Moorhead, William St Leger, 209

INDEX

Morgagni, 2, 257
'Mother and Child' scheme, 264–5
Murchison, Charles, 86
Murdoch, Anna, 152
Murphy, Fr J., 128
Murray, George R., 162
Murray, Mrs, 68
Murray, Paul, 242
Murray, William, 107
myxoedema, 162–3

narcolepsy, 170
National Children's Hospital, 87, 237
National Eye Hospital, Cuffe St, 109
National Heart, Lung and Blood Institute, 8
nephritis, 267–8, 269
nephrology, 280
Nesbitt, Alexander, 237
Nesbitt, George Edward, 237–43
  blood transfusion, 241–2
  diabetes, 239–40
  early papers, 238–9
  encephalitis, 240–1
  insulin, 242
  laboratory tests, 239
  on modern developments, 237–8
  South Africa, 242–3
neurology, 169–70, 224–6, 233
New England Surgical Society, 233
New Sydenham Society, 228
New York Hospital, 9
North Dublin Union, 182, 190
nosology, 136–7
Nurock, Max, 255
Nurock, Tillie, 255, 262
Nursing Board, 286
nursing education, 16–17

O'Beirne, James, 89, 108
O'Brien, Dr Brendan, 246, 253
O'Brien, Eoin, 271
O'Brien, G. W., 147–8
O'Brien, Mabel, 223
O'Carroll, Joseph, 240
Ó Casaide, Séamus, 58
Ó Coinniallain, Tadhg, 59
O'Connor, Charles, 230
O'Donovan, D.K., 277
O'Dwyer, William Francis, 8, 277–89
  chair of medicine, 283–4
  Charitable Infirmary, 278–9
  medical education, 287–8

nephrology, 280
renal dialysis, 279–80, 280–1
renal unit, 282–4
research, 288–9
O'Farrell, P. T., 221
O'Flanagan, Harry, 5
O'Halloran, Sylvester, 2, 3, 5
O'Keefe, C., 113
O'Loughlin, Tim, 174
ophthalmology, 226
Oppenheim, Hermann, 226
Ord, W. M., 172
O'Reilly, Richard, 108
Ormsby, Sir Lambert, 158, 175, 181
Orpen, Dr, 20, 112, 119
Osborne, Jonathan, 95, 224, 231
O'Shaughnessy, William, 142, 143
Osler, Sir William, 20, 103, 172, 184, 213, 257
O'Sullivan, Seán, 206

Pachon, 256
paediatrics, 20–1, 120–2, 205–6
Paine, Tom, 54–6
Paisley, John, 24
Papavoine, 27
Pardee, H. E. B., 259
Parke, Edward, 4
Parke, T. H., 186
Parkinson, James, 226
Parkinson, John, 259
Park Street Medical School, 77, 87, 97, 119
Parr, Dr, 26
Parry, Caleb Hillier, 172
Parsons, Alfred, 184, 250, 251–2
Pasteur, Louis, 2, 144–5, 157, 160, 188, 206
Pathological Society of Dublin, 89, 90, 168, 171
Patterson, Frank, 279
Patterson, William, 27
Peacock, 257
Peebles, Dr, 31
Percival, Edward, 17–18, 19, 33
Peter Street School, 82, 101–5, 110–11, 112
Petty, Sir William, 201
phosphorescence, 89–90
Picknell, Mary Anne, 49, 66
Pitcairn, David, 257
Pitt Street Institute, 87, 120
Pius XII, Pope, 128

Plummer, 173
Plunket, William, 66
P&O Steam Navigation Company, 151, 155
Poiseuille, 238
population studies, 60–1
Porter, George, 5, 181
Porter, William Henry, 73
Portobello Nursing Home, 259–60
practical therapeutics, 160–1
preventive medicine, 122–3
Price, Dorothy, 253
Price, Dr, 116
Pringle, Seton Sidney, 224, 246, 251
private hospitals, 183–4
public health, 194–6, 197–203
Purser, Francis Carmichael, 223–35, 228, 242
   aphasia, 226–8
   clinical neurology, 225–6
   early career, 223–4
   education, 223
   Mercer's Hospital, 224
   professor of neurology, 233
   publications, 228–9, 231–3
   rat-bite fever, 230–1
   sciatica, 233–4
   shell-shock, 229–30
Purser, John Mallet, 162, 223
Purser, Louis Claude, 223
Purser, Sarah, 223
Purser, William Edward, 223

Quarterly Journal of Medicine, 258
Queen's University of Ireland, 4
Quin, Charles William, 25
Quinn, Mai Beatrice, 209

Radcliffe, John, 146–7
Radio Eireann, 272–3, 274
rat-bite fever, 230–1
Read, Alexander, 101, 102
Reid, Seaton, 152
Renal Association, the, 284
renal dialysis, 278–80, 280–1, 289
Renny, George, 34
Reverdins, 172
Reynolds, James Emerson, 173
Reynolds, Russell, 171
rheumatic heart disease, 246–7
rheumatism, 148
Richmond, Whitworth and Hardwicke
   Hospitals, 223, 228
Richmond Hospital, 14, 30, 84, 131, 158, 223, 228, 242, 263, 267, 273, 284
   Abrahamson, 260–2
   Nesbitt, 237
   school, 77
Ridley, Ellie, 186
rising, 1798, 12–13
Ritchie Russell and Espir, 227
Robertson, Douglas A., 226
Robinson, Alexander, 151
Roger, Henri, 257
Rogers, Joseph, 201
Rollo, John, 83
Romberg, Moritz H., 170, 225–6
Roney, Thomas, 73
Rotunda Lying-in Hospital, 14, 87, 100, 245, 256, 267, 273
Royal Academy of Medicine in Ireland, *see* Academy of Medicine
Royal Army Medical Corps, 210–11, 228, 241
Royal City of Dublin Hospital, Baggot St, 151, 158, 209
   Benson, 132–3, 146, 148
   Marsh, 89
   opened, 109
   Synge, 245, 246, 247, 248, 251, 253
Royal College of Physicians of Ireland, 8, 97, 111, 160, 234
   Abrahamson, 256, 263–5
   Foot, 173, 174
   Little, 164–5
   Medical Society, 154
   Moore, 187
Royal College of Surgeons in Ireland, 3, 82, 100–2, 119, 173, 197
   Abrahamson, 258, 260
   amalgamations, 173, 179
   Benson, 133–6, 148
   Kirby, 102–108
   Little, 151, 155
   Marsh, 87–9
   Maunsell, 122
   Moorhead, 212
   museum, 107–8
   Nesbitt, 242
   O'Dwyer, 283–7, 288
   presidency, 131
   surgical education by-law, 89, 111–12
   Synge, 245
   Thompson, 273–5

INDEX

Royal Dublin Society, 155, 194
Royal Hospital for Incurables, 14
Royal Institute of Health, 201
Royal Institute of Public Health, 195–6
Royal Irish Academy, 89–90, 147
Royal Irish Yacht Club, 218
Royal Society of Medicine in Ireland
  Synge, 248, 250
Royal University of Ireland, 4
Royal Victoria Eye and Ear Hospital, 149
Royal Zoological Society, 147
rugby, 242
Rumley, Mr, 105
Rush, Benjamin, 257
Russell, Thomas, 51, 58
Rutty, Thomas, 196, 197, 201
Ruz, 121

St Clair, Dr, 24–5
St James's Hospital, 250
St Laurence's Hospital, 267–8, 289
St Lô hospital, Normandy, 269–73
St Luke, Guild of, 1
St Mary Magdalene, Guild of, 1
St Vincent's Hospital, 89, 159, 204, 210, 221, 277
SS Peter and Bridget Hospital, 102, 104
Sanderson, Dr John Burdon, 157
Sattler, 172
Saurin, William, 71
Savory, William, 219
Schafer, Edward, 172–3
Schaudin, F. R., 237
Schleiden, M. J., 225
Schwann, T., 225
sciatica, 233–4
Scott, J. Alfred, 163, 233
Second World War, 269–73, 278, 281
Shanley, John, 220
Shaw, H. Batty, 239
Shekelton, John, 19, 132
shell-shock, 229–30
Sick and Indigent Roomkeepers Society, 48
Sigerson, George, 228
Sir Patrick Dun's Hospital, 14, 30, 209, 210, 245
Smart, Dr, 142
Smith, Aquilla, 185
Smith, Adam, 6
Smith, Professor R. W., 219
Smith, Stephen Catterson, 148
Smith, Walter, 219

Smyly, Philip, 4, 95, 181, 192
Snow, John, 143
Soemmering, S. T., 139
Solomons, Dr Michael, 283
South Africa, 243
Spear, Dr, 68
Spurzheim, J. C., 225
Starling, Ernest H., 173
state medicine, 197–203, 264–5
Stedman, Thomas L., 192
Stelfox, Arthur Wilson, 167
Stellwag, 171
Stephen, 231
Stephens, Rev. Walter, 60
Stephens, William, 224
Stevenson, Walter, 185
Stokes-Adams syndrome, 19–20
Stoker, William Thornley, 158, 160
Stokes, Adrian, 78–9, 209–10
Stokes, Gabriel, 47–8, 78
Stokes, George Gabriel, 77
Stokes, Henry, 78–9, 241–2
Stokes, Henry John, 78
Stokes, Margaret, 78
Stokes, Whitley, 15, 47–79, 84, 87, 114, 120–1, 122, 232, 256
  birth and ancestry, 47–8
  chair of medicine, 71–2
  contagion, 145
  family of, 78–9
  King's Professor, 65–6
  medical writings, 67–71
  non-medical writings, 54–9
  number of lectures, 75–7
  polymath, 48–50
  population and resources, 59–62
  Regius Professor, 77
  TCD visitation, 51–4
  United Irishmen, 50–1
  verses, 62–5
Stokes, Whitley (younger), 78
Stokes, Sir William, 18–19, 39, 71, 95, 97, 158, 160, 184, 185, 190, 191, 206, 219
  career of, 78
  Meath Hospital, 39, 75, 76, 77, 179
  and Moore, 180–1
  Park St School, 119
  publications, 187, 257
Stoney, Richard Atkinson, 206
Stuart, Mary, 38–9
Studies, 249–50
Surgical Society of Ireland, 158–60

303

Swift, Theophilus, 65–6
Sydenham, Thomas, 28, 34, 136, 138
Sydenham's chorea, 82–3
Synge, Edward, 245
Synge, J. L., 250
Synge, Victor Millington, 245–53, 260
   appointments, 245
   diphtheria and heart disease, 246–7
   disappointed of PRCPI, 249
   holistic medicine, 252–3
   medical education, 249–50
   obituaries by, 250–2
   presidential address, 247–9
   publications, 246

tabes dorsalis, 169–70, 225, 226
Tagert, Mr, 114
Taylor, Dr Thomas, 60–1
Temple Street Children's Hospital, 277
Theatre of Anatomy, 101–5
Thompson, Alan Herbert, 267–75
   chair of medicine, 273–5
   publications, 267–9
   St Lô hospital, 269–73
Thompson, Geoffrey, 267, 270
Thompson, Sylvia, 273, 275
Tiedemann, 139
Tierney, Sir Matthew, 142
Todd, Charles Hawkes, 19, 39, 103, 131
   dissecting-room deaths, 131–2
Todd, Rev. James Henthorn, 39
Todd, Robert Bentley, 39, 78, 131, 225
Todderick, G. F., 15
Todhunter, John, 168, 181, 185
Toksvig, Signe, 259–60
Townsend, Richard, 39
Townsend Street Hospital, 143
Trades Union Act, 1941, 265
Traill, Antony, 245
Traill, Robert, 245
Traube, Ludwig, 19, 153
Trinity College Dublin, 1, 4, 103, 111, 127, 151, 164, 167, 197. *see also* Biological Society
   Abrahamson, 255
   Foot, 168
   Kirby, 100
   Moore, 180–1
   Moorhead, 209
   Nesbitt, 237
   neurology chair, 233
   Purser, 223, 234

state medicine diploma, 180–1
Stokes, 65–6
Thompson, 267
visitation, 51–4
Trousseau, 42, 170
tuberculosis, 190–1, 201
Tuffnell, Thomas Joliffe, 144, 274
Tyndall, John, 145, 157
typhoid fever, 153–5, 202–3
typhus, 29–33, 68–71, 182–3, 188, 202–3
Tyrrell, Professor H. J., 146

Underwood, John, 197
United Irishmen, 50–1, 57–8
   TCD visitation, 51–4
United States of America, 173, 216–17, 240
University College Dublin, 277, 280
University of British Columbia, 9
University of Dublin. *see* Trinity College Dublin
University of Edinburgh, 11

Vaquez, 256
venous pulsation, 132–3
Vesalius, Andreas, 2, 280
Victoria, Queen, 78, 143, 164, 186
Vierordt, 238
Vieussens, Raymond, 257
Virchow, R., 135, 190
vivisection, 225
Voltaire, 2
von Basch, 238
Von Basedow, 172
von Economo, C., 241
von Graefe, Albrecht, 171, 226
von Haller, Albrecht, 257

Wade, Walter, 6
Walker, John, 65, 100
Walkerites, 65, 100
Wallace, Alfred Russell, 126
Wallace, William, 108, 278
Walsh, A. J., 103
Walsh, Anthony, 279
Walshe, F. M. R., 226
Wassermann, A. von, 237
water supply, 202–3
Watson, Dr, 24
Webb, D. A., 250–1
Wernicke, Carl, 227
West, George Foster, 117

INDEX

Westphal, Carl, 226
Wharton, J. H., 181
Wheeler, Sir William, 160, 251
White, Francis, 109
White, R. Persse, 181
Whitla, Sir William, 164, 219
Whitworth Hospital, 28, 30–1, 84, 223, 228
    dysentery, 33–4
    Thompson, 267–8, 269
Whytt, Robert, 24, 26–7, 121
Widal, 255
Widdess, J. D. H., 16, 122–3, 133–4, 260
Wilde, Sir William, 19, 87–8, 147, 201

Wilkinson, 269
Willis, 83
Wilmot, Samuel, 108
Withering, William, 25
Wolfe Tone, Theobald, 48, 50, 53–4
women, as doctors, 4–5
Woodcock, Joe, 279

Yeats, W. B., 185
Yeo, Gerald, 168, 181
Young, Andrew, 75

Zinsser, Hans, 144
zymotic disease, 157–8, 188

Departmen

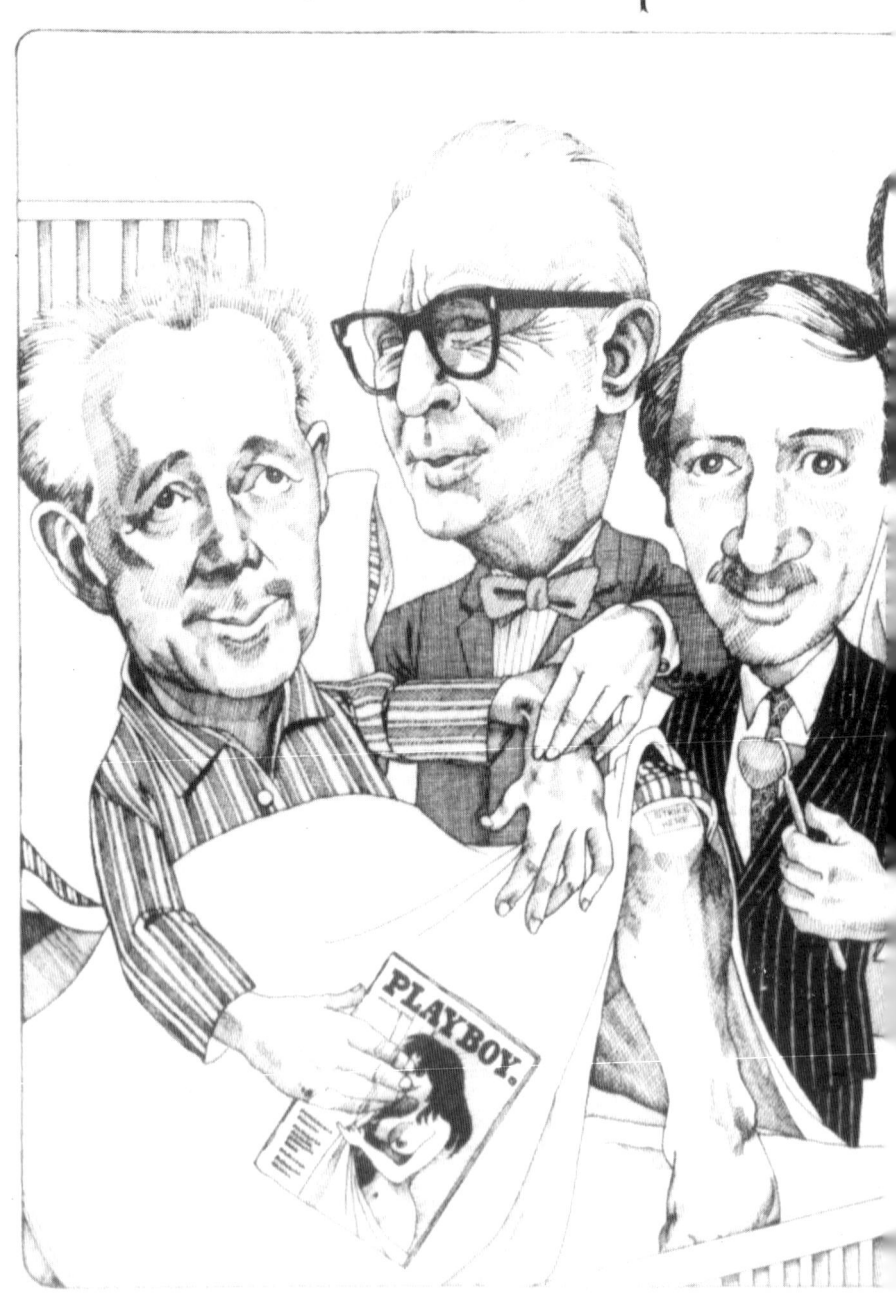

The Department of Medicine of the Royal College of Surgeons in Ireland in Mervyn Abrahamson, Tommy Ryan, Jim Devlin, Stephen Doyle, Max Ryan (c